Politics and Health Care

The Milbank Readers
John B. McKinlay, general editor

Politics and Health Care

Milbank Reader 6

edited by John B. McKinlay

The MIT Press
Cambridge, Massachusetts
London, England

Printed and bound in the United States of America

Library of Congress Cataloging in Publication Data

Main entry under title:
Politics and health care.

   (The Milbank reader series; 6)
   Bibliography: p.
   Includes index.
   1. Medical policy—United States—Addresses, essays, lectures.
2. Medical policy—Addresses, essays, lectures. I. McKinlay, John B.
II. Series. [DNLM: 1. Health services—United States—Collected works.
2. Government—United States—Collected works. 3. Policy making—
Collected works. W 84 AA1 P7]
RA395.A3P628   362.1′042′0973   81–12414
ISBN 0–262–63082–6 (pbk.)   AACR2
      0–262–13181–1 (hard)

Contents

Foreword

During 1973–74, the Milbank Memorial Fund, in conjunction with Prodist (New York), produced four edited volumes that drew together and organized published papers from the well-known and respected *Milbank Memorial Fund Quarterly*. In producing these four initial resource books (*Research Methods in Health Care, Politics and Law in Health Care Policy, Economic Aspects of Health Care*, and *Organizational Issues in the Delivery of Health Services*), the Fund had attempted to respond to heavy and continuing requests for accessibility and economy of the Milbank papers. The success of the four books exceeded even the most optimistic expectations, and all are now, unfortunately, out of print. They were adopted as course texts by many different health-related disciplines, were used widely throughout North America and abroad, were acquired by many university and professional libraries and were favorably reviewed in internationally respected professional journals.

The foreword to the earlier series noted that we always "planned to keep this series active and responsive to changing needs. Suggestions for future volumes will be welcome." Since their release, there have been numerous inquiries, requests, and suggestions for further volumes dealing with new and emerging issues concerning health care and social policy. The titles included in this second wave of edited volumes attempt to respond again to this widespread enthusiasm and need.

A venture of this nature has several obvious limitations. First of all, the universe from which the contributions were selected was limited to the *Milbank Memorial Fund Quarterly/Health and Society* and to several books produced by the Fund as a result of round-table meetings on particular health-care issues. However, more than enough rich material by eminent scholars was available for at least the present volumes. For the editor, a major problem was to decide which of several excellent papers had to be omitted (for reasons of economy, coverage, datedness, etc.) rather than what was available for inclusion in each volume. It should be emphasized that all of the authors represented here have progressed in their thinking and have advanced their work in other journals and books since original publication of the papers. Some have altered their theoretical orientation and some even their substantive interests. Wherever possible the editor has selected contributions published since the early 1970s. Indeed, most of the articles were first published within the last three or four years. Articles that were widely recognized as classic statements were selected from earlier years. Finally, several contributions dealt with a breadth of issues and were of sufficient quality to warrant their inclusion in more than one volume. Since each volume is likely to appeal to somewhat different readerships, this duplication was not considered problematic but rather enhanced the treatment of some health-care issues and the value of each volume.

It is hoped that this new series will help teachers, researchers, policymakers, public administrators, and especially students to overcome an ever-increasing problem: namely, how to gain easy and economical access to the rich resources contained in recent Milbank Memorial Fund publications.

Introduction

The papers in this volume are organized into four sections for the convenience of the reader. The first section deals with some aspects of the role of the state in health care. Daniel Wikler considers what the government's role should be in promoting the kinds of personal behavior that lead to long life and good health. He suggests that mild measures of health education and exhortation may be ineffective and imposition of stronger coercive actions may be generally unacceptable. Wikler seeks to identify the moral principles underlying a reasoned judgment on whether stronger methods might justifiably be used by the state, and if so, what limits ought to be observed. The philosophical and social principles involved are extremely complex and threats to freedoms may be averted through a sound understanding of the moral justification for any state intrusion. The complementary paper by David Courtwright shows that historically the most important rationale for coercive public health measures by the state has been the prevention of disease and harm to others. However, as noncommunicable diseases induced in large part by life-styles and personal habits account for higher rates of death and disability, state restrictions on individual behavior appear to be based now on a new argument—social costs. Indirect monetary effects are being substituted for direct health effects. Courtwright argues that since we lack precise measurement of net costs, any kind of state coercion should be approached with extreme caution.

The second section deals with aspects of federal policy. In the first paper, James Blumstein and Michael Zubkoff attempt to view issues of health policy within an analytic framework that they believe could be useful for those involved in policy formulation and implementation. They argue that insufficient attention has been paid to first principles of policy analysis and, as a consequence, some previous and proposed policy instruments have not and would not successfully address the problems identified. They believe that policy must accommodate itself to the realities of the economic market and that additional attention must be given to governmental initiatives that promote increased effectiveness of the market as a device of social ordering. They recognize that regulation should have a place in any comprehensive national health strategy but government intervention ought to follow from theoretical analysis and should encourage market perfection wherever feasible and appropriate. The paper by Victor Rodwin offers a valuable cross-national experience and shows that in France, as in the United States and elsewhere, the problems of controlling health care costs are seemingly intractable. He argues that the incongruity of private provision with public financing can be traced to adherence to competing and even contradictory policies—solidarity and liberal pluralism. It is argued that this marriage of ideologies has been extremely costly, and efforts to stem rising health care costs have resulted in political stalemate.

The next two papers deal with some ways in which the problem of inflation has permitted an ever increasing role for the federal government in health care. Louise Russell argues that proposals for combatting health sector inflation can be grouped under two headings, regulation and the restructuring of insurance. Increased regulation of the health sector is probably unavoidable, but past experience does not suggest any models for successful regulation of prices and costs. She suggests that the principle behind proposals to change the structure of insurance is that some financial incentives must be built into the framework that shapes the decisions of participants in the health sector. It appears that these incentives may be able to substitute for regulation in some areas but may serve as a way of reinforcing regulation in others. Theodore Marmor and his colleagues suggest that the economic market will systematically underproduce public goods and that this economic theory is often used as a justification for governmental intervention. The authors argue, however, that moving from the economic marketplace to the political marketplace does not necessarily solve the problems. In the absence of some concentrated interest the political market is unlikely to adopt a policy simply because it constitutes a public good. The political market, like the economic one, tends to systematically underproduce public goods and overproduce bad ones, and it appears that the political process is unlikely to right the distributive wrongs of the economic marketplace when a similar set of actors dominates both. This fundamental problem is illustrated through a review of the history of medical inflation and governmental response or lack of response to it.

The next three papers consider federal policy in relation to health maintenance organizations. John Iglehart's paper discusses the federal government's interest in promoting the development of HMOs as a unique experiment in venture capitalism. HMOs involve an activity that requires some reconciliation of the sometimes competing goals and procedures of government and private business. Within the context of the Department of Health and Human Services, which appears to favor regulatory approaches, the Office of Health Maintenance Organizations (OHMO) suggests some marketplace solutions to problems in the production, distribution, and financing of health care. Richard McNeil and Robert Schlenker consider the role of three forces that appeared to influence the development of HMOs during the early 1970s: legal restrictions, market conditions, and the federal government's policy stance. The authors suggest that the rapid increase in the number of HMOs in the 1970s was primarily due to favorable market conditions in certain areas of the country combined with a highly encouraging federal policy toward HMOs. Contrary to earlier beliefs, legal restrictions do not appear to have been a serious barrier to HMO development. In 1973–74, new legislation was enacted at both the federal and state levels, ostensibly to encourage HMO development. The authors' review of this legislation suggests that while it does remove many of the old legal requirements, which apparently were not serious barriers to HMO development, the new legislation imposes a host of new conditions and requirements on HMO participation in the health-care marketplace. Ironically, some of these new features appear to actually impede the operation of the very market forces that encouraged earlier HMO growth. Donald Moran considers the recent policy fad that seeks to inject competition into the market for health care financing. He argues that pushing pro-competition legislation through Congress may have unanticipated consequences for its proponents. Given these and other political considerations, Moran suggests it may be preferable to turn to an accommodation of interests that provides some constraints on adverse selection and free riders, some constraints on plan innovation and product differentiation, some bias against fee-for-service solo practitioners, and some risk that, left to themselves in an open system, the American people may spend more, rather than less, on health care.

In the next two papers, the impact of federal policy on different aspects of health care is considered. Stephen Rose argues that deinstitutionalization as a public policy promised to be a major departure from previous psychiatric practice. Policy makers advanced a bold new approach for care in the community while decrying traditional medical paradigms and the custodial warehousing of mental patients. Community mental centers were to be the heart of a new national initiative. However the rhetoric of reform failed to coalesce the activities among varying federal and state interests and systems. Overall, the intended beneficiaries may have become unfortunate victims. Anne-Marie Foltz examines why Congress's first major program for comprehensive health care to needy children took five years to begin even partial operation. Through a careful review of the 1967 programs' legislative history, it appears that Congress paid little attention to Early and Periodic Screening, Diagnosis and Treatment (EPSDT), and that it was left ambiguous whether Health or Welfare would administer it. The costs were never clearly stated and the eligibility and scope of services to be provided remained vague. Despite pressure from welfare rights interest groups, these ambiguities delayed the preparation of regulation and guidelines that never did succeed in resolving the question of overlapping jurisdiction and costs. In addition, the resistance of many states to pay for the program further delayed its implementation.

In the third section, Theodore Marmor and James Morone discuss ways in which the health planning legislation of 1974, which established Health Systems Agencies (HSAs), represented an important attempt to break patterns of decision making in public choices. It appears that one widely heralded strategy for controlling contemporary medical care—consumer involvement through accountability, representation and participation—is flawed by the failure to recognize that political markets are always imbalanced because of unequal interests and disproportionate resources. They ask how broad diffuse interests can be represented when all the incentives point to domination by a minority of intensely interested producers. They recognize that solutions favored at the local level may not best serve the entire nation. They suggest adjustment of mechanisms both internal to HSAs and external to them, but recognize that their mandate reaches far beyond possibility of accomplishment. The final paper by Rudolf Klein draws on cross-national experience with Britain's National Health Service, and suggests that there is a conflict between different social values and policy aims and that progress toward achieving more community or worker control is constrained by the pursuit of other desired objectives. He observes that the egalitarian ideology of the National Health Service emphasizes central control to achieve a nationally equitable distribution of resources. Moreover, the emphasis on coordination between National Health Service and other social services appears to limit freedom of action. It is suggested that democracy as accountable policy making on the national scale may be incompatible with democracy as a direct control, whether by the community or by workers. To encourage participation means accepting diversity in the provision of health care and the multiplication of small, self-governing units. Similarly, worker control is professional autonomy writ large and may, therefore, conflict with community control.

John B. McKinlay

I The Role of the State in Health Care

Millbank Memorial Fund Quarterly/*Health and Society, Vol. 56, No. 3, 1978*

Persuasion and Coercion for Health

Ethical Issues in Government Efforts to Change Life-Styles

DANIEL I. WIKLER

Center for Health Sciences, University of Wisconsin

WHAT SHOULD be the government's role in promoting the kinds of personal behavior that lead to long life and good health? Smoking, overeating, and lack of exercise increase one's chances of suffering illness later in life, as do many other habits. The role played by life-style is so important that, as stated by Fuchs (1974): "The greatest current potential for improving the health of the American people is to be found in what they do and don't do for themselves." But the public has shown little spontaneous interest in reforming. If the government uses the means at its disposal to remedy the situation, it may be faced with problems of an ethical nature. Education, exhortation, and other relatively mild measures may not prove effective in inducing self-destructive people to change their behavior. Attention might turn instead to other means, which, though possibly more effective, might also be intrusive or otherwise distasteful. In this essay, I seek to identify the moral principles underlying a reasoned judgment on whether stronger methods might justifiably be used, and, if so, what limits ought to be observed.

0026-3745-78-5603-0303-36/$01.00/0 © 1978 Milbank Memorial Fund

1

Daniel I. Wikler

Background To Government Involvement
in Life-Style Reform

This inquiry occurs at a time when the government is widening its scope of involvement in life-style reform. Major prospective health policy documents of both the United States (Department of Health Education, and Welfare, 1975) and Canadian governments (documented by Lalonde, 1974) have announced a change of orientation in this direction. Behind this shift is a host of factors, one of which is the pattern of disease in which an increasing share of ill health is attributed to chronic illnesses and accidental injuries that are aggravated by living habits. This development has caused increased interest in preventive behavioral change, and has been abetted by the current wave of "therapeutic nihilism," an attitude that questions medical intervention and is more friendly to health efforts that begin and end at home.

That life-style reform should be undertaken by the *government,* rather than by private individuals or associations, is part of the general emergence of the government as health-care provider. Encouragement of healthful living may also have a budgetary motive. Government officials may find that life-style reform is one of the most cost-effective ways of delivering health, especially if more effective change-inducing techniques are developed.[1] Indeed, the present cost-containment crisis may propel life-style reform to a central place in health planning before the necessary scientific and policy thinking has taken place.

Further pressure on the government to take strong steps to change unhealthy life-styles might come from those who live prudently. All taxpayers have a stake in keeping federal health costs down, but moderate persons may particularly view others' self-destructive life-styles as a kind of financial aggression against them. They may be expected to intensify their protest in the event of a national health insurance plan or national health service.

Involvement of the government in legislating healthful patterns of living is not wholly new; there have been public health and labor

---

[1]Though there is much dispute over the effectiveness of many health-promotion measures, efficient techniques may be developed in step with the progress of behavioral medicine generally. See Ubell (1972), Pomerleau, Bass, and Crown, (1975), and Haggerty (1977).

laws for a long time. Still, with the increased motivation for government action in life-style reform, it is time to reflect on the kinds of interventions the public wants and should have to accept. Various sorts of behavior change measures need to be examined to see if they might be used to induce healthier living. But that is not enough; goals must also be identified and subjected to ethical examination.[2]

The discussion below will examine a small number of possible goals of government life-style reform, and follow with a survey of the principal kinds of steps now contemplated. The approach will be to devote attention to those behavior change measures that are likely to be unpleasant and unwelcome. Since most techniques now used or contemplated for future use do not have such properties, there is little need to justify or focus on them. The reader should also note that each possible policy goal will be discussed in isolation from others. Although in actuality most government programs would probably be expected to serve several purposes at once, and some might be justified by the aggregate but not by one end alone, it is best for our purposes to consider one goal at a time so as to determine the contribution of each. Finally, my analysis should be understood as independent of certain political currents with which my views might be associated. There is some danger that attention to health-related personal behavior will distract the government and public from examining other sources of illness, such as unsafe working conditions, environmental health hazards, and even social and commercial

---

[2] I am not attempting to determine what the actual goals of the government are in intervening in life-style; indeed, it may make little sense to speak of specific goals at all. (See MacCallum (1966).) The rationale for legislation as voiced by the legislature may have the purpose of establishing the legal basis for the legislation rather than that of exhibiting the legislators' goals in passing the measures or of identifying the need to which the measure was a response.

For example, a bill requiring motorcyclists to wear helmets might be accepted by the public on paternalistic grounds, but the personal motivation of the legislators may have been harassment of the cyclists. And the measure might be upheld in court as a legitimate attempt to prevent the public from being saddled with the cost of caring for injured cyclists who could not afford to pay for medical care.

My inquiry into the goals of a proposed health policy has the sole purpose of determining whether the goal of the policy and the means to it are legitimate. Thus, if it is decided that such a helmet law is unwarranted, even on the paternalistic grounds which seem most applicable, it will not concern us that the law could be cleared through the courts by nimble use of the possibility of the cyclists becoming public charges. This is not to denigrate the use of such methods in the practice of legislation and legal challenge; but these pursuits are different from those undertaken here.

determinants of the injurious behavior. Further, undue stress upon
the individual's role in the cause of illness could lead to a "blame-
the-victim" mentality, which could be used as a pretext for failing to
make curative services available. Although these matters are essentially external to the issue of reform of unhealthy living habits, they
pose ethical questions of equal or greater moral gravity.

Goals of Health Behavior Reform

I propose to discuss three possible goals of health behavior reform
with regard to their appropriateness as goals of government
programs and the problems arising in their pursuit. The first goal
can be simply stated: health should be valued for its own sake.
Americans are likely to be healthier if they can be induced to adopt
healthier habits, and this may be reason enough to try to get them to
do so. The second goal is the fair distribution of the burdens caused
by illness. Those who become ill because of unhealthy life-styles may
require the financial support of the more prudent, as well as the sharing of what may be scarce medical facilities. If this is seen as unfair
to those who do not make themselves sick, life-style reform measures
will also be seen as accomplishing distributive justice. The third goal
is the maintenance and improvement of the general welfare, for the
nation's health conditions have their effects on the economy, allocation of resources, and even national security.

Health as a Goal in Itself: Beneficence and Paternalism

Much of the present concern for the reform of unhealthy life-styles
stems from concern over the health of those who live dangerously.
Only a misanthrope would quarrel with this goal. There are several
steps that might immediately be justified: the government could
make the effects of unhealthy living habits known to those who practice them, and sponsor research to discover more of these facts. The
chief concern over such efforts might be that the government would
begin its urgings before the facts in question had been firmly established, thus endorsing living habits that might be useless or
detrimental to good health.

    Considerably more debate, however, would arise over a decision
to use stronger methods. For example, a case in point might be a

government "fat tax," which would require citizens to be weighed and taxed if overweight. The surcharges thus derived would be held in trust, to be refunded with interest if and when the taxpayers brought their weight down.[3] This pressure would, under the circumstances, be a bond imposed by the government upon its citizens, and thus can be fairly considered as coercive.

The two signal properties of this policy would be its aim of improving the welfare of obese taxpayers, and its presumed unwelcome imposition on personal freedom. (Certain individual taxpayers, of course, might welcome such an imposition, but this is not the ordinary response to penalties.) The first property might be called "beneficence," and it is generally a virtue. But the second property becomes paternalism;[4] and its status as a virtue is very much in doubt. "Paternalism" is a loaded word, almost automatically a term of reprobation. But many paternalistic policies, especially when more neutrally described, attract support and even admiration. It may be useful to consider what is bad and what is good about paternalistic practices, so that we might decide whether in this case the good outweighs the bad. For detailed discussions of paternalism in the abstract, see Feinberg (1973), Dworkin (1971), Bayles (1974), and Hodson (1977).

What is good about some paternalistic interventions is that people are helped, or saved from harm. Citizens who have to pay a fat tax, for example, may lose weight, become more attractive, and live longer. In the eyes of many, these possible advantages are more than offset by the chief fault of paternalism, its denying persons the chance to make their own choices concerning matters that affect them. Self-direction, in turn, is valued because people usually believe themselves to be the best judges of what is good for them, and because the choosing is considered a good in itself. These beliefs are codified in our ordinary morality in the form of a moral right to noninterference so long as one does not adversely affect the interests of

---

[3]This measure was concocted for the present essay, but it shares its important features with others which have been actually proposed.

[4]"Coercive beneficence" is not a fully correct definition of paternalism; but I will not attempt to give adequate definition here (see Gert and Culver, 1976). The term itself is unnecessarily sex-linked; "Parentalism" carries the same meaning without this feature. However, "paternalism" is a standard term in philosophical writing, and a change from it invites confusion.

others. This right is supposed to shield an individual's "self-regarding" actions from intervention by others, even when those acts are not socially approved ones and even when they promise to be unwise.

At the same time, the case for paternalistic intervention on at least some occasions seems compelling. There may be circumstances in which we lose, temporarily or permanently, our capacity for competent self-direction, and thereby inflict harm upon ourselves that serves little purpose. Like Ulysses approaching the Sirens, we may hope that others would then protect us from ourselves. This sort of consideration supports our imposed guardianship of children and of the mentally retarded. Although these persons often resent our paternalistic control, we reason that we are doing what they would want us to do were their autonomy not compromised. Paternalism would be a benefit under the sort of social insurance policy that a reasonable person would opt for if considered in a moment of lucidity and competence (Dworkin, 1971).

Does this rationale for paternalism support governmental coercion of competent adults to assure the adoption of healthy habits of living? It might seem to, at first sight. Although these adults may be generally competent, their decision-making abilities can be compromised in specific areas. Individuals may be ignorant of the consequences of their acts; they may be under the sway of social or commercial manipulation and suggestion; they may be afflicted by severe psychological stress or compulsion; or be under external constraint. If any of these conditions hold, the behavior of adults may fail to express their settled will. Those of us who disavow any intention of interfering with free and voluntary risk-taking may see cause to intervene when a person's behavior is not under his or her control.

Paternalism: Theoretical Problems. There are a number of reasons to question the general argument for paternalism in the coercive eradication of unhealthful personal practices. First, the analogy between the cases of children and the retarded, where paternalism is most clearly indicated, and of risk-taking adults is misleading. If the autonomy of adults is compromised in one or more of the ways just mentioned, it might be possible to restore that autonomy by attending to the sources of the involuntariness; the same cannot ordinarily be done with children or the retarded. Thus, adults who are destroying their health because of ignorance may be educated; adults acting under constraint may be freed. If restoration of autonomy is a realistic project, then paternalistic interference is unjustified. The two kinds of interventions are aimed at the same target, *i.e.,* harmful behavior not freely and competently chosen. But they accomplish the result differently. Paternalistic intervention blocks the harm; education and similar measures restore the choice. The state or health planners would seem obligated to use this less restrictive alternative if they can. This holds true even though the individuals might still engage in their harmful practices once autonomy is restored. This would not call for paternalistic intervention, since the risk would be voluntarily shouldered.

It remains true, however, that autonomy sometimes cannot be restored. It may be impossible to reach a given population with the information they need; or, once reached, the persons in question may prove ineducable. Psychological compulsions and social pressures may be even harder to eradicate. In these situations, the case for paternalistic interference is relatively strong, yet even here there is reason for caution. Persons who prove incapable of absorbing the facts about smoking, for example, or who abuse drugs because of compulsion or addiction, may retain a kind of second-order autonomy. They can be told that they appear unable to accept scientific truth, or that they are addicted; and they can then decide to reconsider the facts or to seek a cure. In some cases these will be decisions that the individuals are fully competent to carry out; paternalistic intervention would unjustly deny them the right to control their destinies. Coercion would be acceptable only if this second-order decision were itself constrained, compelled, or otherwise compromised—which, in the case of health-related behavior, it may often be.

A second reason for doubting the justifiability of paternalistic interference concerns the subjectivity of the notion of harm. The same experience may be seen as harmful by one person and as beneficial by another; or, even more common, the goodness (or badness) of a given eventuality may be rated very differently by different persons. Although we as individuals are often critical of the importance placed on certain events by others, we nevertheless hesitate to claim special authority in such matters. Most of us subscribe to the pluralistic ethic, for better or for worse, which has as a central tenet the proposition that there are multiple distinct, but equally valid, concepts of good and of the good life. It follows that we must use personal preferences and tastes to determine whether our health-related practices are detrimental.

Unfortunately, it is often difficult to defer the authority of others in defining harm and benefit. It is common to feel that one's own preferences reflect values that reasonable people adopt; one can hardly regard oneself as unreasonable. To the extent that government planners employ their own concepts of good in attempting to change health practices for the public's benefit, the social insurance rationale for paternalism is clearly inapplicable.

A third reason for criticism of paternalism is the vagueness of the notion of decision-making disability. The conscientious paternalist intervenes only when the self-destructive individual's autonomy is compromised. It is probably impossible, however, to specify a compromising condition. To be sure, there are cases in which the lack of autonomy is evident, such as that of a child swallowing dangerous pills in the belief that they are candy. But the sorts of practices that would be the targets of coercive campaigns to reform health-related behavior are less dramatic and their involuntary quality much less certain. Since the free and voluntary conditions of health-related practice cannot be specified in advance, there is obviously considerable potential for unwarranted interference with fully voluntary choices.

Indeed, the dangers involved in disregarding individuals' personal values and in falsely branding their behavior involuntary are closely linked. In the absence of independent criteria for decision-making disability, the paternalist may try to determine disability by seeing whether the individual is rational, *i.e.,* whether he or she competently pursues what is valuable. An absence of rationality may be reason to suspect the presence of involuntariness and hence grounds for paternalism. The problem, however, is that this test for rationality—whether the chosen means are appropriate for the individual's personal ends—is not fully adequate. Factors that deprive an individual of autonomy—such as compulsion or constraint—not only affect a person's ability to calculate means to ends but also induce ends that are in some sense foreign. Advertisements, for example, may instill desires to consume certain substances whose pleasures would ordinarily be considered trifling. Similarly, ignorance may induce people to value a certain experience because they believe it will lead to their attainment of other ends. Alcoholics, for example, may value intoxication because they think it will enhance their social acceptance. The paternalist on the lookout for non-autonomous, self-destructive behavior will be interested not only in irrational means but also uncharacteristic, unreasonable values.

The difficulty for the paternalist at this point is plain. The desire to interfere only with involuntary risk-taking leads to designating individuals for intervention whose behavior proceeds from externally-instilled values. Pluralism commits the paternalist to use the persons' own values in determining whether a health-related practice is harmful. What is needed is some way of determining individuals' "true" personal values; but if these cannot be read off from their behavior, how can they be known?

In certain individual cases, a person's characteristic preferences can be determined from wishes expressed before losing autonomy, as was Ulysses' desire to be tied to the mast. But this sort of data is hardly likely to be available to government health planners. The problem would be at least partially solved if we could identify a set of goods that is basic and appealing, and that nearly all rational persons value. Such universal valuation would justify a presumption of involuntariness should an individual's behavior put these goods in jeopardy. On what grounds would we include an item on this list? Simple popularity would suffice: if almost everyone likes something, such approval probably stems from a common human nature, shared by even those not professing to like that thing. Hence we may suspect, that, if unconstrained, they would like it also. Alternatively, there may be experiences or qualities that, while not particularly appealing in themselves, are preconditions to attaining a wide variety of goods that people idiosyncratically value. Relief from pain is an example of the first sort of good; normal-or-better intelligence is an instance of the latter.

The crucial question for health planners is whether *health* is one of these primary goods. Considered alone, it certainly is: it is valued for its own sake; and it is a means to almost all ends. Indeed, it is a necessary good. No matter how eccentric a person's values and tastes are, no matter what kinds of activities are pleasurable, it is impossible to engage in them unless alive. Most activities a person is likely to enjoy, in fact, require not only life but good health. Unless one believes in an afterlife, the rational person must rate death as an incomparable calamity, for it means the loss of everything.

But the significance of health as a primary good should not be overestimated. The health planner may attempt to argue for coercive reform of health-destructive behavior with a line of reasoning that recalls Pascal's wager.[5] Since death, which precludes all good experience, must receive an enormously negative valuation, contemplated action that involves risk of death will also receive a substantial negative value after the good and bad consequences have been considered. And this will hold true even if the risk is small, since even low probability multiplied by a very large quantity yields a large quantity. Hence anyone who risks death by living dangerously must, on this view, be acting irrationally. This would be grounds for suspecting that the life-threatening practices were less than wholly voluntary and thus created a need for protection. Further, this case would not require the paternalistic intervenor to turn away from pluralistic ideals, for the unhealthy habits would be faulted not on the basis of deviance from paternalistic values, but on the apparent lapse in the agent's ability to understand the logic of the acts.

This argument, or something like it, may lie behind the willingness of some to endorse paternalistic regulation of the life-styles of apparently competent adults. It is, however, invalid. Its premises may sometimes be true, and so too may its conclusion, but the one does not follow from the other. Any number of considerations can suffice to show this. For example, time factors are ignored. An act performed at age 25 that risks death at age 50 does not threaten every valued activity. It simply threatens the continuation of those activities past the age of 50. The argument also overlooks an interplay between the possible courses of action: if every action that carries some risk of death or crippling illness is avoided, the enjoyment of life decreases. This makes continued life less likely to be worth the price of giving up favorite unhealthy habits.[6] Indeed,

[5]The agnostic should adopt the habits which would foster his own belief in God. If he does and God exists, he will receive the infinite rewards of paradise; if he does and God does not exist, he was only wasting the efforts of conversion and prayer. If he does not try to believe in God, and religion is true, he suffers the infinitely bad fate of hell; whereas if God does not exist he has merely saved some inconvenience. Conversion is the rational choice even if the agnostic estimates the chances of God's existing as very remote, since even a very small probability yields a large index when multiplied against an infinite quantity.

[6]Readers of the previous footnote might note that a similar difficulty attends Pascal's wager. If the agnostic took steps to foster belief in every diety for which the chance of existing was greater than zero, the inconvenience suffered would be considerable, after all. Yet such would be required by the logic of the wager.

although it may be true that death would deny one of all chances for valued experiences, the experiences that make up some people's lives have little value. The less value a person places on continued life, the more rational it is to engage in activities that may brighten it up, even if they involve the risk of ending it. Craig Claiborne (1976), food editor of *The New York Times,* gives ebullient testimony to this possibility in the conclusion of his "In Defense of Eating Rich Food":

> I love hamburgers and chili con carne and hot dogs. And foie gras and sauternes and those small birds known as ortolans. I love banquettes of quail eggs with hollandaise sauce and clambakes with lobsters dipped into so much butter it dribbles down the chin. I like cheesecake and crepes filled with cream sauces and strawberries with crème fraîche . . .
>
> And if I am abbreviating my stay on this earth for an hour or so, I say only that I have no desire to be a Methuselah, a hundred or more years old and still alive, grace be to something that plugs into an electric outlet.

The assumption that one who is endangering one's health must be acting irrationally and involuntarily is not infrequently made by those who advocate forceful intervention in suicide attempts; and perhaps some regard unhealthy life-styles as a sort of slow suicide. The more reasonable view, even in cases of imminent suicide, seems rather to be that *some* unhealthy or self-destructive acts are less-than-fully voluntary but that others are not. Claiborne's diet certainly seems to be voluntary, and suggests that the case for paternalistic intervention in life-style cannot be made on grounds of logic alone. It remains true, however, that much of the behavior that leads to chronic illness and accidental injury is not fully under the control of the persons so acting. My thesis is merely that, first, this involuntariness must be shown (along with much else) if paternalistic intervention is to be justified; and, second, this can only be determined by case-by-case empirical study. Those who advocate coercive measures to reform life-styles, whose motives are purely beneficent, and who wish to avoid paternalism except where justified, might find such study worth undertaking.

Any such study is likely to reveal that different practitioners of a given self-destructive habit act from different causes. Perhaps one obese person overeats because of an oral fixation over which he has no control, or in a Pavlovian response to enticing television food advertisements. The diminished voluntariness of these actions lends support to paternalistic intervention. Claiborne has clearly thought matters through and decided in favor of a shorter though gastronomically happier life; to pressure him into changing so that he may live longer would be a clear imposition of values and would lack the justification provided in the other person's case.

The trouble for a government policy of life-style reform is that a given intervention is more likely to be tailored to practices and habits than to people. Although we may someday have a fat tax to combat obesity, it would be surprising indeed to find one that imposed charges only on those whose obesity was due to involuntary factors. It would be difficult to reach agreement on what constituted diminished voluntariness; harder still to measure it; and perhaps administratively impractical to make the necessary exceptions and adjustments. We may feel, after examining the merits of the cases, that intervention is justified in the compulsive eater's life-style but not in the case of Claiborne. If the intervention takes the form of a tax on obesity *per se,* we face a choice: Do we owe it to those like Claiborne *not* to enforce alien values more than we owe it to compulsive overeaters to protect them from self-destruction? The general right of epicures to answer to their own values, a presumptive right conferred by the pluralistic ethic spoken of earlier, might count for more than the need of compulsive overeaters to have health imposed on them, since the first violates a right and the second merely confers a benefit. But the situation is more complex than this. The compulsive overeater's life is at stake, and this may be of greater concern (everything else being equal) than the epicure's pleasures. Then, too, the epicure is receiving a compensating benefit in the form of longer life, even if this is not a welcome exchange. And there may be many more compulsive overeaters than there are people like Claiborne. On the other hand, the positive causal link between tax and health for either is indirect and tenuous, while the negative relation between tax and gastronomic pleasure is relatively more substantial. (For a fuller discussion of this type of trade-off, see Bayles [1974].) Perhaps the firmest conclusion one may draw from all this is that a thoroughly reasoned moral rationale for a given kind of intervention can be very difficult to carry out.

Paternalism: Problems in Practice. Even if we accept the social insurance rationale for paternalism in the abstract, then, there are theoretical reasons to question its applicability to the problem of living habits that are injurious to health. It is still possible that in some instances these doubts can be laid to rest. We may have some non-circular way of determining when self-destructive behavior is involuntary; we may have knowledge of what preferences people would have were their behavior not constrained; and there may be no way to restore their autonomy. While at least a *prima facie* case for paternalistic intervention would exist under such circumstances, I think it is important to note several practical problems that could arise in any attempt to design and carry out a policy of coercive life-style reform.

First, there is the distinct possibility that the government that takes over decision-making power from partially-incompetent individuals may prove even less adept at securing their interests than they would have been if left alone. Paucity of scientific data may lead to misidentification of risk factors. The primitive state of the art in health promotion and mass-scale behavior modification may render interventions ineffective or even counterproductive. And the usual run of political and administrative tempests that affect all public policy may result in the misapplication of such knowledge as is available in these fields. These factors call for recognizing a limitation on the social insurance rationale for paternalism. If rational persons doubt that the authorities who would be guiding their affairs during periods of their incompetence would themselves be particularly competent, they are unlikely to license interventions except when there is a high probability of favorable cost-benefit trade-off. This yields the strongest support for those interventions that prevent very serious injuries, and in which the danger posed is imminent (Feinberg, 1973).

These reflections count against a rationale for government involvement in vigorous health promotion efforts, as recently voiced by the Secretary of Health, Education, and Welfare (1975) and found elsewhere (McKeown and Lowe, 1974). Their statements that smoking and similar habits are "slow suicide" and should be treated as such make a false analogy, precisely because suicide often involves certain imminent dangers of the most serious sort in situations in which there cannot be time to determine whether the act is voluntary. This is just the sort of case that the social insurance policy here described would cover; but this would not extend to the self-destruction that takes 30 years to accomplish.

Second, there is some possibility that what would be advertised as concern for the individual's welfare (as that person defines it) would turn out to be simple legal moralism, *i.e.,* an attempt to impose the society's or authorities' moral prescriptions upon those not following them. In Knowles's call for life-style reform (1976) the language is suggestive:

> The next major advances in the health of the American people will result from the assumption of individual responsibility for one's own health. This will require a change in lifestyle for the majority of Americans. The cost of sloth, gluttony, alcoholic overuse, reckless driving, sexual intemperance, and smoking is now a national, not an individual responsibility.[7]

All save the last of these practices are explicit *vices*; indeed, the first two—sloth and gluttony—use their traditional names. The intrusion of non-medical values is evidenced by the fact that of all the living habits that affect health adversely, only those that are sins (with smoking excepted) are mentioned as targets for change. Skiing and football produce injuries as surely as sloth produces heart disease; and the decision to postpone childbearing until the thirties increases susceptibility to certain cancers in women (Medawar, 1977). If it is the unhealthiness of "sinful" living habits that motivates the paternalist toward reform, then ought not other acts also be targeted on occasions when persons exhibit lack of self-direction? The fact that other practices are not ordinarily pointed out in this regard provides no *argument* against paternalistic life-style reform. But those who favor pressuring the slothful to engage in physical exercise might ask themselves if they also favor pressure on habits which, though unhealthy, are not otherwise despised. If enthusiasm for paternalistic intervention slackens in these latter cases, it may be a signal for reexamination of the motives.

A third problem is that the involuntariness of some self-destructive behavior may make paternalistic reform efforts ineffective. To the extent that the unhealthy behavior is not under the control of the individual, we cannot expect the kind of financial threat involved in a

---

[7]Elsewhere, however, Dr. Knowles emphasizes that "he who hates sin, hates humanity" (Knowles, 1977). Knowles's argument in the latter essay is primarily non-paternalistic.

"fat tax" to exert much influence. Paradoxically, the very conditions under which paternalistic intervention seems most justified are those in which many of the methods available are least likely to succeed. The result of intervention under these circumstances may be a failure to change the life-threatening behavior, and a needless (and inexcusable) addition to the individual's woes through the unpleasantness of the intervention itself. A more appropriate target for government intervention might be the commercial and/or social forces that cause or support the life-threatening behavior.

Although the discussion above has focused on the problems attendant to a paternalistic argument for coercive health promotion programs, I have implicitly outlined a positive case for such interventions as well. A campaign to reform unhealthy habits of living will be justified, in my view, so long as it does not run afoul of the problems I have mentioned. It may indeed be possible to design such a program. The relative weight of the case against paternalistic intervention can be lessened, in any case, by making adjustments for the proportion of intervention, benefit, and intrusion. Health-promotion programs that are only very mildly coercive, such as moderate increases in cigarette taxes, require very little justification; non-coercive measures such as health education require none at all. And the case for more intrusive measures would be stronger if greater and more certain benefits could be promised. Moreover, even if the paternalistic rationale for coercive reform of health-related behavior fails completely, there may be other rationales to justify the intrusion. It is to these other sorts of arguments that I now turn.

Fair Distribution of Burdens

The problem of health-related behavior is sometimes seen as a straight-forward question of collective social preference:

> The individual must realize that a perpetuation of the present system of high cost, after-the-fact medicine will only result in higher costs and greater frustration ... This is his primary critical choice: to change his personal bad habits or stop complaining. He can either remain the problem or become the solution to it; Beneficent Government cannot—indeed, should not—do it for him or to him. (Knowles, 1977)

A good deal of the controversy is due, however, not to any one person's distaste for having to choose between bad habits and high costs, but rather some people's distaste for having to accept both high costs and someone *else's* bad habits. In the view of these persons, those who indulge in self-destructive practices and present their medical bills to the public are free riders in an economy kept going by the willingness of others to stay fit and sober. Those who hold themselves back from reckless living may care little about beneficence. When they call for curbs on the expensive health practices of others, they want the government to act as their agent primarily out of concern for their interests.

The demand for protection from the costs of calamities other people bring upon themselves involves an appeal to fairness and justice. Both the prudent person and the person with unhealthy habits, it is thought, are capable of safe and healthy living; why should the prudent have to pay for neighbors who decide to take risks? Neighbors are certainly not permitted to set fire to their houses if there is danger of its spreading. With the increasing economic and social connectedness of society, the use of coercion to discourage the unhealthy practices of others may receive the same justification. As the boundary between private and public becomes less distinct, and decisions of the most personal sort come to have marked adverse effects upon others, the state's protective function may be thought to give it jurisdiction over any health-related aspect of living.

This sort of argument presupposes a certain theory of justice; and one who wishes to take issue with the rationale for coercive intervention in health-related behavior might join the debate at the level of theory. Since this debate would be carried out at a quite general level, with only incidental reference to health practices, I will accept the argument's premise (if only for argument's sake) and comment only upon its applicability to the problem of self-destructive behavior. A number of considerations lead to the conclusion that the fairness argument as a justification of coercive intervention, despite initial appearances, is anything but straightforward. Underlying this argument is an empirical premise that may well prove untrue of at least some unhealthy habits: that those who take chances with their health *do* place a significant financial burden upon society. It is not enough to point to the costs of medical care for lung cancer and other diseases brought on by individual behavior. As Hellegers (1978) points out, one must also determine what the individual would have died of had he not engaged in the harmful practice, and subtract the cost of the care which that condition requires. There is no obvious reason to suppose that the diseases brought on by self-destructive behavior are costlier to treat than those that arise from "natural causes."

Skepticism over the burden placed on society by smokers and other risk-takers is doubly reinforced by consideration of the nonmedical costs and benefits that may be involved. It may turn out, for all we know prior to investigation, that smoking tends to cause few problems during a person's productive years and then to kill the individual before the need to provide years of social security and pension payments. From this perspective, the truly burdensome individual may be the unreasonably fit senior citizen who lives on for 30 years after retirement, contributing to the bankruptcy of the social security system, and using up savings that would have reverted to the public purse via inheritance taxes had an immoderate life-style brought an early death. Taken at face value, the fairness argument would require taxes and other disincentives on *non*-smoking and other healthful personal practices which in the end would sap the resources of the healthy person's fellow citizens. Only detailed empirical inquiry can show which of these practices would be slated for discouragement were the argument from fairness accepted; but the fact that we would find penalties on healthful behavior wholly unpalatable may weaken our acceptance of the argument itself.

A second doubt concerning the claim that the burdens of unhealthy behavior are unfairly distributed also involves an unstated premise. The risk taker, according to the fairness argument, should have to suffer not only the illness that may result from the behavior but also the loss of freedom attendant to the coercive measures used in the attempt to change the behavior. What, exactly, is the cause cited by those complaining of the financial burdens placed upon society by the self-destructive? It is not simply the burden of caring and paying for care of these persons when they become sick. Many classes of persons impose such costs on the public besides the self-destructive. For example, diabetics, and others with hereditary dispositions to contract diseases, incur unusual and heavy expenses, and these are routinely paid by others. Why are these costs not resisted as well?

One answer is that there *is* resistance to these other costs, which partly explains why we do not yet have a national health insurance system. But even those willing to pay for the costs of caring for diabetics, or the medical expenses of the poor, may still bridle when faced by the needs of those who have compromised their own health. Is there a rationale for resisting the latter kinds of costs while accepting the former? One possible reason to distinguish the costs of the person with a genetic disease from those of the person with a life-style-induced disease is simply that one can be prevented and the other cannot. Health behavior change measures provide an efficient way of reducing the overall financial burden of health care that society must shoulder, and this might be put forward as the reason why self-destructive presons may have their presumptive rights compromised while others with special medical expenses need not.

But this is not the argument we seek. The medical costs incurred by diseases caused by unhealthy life-styles may be preventable, if our behavior-modifying methods are effective; but this fact shows only that there is a utilitarian opportunity for reducing costs and saving health-care dollars. It does *not* show that this opportunity makes it right to burden those who lead unhealthy lives with governmental intrusion. If costs must be reduced, perhaps they should be reduced some other way (*e.g.,* by lessening the quality of care provided for all); or perhaps costs should not be lowered and those feeling burdened should be made to tolerate the expense. The fact that money could be saved by intruding into the choice of life-styles of the self-destructive does not *itself* show that it would be particularly fair to do so.

If intrusion is to be justified on the grounds that unhealthy life-styles impose unfair financial burdens on others, then, something must be added to the argument. That extra element, it seems, is *fault.* Instead of the *avoidability* of the illnesses and their expenses, we point to the *responsibility* for them, which we may believe falls upon those who contract them. This responsibility, it might be supposed, makes it unfair to force others to pay the bills and makes it fair for others to take steps to prevent the behaviors that might lead to the illness, even at the cost of some of the responsible person's privacy and liberty.

The argument thus depends crucially on the premise that the person who engages in an unhealthy life-style is responsible for the costs of caring for the illness that it produces. "Responsible" has many senses, and this premise needs to be stated unambiguously. Since responsibility was brought into the argument in hopes of contrasting life-style-related diseases from others, it seems to involve the notions of choice and voluntariness. If the chronic diseases resulting from life-style were not the result of voluntary choices, then there could be no assignment of responsibility in the sense in which the term is being used. This would be the case, for example, if a person contracted lung cancer from breathing the smog in the atmosphere rather than from smoking. But what if it should turn out that even a person's smoking habit were the result of forces beyond the smoker's control? If the habit is involuntary, so is the illness; and the smoker in this instance is no more to be held liable for imposing the costs of treatment than would, say, the diabetic. Since much self-destructive behavior is the result of suggestion, constraint, compulsion, and other factors, the applicability of the fairness argument is limited.

Even if the behavior leading to illness is wholly voluntary, there is not necessarily any justification for intervention *by the state*. The only parties with rights to reform life-styles on these grounds are those who are actually being burdened by the costs involved. A wealthy man who retained his own medical facilities would not justifiably be a target of any of these interventions, and a member of a prepaid health plan would be liable to intervention primarily from others in his payments pool. He would then, of course, have the option of resigning and continuing his self-destructive ways; or he might seek out an insurance scheme designed for those who wish to take chances but who also want to limit their losses. These insured parties would join forces precisely to pool risks and remove reasons for refraining from unhealthy practices; preventive coercion would thus be out of the question. Measures undertaken by the government and applied indiscriminately to all who indulge in a given habit may thus be unfair to some (unless other justification is provided). The administrative inconvenience of restricting these interventions to the appropriate parties might make full justice on this issue too impractical to achieve.

This objection may lose force should there be a national health insurance program in which membership would be mandatory. Indeed, it might be argued that existing federal support of medical education, research, and service answers this objection now. But this only establishes another ground for disputing the responsibility of the self-destructive individual for the costs of his medical care. To state this objection, two classes of acts must be distinguished: the acts constituting the life-style that causes the disease and creates the need for care; and the acts of imposing financial shackles upon an unwilling public. Unless the acts in the first group are voluntary, the argument for imposing behavior change does not get off the ground. Even if voluntary, those acts in the second class might not be. Destructive acts affect others only because others are in financial relationships with the individual that cause the medical costs to be distributed among them. If the financial arrangement is mandatory, then the individual may not have *chosen* that his acts should have these effects on others. The situation will have been this: an individual is compelled by law to enter into financial relationships with certain others as a part of an insurance scheme; the arrangement causes the individual's acts to have effects on others that the others object to; and so they claim the right to coerce the individual into desisting from those acts. It seems difficult to assign to this individual responsibility for the distribution of financial burdens. He or she may (or may not) be responsible for getting sick, but not for having the sickness affect others adversely.

This objection has certain inherent limitations in its scope. It applies only to individuals who are brought into a mandatory insurance scheme against their wishes. Those who join the scheme gladly may perhaps be assigned responsibility for the effect they have on others once they are in it; and certainly many who will be covered in such a plan will be glad of it. Further, the burden imposed under such a plan does not occur until persons who have made themselves sick request treatment and present the bill to the public. Only if treatment is mandatory and all financing of care taken over by the public can the imposition of burden be said to be wholly involuntary.

In any case, certain adjustments could be made in a national health insurance plan or service that would disarm this objection. Two such changes are obvious: the plan could be made voluntary, rather than mandatory; and/or the public could simply accept the burdens imposed by unhealthy life-styles and refrain from attempts to modify them. The first of these may be impractical for economic reasons (in part because the plan would fill up with those in greatest need, escalating costs), and the second only ignores the problem for which it is supposed to be a solution.

There is, however, a response that would seem to have more chance of success: allowing those with unhealthy habits to pay their own way. Users of cigarettes and alcohol, for example, could be made to pay an excise tax, the proceeds of which would cover the costs of treatment for lung cancer and other resulting illnesses. Unfortunately, these costs would also be paid by users who are not abusers: those who drink only socially would be forced to pay for the excesses of alcoholics. Alternatively, only those contracting the illnesses involved could be charged; but it would be difficult to distinguish illnesses resulting from an immoderate life-style from those due to genetic or environmental causes. The best solution might be to identify persons taking risks (by tests for heavy smoking, alcohol abuse, or dangerous inactivity) and charge higher insurance premiums accordingly. This method could be used only if tests for these behaviors were developed that were non-intrusive and administratively manageable.[8] The point would be to have those choosing self-destructive life-styles assume the true costs of their habits. I defer to economists for devising the best means to this end.[9]

This kind of policy has its good and bad points. Chief among the favorable ones is that it allows a maximum retention of liberty in

---

[8]It may be that the only way to separate smokers and drinkers taking risks from those not taking risks is to wait until illness develops or fails to develop. Perhaps smokers could save their tax seals and cash them in for refunds if they reach 65 without developing lung cancer!

[9]The reader may sense a paradox by this point. Taxes on unhealthy habits would avoid inequities involved in life-style reform measures, such as taxes on unhealthy habits. And it is true that some of the steps that might be taken to permit those with unhygienic life-styles to assume the costs incurred might resemble those that could be used to induce them to give the habits up. Despite this, and despite the fact that the two kinds of programs might even have the same effects, I believe that they can and ought to be distinguished. The imposition of a fat tax has a behavior change as its goal. It is this goal that made it a topic for discussion in this paper. It would not be imposed to cover the costs of diseases stemming from unhealthy life-styles—indeed, as the reader will recall, the funds obtained through the tax were to be kept in trust and returned later if and when the behavior changed. In contrast, the taxes being mentioned as part of a "pay-as-you-go" plan would not be imposed as a means to changing behavior. Such a proposal would constitute one way of financing health costs, a topic I am not addressing in the present paper. These taxes would, of course, tend to discourage the behavior in question; but this (welcome) effect would not be their purpose nor provide their rationale (more precisely, *need* not be their purpose). Any program, of course, can serve multiple needs simultaneously. The "pay-as-you-go" tax would succeed as a program even if no behavior change occurred, and the behavior-modifying tax would succeed if behavior did change even if no funds were raised. In any case, surcharges and taxes would be but a few methods among many that might be used to induce behavior change; while they could constitute the whole of a policy aimed to impose costs upon those incurring them.

a situation in which liberty carries a price. Under such a policy, those who wished to continue their self-destructive ways without pressure could continue to do so, provided that they absorbed the true costs of their practices themselves. Should they not wish to shoulder these costs, they could submit to the efforts of the government to induce changes in their behavior. If the rationale for coercive reform is the burden the unhealthy life-styles impose on others, this option seems to meet its goals; and it does so in a way that does not require loss of liberty and immunity from intrusions. Indeed, committed immoderates might have reason to welcome the imposition of these costs. Although their expenses would be greater, they would thereby remove at one stroke the most effective device held by others to justify meddling with their "chosen" life-styles (Detmer, 1976).

The negative side of this proposal stems from the fact that under its terms the only way to retain one's liberty is to pay for it. This, of course, offers very different opportunities to rich and poor. This inequality can be assessed in very different ways. From one perspective, the advantage money brings to rich people under this scheme is the freedom to ruin their own health. Although the freedom may be valued intrinsically (*i.e.,* for itself, not as a means to some other end), the resulting illness cannot; perhaps the poor, who are denied freedom but given a better chance for health, are coming off best in the transaction. From another perspective, however, it seems that such a plan simply adds to the degradation already attending to being poor. Only the poor would be forced to submit to loss of privacy, loss of freedom from pressure, and regulation aimed at behavior change. Such liberties are what make up full citizenship, and one might hold that they ought not to be made contingent on one's ability to purchase them.[10]

---

[10]It might be possible to devise charges that would be assessed proportionately to income, so that the "bite" experienced by rich and poor would be about the same. This has not been the pattern in the past: all pay the same tax on a pack of cigarettes. In any case, this adjustment is in no way mandated by the fairness argument. The purpose of the charges would be to permit self-destructive individuals to "pay their own way" and hence remain free to indulge in favored habits. Reducing the amounts charged to low-income persons fails to realize that end; the costs of medical treatment for the poor are not any lower than for the rich. Indeed, being poor may increase the likelihood that the costs of treatment would have to be borne by the public. This suggests a scheme in which charges are assessed *inversely* proportional to income.

The premise that illnesses caused by unhealthy habits impose financial burdens on society, then, does not automatically give cause for adopting strong measures to change the self-destructive behavior. Still, it *may* do so, if the underlying theory of justice is correct and if its application can skirt the problems mentioned here. Besides, justification for such programs may be derived from other considerations.

Indeed, there is one respect in which the combined force of the paternalistic rationale and the fairness argument is greater than the sum of its parts. The central difficulty for the fairness argument, mentioned above, is that much of the self-destructive behavior that burdens the public is not really the fault of the individual; various forces, internal and external, may conspire to produce such behavior independently of the person's will. Conversely, a problem for the paternalist is that much of the harm from which the individual would be "protected" may be the result of free, voluntary choices, and hence beyond the paternalist's purview. The best reason to be skeptical of the first rationale, then, is doubt over the *presence* of voluntariness; the best reason to doubt the second concerns the *absence* of voluntariness. Whatever weighs against the one will count for the other.

The self-destructive individual, then, is caught in a theoretical double-bind: whether the behavior is voluntary or not, there will be at least *prime facie* grounds for coercive intervention. The same holds true for partial voluntariness and involuntariness. This consideration is of considerable importance for those wanting to justify coercive reform of health-related behavior. It reduces the significance of the notion of voluntariness in the pro-intervention arguments, and so serves to lessen concern over the intractable problems of defining the notion adequately, and detecting and measuring its occurrence.

Public Welfare

Aside from protecting the public from unfair burdens imposed by those with poor health habits, there may be social benefits to be realized by inducing immoderates to change their behavior. Health behavior change may be the most efficient way to reduce the costs of health care in this country, and the benefits derived may give reason to create some injustices. Further, life-style reform could yield some important collective benefits. A healthier work force means a stronger economy, for example, and the availability of healthy soldiers enhances national security.

There may also be benefits more directly related to health. If the supply of doctors and curative facilities should prove relatively inelastic, or if the economy would falter if too much of our resources were diverted to health care, it may be impossible to increase access to needed medical services. The social goal of adequate treatment for all would then not be realizable unless the actual need for medical care were reduced. Vigorous government efforts to change life-styles may be seen as the most promising means to this end.

The achievement of these social goals—enhanced security, improved economic functioning, and universal access to medical care—could come at the price of limits to the autonomy of that segment of society that indulges in dangerous living. If we do not claim to find fault with them, it would be unreasonable to insist that the immoderate *owed* the loss of some of their liberties to society as a part of some special debt—while continuing to exempt from special burden those with involuntary special needs due to genes or body chemistry. The reason for society to impose a loss upon the immoderate rather than upon the diabetic would be, simply, that it stood to benefit more by doing so.

Whether it is permissible to pursue social goods by extracting benefits from disadvantageously situated groups within society is a matter of political ideology and justice. Our society routinely compromises certain of its citizens' interests and privileges for the public good; others are considered inviolate. The question to be decided is whether the practices that we now know to be dangerous to health merit the protection given by the status of right. The significance of this status is that considerations of utility must be very strong before curbing the practice can be justified. Unfortunately, I see no decisive argument that shows that smoking, sloth, and other dangerous enjoyable pastimes are or are not protected by rights. It is worth mentioning, however, that many behaviors of interest to health planners are almost certainly of too trivial significance to aspire to such protection; freedom to drive at 65 miles per hour rather than 55 is an example, as is the privilege of buying medicine in non-childproof containers. Consideration of social utility would seem to justify much that is being currently overlooked in prevention of injury and illness through behavior change.

Even those whose ideology would not ordinarily warrant government intervention on these grounds might make an exception for reform of unhealthy habits. Even if the real motivation for the reform efforts were to achieve the social goals mentioned above, some of the intervention might in fact be justifiable on paternalistic grounds; and even the intervention that is not thus justified confers some benefit in the form of promise of better health.

Means of Health Behavior Reform

Two questions arise in considering the ethics of government attempts to bring about healthier ways of living. The first question is: Should coercion, intrusion, and deprivation be used as methods for inducing change? The other question is: How do we decide whether a given health promotion program is coercive, intrusive, or inflicts deprivations? These questions are independent of each other. Two parties who agreed on the degree of coerciveness that might be justifiably employed in a given situation might still assess a proposed policy differently in this regard, and hence reach different conclusions on whether the policy should be put into effect.

Disagreement over the degree of coerciveness of health behavior change programs is to be expected, not least because of the vagueness of the notion of coercion itself. Some of the most difficult problems addressed in the philosophical literature (Nozick, 1969; Held, 1972; Bayles, 1972; and Pennock, 1972) arise in the present context: What is the difference between persuasion and manipulation? Can offers and incentives be coercive, or is coerciveness a property only of threats? And can one party be said to have coerced another even if the latter manages to accomplish that which the first party tried to prevent?

The answers to these and similar queries will affect the evaluation of various kinds of health promotion measures.

Health Education

Health education seems harmless. Education generally provides information and this generally increases our power, since it enhances the likelihood that our decisions will accomplish our ends. For the most part, there is no inherent ethical problem with such programs, and they do not stand in need of moral justification. Still, there are certain problems with some health education programs, and these should be mentioned.

Health education *could* be intrusive. Few could object to making information available to those who seek it out. But if "providing information" were taken to mean making sure that the public attained a high level of awareness of the message, the program might require an objectionably high level of exposure. This is primarily an esthetic issue, and is unlikely to cause concern.

Can education be coercive? Information can be used as a tool for one party to get another to do its bidding, just as threats can. But the method is different: Instead of changing the prospective consequences of available actions, which is what a threat does, education alerts one to the previously unrecognized consequences of one's acts. Educators who hope to increase healthful behavior will disseminate only information that points in that direction; they cannot be expected to point out that, in addition to causing deterioration of the liver, alcohol helps certain people feel relaxed in social settings. It is difficult to know whether to regard this selective informing as manipulative. Theoretically, at least, people are free to seek out the other side on their own. Such measures acquire more definite coercive coloration when they are combined with suppression of the other side; "control over the means of persuasion" is another option open to reformers.[11]

The main threat of coerciveness in health education programs, in my opinion, lies in the possibility that such programs may turn from providing information to manipulating attitude and motivation. Education, in the sense of providing information, is a means of inducing belief and knowledge. A review of the literature indicates, however, that when health education programs are evaluated, they are not judged successful or unsuccessful in proportion to their success in *inducing belief.* Rather, evaluators look at *behavior change,* the actions which, they hope, would stem from these beliefs. If education programs are to be evaluated favorably, health educa-

---

[11]Though this most clearly recalls the banning of liquor and cigarette advertising from the airwaves, I do not believe that the suppression of information was generally involved. The advertisements did not stress the delivery of information. The quoted phrase is Michael Walzer's (1978).

tors may be led to take a wider view of their role (Rosenstock, 1960). This would include attempts to motivate the public to adopt healthy habits, and this might have to be supplied by covert appeals to other interests ("smokers are unpopular," and so on). Suggestion and manipulation may replace information as the tools used by the health educators to accomplish their purpose. (American Public Health Association, 1975; Haefner and Kirscht, 1970; and Milio, 1976). Indeed, health education may call for actual and deliberate *mis*information: directives may imply or even state that the scientific evidence in favor of a given health practice is unequivocal even when it is not (a problem noted by Lalonde, 1974).

A fine line has been crossed in these endeavors. Manipulation and suggestion go well beyond providing information to enhance rational decision making. These measures bypass rational decision-making faculties and thereby inflict a loss of personal control. Thus, health education, except when restricted to information, requires some justification. The possible deleterious effects are so small that the justification required may be slight; but the requirement is there. Ethical concerns for this kind of practice may become more pressing as the educational techniques used to induce behavior change become more effective.[12]

Incentives, Subsidies, and Taxes

Incentive measures range from pleasantly noncoercive efforts such as offering to pay citizens if they will live prudently, to coercive measures such as threatening to fine them if they do not. Various

---

[12]See Ubell (1972). It might be objected that the kind of manipulation I am speaking of is practiced continuously by commercial advertisers, and that no justification is provided by or demanded from them. It certainly is true that these techniques are used, but this does not show that there is not a need for justification when they are used in the course of a government health promotion campaign. The fact that the commercials are tolerated may indicate not that the manipulative techniques are themselves unobjectionable, but rather that private interests enjoy First Amendment freedom from regulation in their attempts to communicate with the public. The rationale for this freedom—if it exists—may not apply to government communications. The government *per se* is not an entity with interests which must be protected by rights in society; and the same holds true (officially, at least) of health education advocates, when agents of the government.

noncoercive measures designed to facilitate healthful life-styles might include: providing jogging paths and subsidizing tennis balls. Threats might include making all forms of transportation other than bicycling difficult, and making inconvenient the purchase of food containing saturated fats.

Generally speaking, justification is required only for coercive measures, not for incentives. However, the distinction is not as clear as it first appears. Suppose, for example, that the government wants to induce the obese to lose weight, and that a mandatory national health insurance plan is about to go into effect. The government's plan threatens the obese with higher premiums unless they lose their excess weight. Before the plan is instituted, however, someone objects that the extra charges planned for eager eaters make the program coercive. No adequate justification is found. Instead of calling off the program, however, some subtle changes are made. The insurance scheme is announced with higher premiums than had been originally planned. No extra charges are imposed on anyone; instead, discounts are offered to all those who avoid overweight. Instead of coercion, the plan now uses positive incentives; and this does not require the kind of justification needed for the former plan. Hence the new program is allowed to go into effect.

The effect of the rate structure in the two plans is, of course, identical: The obese would pay the higher rate, the slender the lower one. It seems that the distinction between coercion and incentive is merely semantic. But this is the wrong conclusion. There is a real difference, upon which much ethical evaluation must rest; the problem is in stating what that difference amounts to. A partial answer is that a given measure cannot be judged coercive or noncoercive without referring to a background standard from which the measure's effects diverge favorably or unfavorably. Ultimately, I believe, the judgment required for the obesity measure would require us to decide what a fair rate would have been for the insurance; any charges above that fair rate would be coercive, and any below, incentive. (For an account of this complex subject, see Nozick, 1969). The rate the government plans to charge as the standard premium might not be the fair rate; and this shows that one cannot judge the coerciveness of a fee structure merely by checking it for surcharges.

Even if we are able to sort the coercive from the incentive measures, however, we may have reason to hesitate before allowing the government unlimited use of incentives. A government in a position to make offers may not necessarily coerce those it makes the offers to, but is relatively more likely to get its way; in this sense its power increases. Increased government power over life-styles would seem generally to require some justification. In particular, there is inevitably some danger that, given the present scientific uncertainty over the effects of many habits, practices might be encouraged that would contribute nothing to health or even be dangerous. A further problem with financial incentives is that if they are to affect the behavior of the rich they must be sizable; and this may redistribute wealth in a direction considered unjust on other grounds.

The imposition of financial penalties as a means of inducing behavior raises questions that have been touched on above. The chief issue, of course, is the deprivation this method inflicts. Even where justifiably applied to induce behavior change, no *more* deprivation ought to be used than is necessary; but there are administrative difficulties in trying to obey this limitation. Different persons respond to different amounts of deprivation—again, the rich man will absorb costs that would deter the poor one. A disincentive set higher than that needed to induce behavior change would be unfair; a rate set too low would be ineffective. The amount of deprivation inflicted ought, then, to be tailored to the individual's wealth and psychology. This may well be administratively impossible, and injustice would result to the degree that these differences were ignored.

Regulative Measures

The coercive measures discussed above concentrate on applying influence on individuals so that their behavior will change. A different way of effecting a reform is to deprive self-destructive individuals of the means needed to engage in their unhealthy habits. Prohibition of the sale of cigarettes would discourage smoking at least as effectively as exhortations not to smoke or insurance surcharges for habitual tobacco use. Yet, these regulative measures are surely as coercive, although they do not involve direct interaction with the individuals affected. They are merely one more way of intervening in an individual's decision to engage in habits that may cause illness. As such, they are clearly in need of the same or stronger justification as those involving threats, despite the argument that these measures are taken only to combat an unhealthy *environment,* and thus cannot be counted as coercing the persons who have unhealthy ways of living (Terris, 1968). For a discussion of this indirect form of paternalism, see Dworkin (1971). What distinguishes these "environmental" causes of illness from, say, carcinogens in the water supply, is the active connivance of the victims. "Shielding" the "victims" from these external forces must involve making them behave in a way they do not choose. This puts regulative measures in the same category as those applied directly to the self-destructive individuals.

Conclusions

I have been concerned with clarifying what sorts of justification must be given for certain kinds of government involvement in the reform of unhealthy ways of living. It is apparent that more is needed than a simple desire on the part of the government to promote health and/or reduce costs. When the measures taken are intrusive, coercive, manipulative, and/or inflict deprivations—in short, when they are of the sort many might be expected to dislike—the moral justification required may be quite complex. The principles that would be used in making a case for these interventions may have limited scope and require numerous exceptions and qualifications; it is unlikely that they can be expressed as simple slogans such as "individuals must be responsible for their own health" or "society can no longer afford self-destructiveness."

My goal has been to specify the kind of justification that would have to be provided for any coercive life-style reform measure. I have not attempted to reach a judgment of right or wrong. Either of these judgments would be foolhardy, if only in view of the diversity of health-promotion measures that have been and will be contemplated. Yet it might be appropriate to recall a few negative and positive points on life-style reform.

Inherent in the subject matter is a danger that reform efforts, however rationalized and advertised, may become "moralistic," in being an imposition of the particular preferences and values of one (powerful) group upon another. Workers in medicine and related fields may naturally focus on the medical effects of everyday habits and practices, but others may not. From this perspective, trying to induce the public to change its style of living would represent an enormous expansion of the medical domain, a "medicalization of life." The parochial viewpoint of the health advocate can reach absurd limits. A recent presidential address to a prominent professional health organization, for example, came close to calling for abolition of alcohol simply on the grounds that the rate of cirrhosis of the liver had increased by 6 per 100,000 over the last 40 years. In this instance, health is being imposed upon us as a goal from above; perhaps medicine would serve us best if it acted to remove the dangers from the pursuit of other goals.

When the motivation behind life-style reform is concern for tax-payers rather than for self-destructive individuals, problems of a different kind are posed. Insistence that individuals are "responsible" for their own health may stem from a conflation of two different phenomena: an individual's life-style playing a causal role in producing illness, and that individual being at fault and accountable for his or her life-style and illness. The former may be undeniable, but the latter may be very difficult to prove. Unless difficulties in this sort of view are acknowledged, attention may be diverted from the various external causes of dangerous health-related behavior, resulting in a lessening of willingness to aid the person whose own behavior has resulted in illness.

On the positive side, two points made earlier bear repetition. First, although I have emphasized the difficulties in justifying coercive measures to induce life-style change, I have done so in the course of outlining the sort of case that might be made in support. It is entirely possible that such measures might be fair and desirable; at least, this is consistent with the principles I have claimed are relevant to deciding the issue. Second, few of the steps called for in either the professional or lay literature have been very coercive or intrusive in nature. Little of what I have said goes against any of these. Indeed, one hopes that these measures will be funded and used to the extent they are effective. An increase in the number and scope of such research, education, and incentive programs may be the best result of the current attention to the role of life-style in maintaining health. This would serve two goals over which there cannot be serious dispute: enabling people to be as healthy as they want to be, given the costs involved; and reducing overall medical need so as to make room in the health care system for all who still require care.

References

American Public Health Association. 1975. Statement on Prevention. *The Nation's Health* 5(10): 7–13.

Bayles, M.D. 1972. A Concept of Coercion. In Pennock, J.R. and Chapman, J.W., eds., *Coercion.* pp. 16–29. Chicago/New York: Aldine Atherton, Inc.

————. 1974. Criminal Paternalism. In Pennock, J.R. and Chapman, J.W., eds., *The Limits of Law: Nomos XV.* New York: Lieber, Atherton.

Claiborne, C. 1976. In Defense of Eating Rich Food. *The New York Times,* December 8.

Department of Health, Education and Welfare. 1975. *Forward Plan for Health FY 1977–81.* (June). Washington, D.C.: U.S. Government Printing Office.

Dershowitz, A. 1974. Toward a Jurisprudence of "Harm" Prevention. In Pennock, J.R. and Chapman, J.W., eds., *The Limits of Law: Nomos XV.* New York: Lieber-Atherton.

Detmer, D.E. 1976. A Health Policy, Anyone? or What This Country Needs is a Market Health Risk Equity Plan! *The Public Affairs Journal* 6(3): 101–102.

Dworkin, G. 1971. Paternalism. In Wasserstrom, R., ed., *Morality and the Law.* Belmont, Calif.: Wadsworth Publishing Co.

Feinberg, J. 1973. *Social Philosophy.* Englewood Cliffs, N.J.: Prentice-Hall.

Fuchs, V.R. 1974. *Who Shall Live?* New York: Basic Books, Inc.

Gert, G., and Culver C. 1976. Paternalistic Behavior. *Philosophy and Public Affairs* 6(1): 45–57.

Haefner, D.P., and Kirscht, J.P. 1970. Motivational and Behavioral Effects of Modifying Health Beliefs. *Public Health Reports* 85(5): 478–484.

Haggerty, R.J. 1977. Changing Lifestyles to Improve Health. *Preventive Medicine* 6(2): 276–289.

Held, V. 1972. Coercion and Coercive Offers. In Pennock, J.R. and Chapman, J.W., eds, *Coercion.* pp. 49–62. Chicago/New York: Aldine Atherton, Inc.

Hellegers, A. 1978. Personal communication.

Hodson, J. 1977. The Principle of Paternalism. *American Philosophical Quarterly* 14(1): 61–69.

Knowles, J.H. 1976. The Struggle to Stay Healthy. *Time:* August 9.

————. 1977. The Responsibility of the Individual. In Knowles, J.H., ed., *Doing Better and Feeling Worse.* New York: W. W. Norton.

Lalonde, M. 1974. *A New Perspective on the Health of Canadians.* Report (April). Ottawa: Government of Canada.

MacCallum, G.C. 1966. Legislative Intent. *Yale Law Journal* 75(5): 754–787.

McKeown, T., and Lowe, C.R. 1974. *An Introduction to Social Medicine.* Second edition. Oxford: Blackwell's.

Mechanic, D. 1977. Personal communication.

Medawar, T.B. 1977. Signs of Cancer. *New York Review of Books* 24(10): 10–14.

Milio, N. 1976. A Framework for Prevention: Changing Health-Damaging to Health-Generating Life Patterns. *American Journal of Public Health* 66(5): 435–439.

Murphy, J.G. 1974. Incompetence and Paternalism. *Archiv für Rechts und Sozialphilosophie* LX(4): 465–486.

Nozick, R. 1969. Coercion. In Morganbesser, S.; Suppes, P.; and White, M.; eds., *Philosophy, Science and Method: Essays in Honor of Ernest Nagel.* New York: St. Martin's Press.

Pennock, J.R. 1972. Coercion: An Overview. In Pennock, J.R. and Chapman, J.W., eds., *Coercion.* pp. 1–15. Chicago/New York: Aldine Atherton, Inc.

Pomerleau, O., Pass, F., and Crown, V. 1975. Role of Behavior Modification in Preventive Medicine. *The New England Journal of Medicine* 292(24): 1277–1282.

Rosenstock, I.M. 1960. What Research in Motivation Suggests for Public Health. *American Journal of Public Health* 50(3): 295–302.

Terris, M. 1968. A Social Policy for Health. *American Journal of Public Health* 58(1): 5–12.

Ubell, E. 1972. Health Behavior Change: A Political Model. *Preventive Medicine* 1(2): 209–221.

Walzer, M. 1978. Review of C. Lindblom, *Politics and Markets.* In *New York Review of Books,* July 20.

Bibliography: Additional Resource Materials Related To This Field

Barry, P.Z. 1975. Individual Versus Community Orientation in the Prevention of Injuries. *Preventive Medicine* 4: 47–56.

Beauchamp, D.E. 1975. Federal Alcohol Policy: Captive to an Industry and a Myth. *The Christian Century* (September 17): 788–791.

———. 1975. Public Health: Alien Ethic in a Strange Land? *American Journal of Public Health* 65: 1338–1339.

———. 1976. Public Health as Social Justice. *Inquiry* 13: 3–14.

Becker, M.H., Drachman, R.H., and Kirscht, J.P. 1972. Motivations as Predictors of Health Behavior. *Health Services Reports* 87: 852–862.

Belloc, N.B. 1973. Relationship of Health Practices and Morality. *Preventive Medicine* 2: 67–81.

———, and Breslow, L. 1972. Relationship of Physical Health Status and Health Practices. *Preventive Medicine* 1: 409–421.

Biener, K.J. 1975. The Influence of Health Education on the Use of Alcohol and Tobacco in Adolescence. *Preventive Medicine* 4: 252–257.

Breslow, L. 1973. Research in a Strategy for Health Improvement. *International Journal of Health Services* 3: 7–16.

Brody, H. 1973. The Systems View of Man: Implications for Medicine, Science, and Ethics. *Perspectives on Biological Medicine* (Autumn): 71–92.

Brotman, R., and Suffet, F. 1975. The Concept of Prevention and Its Limitations. *The Annals of the American Academy of Political and Social Science* 417: 53–65.

Charrette, E.E. 1976. Life Styles: Controlled or Libertarian? (Letter to the Editor.) *The New England Journal of Medicine* 294: 732.

Cooper, J.D. 1966. A Nonphysician Looks at Medical Utopia. *Journal of the American Medical Association* 197: 105–107.

Dingle, J.H. 1973. The Ills of Man. *Scientific American* 229: 77–84.

Freeman, R.A., Rowland, C.R., Smith, M.C. et al. 1976. Economic Cost of Pulmonary Emphysema: Implications for Policy on Smoking and Health. *Inquiry* 13: 15–22.

Goldstein, M.K., and Stein, G.H. 1976. Regarding RF Meenan's Article "Improving the Public's Health — Some Further Reflections." (Letter to Editor.) *The New England Journal of Medicine* 294: 732.

Greenberg, D.S. 1975. Medicine and Public Affairs: Forward, Cautiously, with the Forward Plan for Health. *The New England Journal of Medicine* 293: 673–674.

Glover, P.L., and Miller, J. 1976. Guidelines for Making Health Education Work. *Public Health Reports* 91: 249–253.

Haddon, W, Jr. 1970. On the Escape of Tigers: An Ecologic Note. *American Journal of Public Health* 60: 2229–2234. (Originally published in *Technology Review* 72 (2), 1970.)

Higginson, J. 1976. A Hazardous Society? Individual versus Community

Responsibility in Cancer Prevention. *American Journal Public Health* 66: 359–366.

Kalb, M. 1975. The Myth of Alcoholism Prevention. *Preventive Medicine* 4: 404–416.

Kass, L.R. 1975. Regarding the End of Medicine and the Pursuit of Health. *The Public Interest* 40 (Summer): 11–42.

McKnight, J. 1975. The Medicalization of Politics. *The Christian Century* (September 17).

Meenan, R.F. 1976. Improving the Public's Health — Some Further Reflections. *The New England Journal Medicine* 294: 45–46.

Ogden, H.G. 1976. Health Education: A Federal Overview. *Public Health Reports* 91: 199–217.

Outka, G. 1974. Social Justice and Equal Access to Health Care. *Journal of Religious Ethics* 2(1): 11–32.

Pennock, J.R., and Chapman, J.W., eds. 1972. *Coercion.* Chicago/New York: Aldine Atherton, Inc.

Pierce, C. 1975. Hart on Paternalism. *Analysis:* 205–207.

Preventive Medicine USA: Health Promotion and Consumer Health Education. 1976. A Task Force Report sponsored by the John E. Fogarty International Center for Advanced Study in the Health Sciences, National Institutes of Health, and The American College of Preventive Medicine, New York: PRODIST.

Rabinowitz, J.T. 1976. Review of *The Limits of Law: Nomos XV,* by Pennock, J.R., and Chapman, J.W., eds. (New York: Lieber-Atherton, 1974.) *Philosophical Review* 85: 244–250.

Regan, D.H. 1974. Justifications for Paternalism. In: Pennock, J.R., and Chapman, J.W., eds. *The Limits of Law: Nomos XV.* New York: Lieber-Atherton.

Roccella, E.J. 1976. Potential for Reducing Health Care Costs by Public and Patient Education. *Public Health Reports* 91: 223–224.

Sade, F. 1971. Medical Care as a Right: A Refutation. *The New England Journal of Medicine* 285: 1288–1292.

Somers, A.R. 1971. Recharting National Health Priorities: A New Canadian Perspective. *The New England Journal of Medicine* 285: 415–416.

Somers, H.N. 1975. Health and Public Policy. *Inquiry* 12: 87–96.

Thomas, L. 1975. Notes of a Biology-Watcher: The Health-Care System. *The New England Journal of Medicine* 293: 1245–1246.

Water Supply. 1976. *The United States Law Week* 44: 2480–2481.

Whalen, R.P. 1977. Health Care Begins with the I's. *The New York Times* (April 17).

White, K.L. 1973. Life and Death and Medicine. *Scientific American* 229: 23–33.

White, L.S. 1975. How to Improve the Public's Health. *The New England Journal of Medicine* 293: 773–774.

Wilson, F.R. 1976. Regarding RF Meenan's article "Improving the Public's Health — Some Further Reflections." Letter to Editor.) *The New England Journal of Medicine* 294: 732–733.

Wriston, H.M. 1976. Health Insurance. *The New York Times* (May 23).

Acknowledgments: The author acknowledges support of the Joseph P. Kennedy, Jr., Foundation and of the Institute of Medicine, National Academy of Sciences; helpful suggestions from Lester Breslow, Don Detmer, Edmund Pellegrino, Michael Pollard, Bernard Towers, members of the Institute's Social Ethics Committee, and *Health and Society's* referees; and numerous points and ideas from Norman Fost, Gerald MacCallum, John Robertson, Norma Wikler, and, particularly, David Mechanic.

Address correspondence to: Daniel I. Wikler, Ph.D., Department of the History of Medicine, University of Wisconsin Center for Health Sciences, 1305 Linden Drive, Madison, Wisconsin 53706.

Public Health and Public Wealth: Social Costs as a Basis for Restrictive Policies

DAVID T. COURTWRIGHT

Department of History,
University of Hartford

HISTORICALLY, THE MOST IMPORTANT RATIONALE for coercive public health measures has been the prevention of disease and injury to others. However, as noncommunicable diseases and accidents have assumed increased importance as causes of morbidity and mortality, and as the connection between noncommunicable diseases and accidents and individual practices such as smoking and drinking has become more apparent, a new line of argument based on social costs has emerged. My purpose is both to describe and evaluate the social-costs argument, to explain why it has become so popular, and to show what must be done to make it consistent with its own utilitarian criterion.

Justifying Coercion

In 1710, a Königsberg servant girl, Barbara Thutin, violated a local public health regulation by appropriating several fomites, or articles belonging to plague victims. Shortly thereafter, she and her master died of the disease. When officials learned of her transgression, the servant girl was exhumed, hanged in her coffin on the gallows, and then publicly burned (Nohl, 1961).

Barbara Thutin's fate is an illustration, admittedly extreme, of the

Milbank Memorial Fund Quarterly/*Health and Society,* Vol. 58, No. 2, 1980
© 1980 Milbank Memorial Fund and Massachusetts Institute of Technology
0160-1997-80-5802-0268-15/$01.00/0

coercive nature of most public health measures. Although society no longer resorts to punitive postmortem mutilation, most public health measures still entail a sanction, usually a fine or imprisonment. One of the first actions taken by New York City's Metropolitan Board of Health, for example, was the regulation of noxious odors emanating from rendering plants. The plant owners resisted, complaining that their "private rights" were being violated, but the board pursued the matter in the courts and eventually was able to secure the conviction of a prominent violator of the law. The offender was clapped into prison for sixty days, and thereafter no open violation of the law was noted (New York City, 1866).

When legislators and public health officials are called upon to justify their actions, they usually respond that such measures are a legitimate exercise of the police power, the recognized authority of the state to preserve the public health, safety, morals, and welfare. The concept of police power does not deny the existence of private rights, but it subordinates them to the well-being of the community. The invocation of the police power is especially compelling in the area of public health, since the irresponsible actions of one person may result in the sickness, injury, or death of another, or possibly trigger an epidemic that threatens the fabric of society itself. It was on this ground that New York City sanitarians sought to control miasmas escaping from rendering plants; a similar justification (if a different etiology) underlies current regulation of kitchens and canneries, the sewerage of cities and towns, and even the defecation of urban dogs. The disease-prevention rationale is also applied to situations where the immediate danger is posed only to the individual. The state, for example, might require immunization of a citizen returning from a region where plague was active. If the citizen protested that he would take his own chances, the common-sense reply would be that plague is never an individual matter, that the returning citizen, if infected, might transmit the disease to others.

Thus, historically, concern for the health and safety of society at large, rather than for protecting the individual from his own folly, has served as the primary justification for coercive public health measures. This pattern is changing, however, as the old reasoning is being supplemented, or in some instances superseded, by a newer and more subtle type of analysis based upon social costs. To understand the increasing popularity of the social-costs argument, it is first necessary to examine the changing orientation of public health itself.

Communicable diseases, once the leading causes of death, have largely been replaced in developed countries by heart disease, cancer, stroke, and accidents. In 1976 these four categories of disease accounted for over 70 percent of all deaths in the United States (Department of Health, Education, and Welfare, 1978). If further, significant progress is to be made in reducing the rates of mortality and morbidity in developed countries, it will be made in the areas of noncommunicable disease and accidents. Broadly speaking, three strategies are available: prevention, early detection, and treatment. Each strategy has its proponents, but there is a consensus among public health professionals, as well as among a growing number of physicians, researchers, politicians, and economists, that the best approach is prevention. Better to reduce exposure to carcinogens, for example, than to rely on such drastic and chancy therapies as surgery, radiation, and chemotherapy.

Effective prevention of the leading noncommunicable diseases and accidents, however, will inevitably involve changes in individual lifestyles. John Knowles, a physician who was one of the most trenchant critics of individual health misbehavior, put the matter thus:

> Prevention of disease means forsaking the bad habits which many people enjoy—overeating, too much drinking, taking pills, staying up at night, engaging in promiscuous sex, driving too fast, and smoking cigarettes—or, put another way, it means doing things which require special effort—exercising regularly, going to the dentist, practicing contraception, ensuring harmonious family life, submitting to screening examinations. (Knowles, 1977:59)

To urge people to adopt such reforms is one thing; to require them by law is quite another. The traditional harm-to-others doctrine, as it is generally applied, is inadequate to justify proscription of personal bad habits. Consider laws penalizing drivers who do not wear seat belts, or bans on alleged consumer carcinogens such as saccharin. What does the state say to the irate motorist or diet cola drinker who demands the right to take his own chances? After all, head injuries and bladder cancers are not contagious; only the individual's health and safety are involved.

Alternative Lines of Response

There are many possible rejoinders to such individual objections—virtually as many, in fact, as there are ethical systems. A Kantian, for example, would offer the categorical imperative as a rationale for compliance, while a Thomist would presumably cite Aquinas on the right and duty of the ruler to promote the welfare of the community (D'Entrèves, 1974:79). In practice, however, public health officials are not given to consideration of the universal implications of human actions, nor are they prone to theological speculation; instead, they have consistently justified their regulations on the narrowest and most secular of grounds. In liberal democracies, this has meant a growing recourse to the quantitative utilitarianism of social-costs analysis; in totalitarian societies, officials have tended—when they have bothered to justify their decisions at all—to couch their arguments in what I would describe as neocameralist terms.

Cameralism was a philosophy that developed in the seventeenth- and eighteenth-century Germanic states; akin to mercantilism, it held that numerous and healthy subjects were a vital source of the monarch's wealth and power. This idea found its culminating expression in Johann Peter Frank's (1976) *A System of Complete Medical Police*, a six-volume treatise printed at intervals over the years 1779–1819, touching on virtually all aspects of human behavior. Writing on such concerns as "the maternal duty to suckle and its influence on the welfare of the state," Frank completely subordinated the individual to society; health was not so much an inalienable right as something one pursued, or was forced to pursue, to foster the strength of the absolutist state. Although monarchical governments have largely disappeared, cameralist notions have lingered, especially in highly nationalistic and totalitarian societies like Nazi Germany. Erich Hesse, a German physician, furnished a good example of this type of reasoning in his 1938 book, *Die Rausch- und Genussgifte,* translated as *Narcotics and Drug Addiction* (Hesse, 1946). He was discussing the rationale of compulsory detoxification programs for morphine addicts:

> The justification . . . hinges on the question: Has a man the right to destroy his own body by poisons? No member of the national community has this right. On the contrary, everyone has the obligation to keep himself fit to the benefit of the community. The community, which gives the individual his chance to live and to make a living, has every right . . . to demand this. (Hesse, 1946:47)

The terminology has altered somewhat ("national community" replaces "monarchy"), but in outline the argument is basically the same: the state is an organic whole, related to individuals in the way a human body is related to its constituent cells. Unhealthy cells mean an unhealthy body, but this is unthinkable, since the well-being—indeed, the very existence of the cells—is inseparable from the fate of the body. Put another way, it is difficult to construct a sturdy *fasces* out of a bundle of rotten sticks. This type of neocameralist argument can easily serve to justify the most restrictive public health policies, even if no direct harm results to others. Saccharin and tobacco are bad for the individual and therefore bad for the state; laws compelling the use of seat belts and motorcycle helmets can be predicated on similar grounds.

There are, however, serious political and philosophical objections to neocameralism. Practically speaking, the United States and many European societies are dominated by consumerism and are characterized, in varying degrees, by acquisitive individualism. In a country like the United States, where life, liberty, and the pursuit of happiness are enshrined in the Declaration of Independence, appeals to end unhealthy but pleasurable practices on the basis of an abstract doctrine of national health are highly unpopular. Beyond the instinctive unwillingness of individual consumers to heed neocameralist injunctions, there is a sophisticated libertarian tradition, urging, as John Stuart Mill wrote in 1859, "that the only purpose for which power can be rightfully exercised over any member of a civilized community, against his will, is to prevent harm to others. His own good, either physical or moral, is not a sufficient warrant" (Mill, 1977:223). Regulation of individual actions that do not cause "perceptible hurt" to others, Mill argued, is inevitably disutilitarian; governmental meddling hampers the development of personality, checks social progress, fosters the tyranny of the majority, and disregards the opinion of the one person—the individual himself—who is in the best position to know what constitutes his own happiness. Mill did not dispute the importance of national strength and well-being, but adopted the issue as his own. "The worth of a State, in the long run," he wrote, "is the worth of the individuals composing it . . . ; a State which dwarfs its men, in order that they may be docile instruments in its hands even for beneficial purposes [,] will find that with small men no great thing can really be accomplished" (Mill, 1977:310). Mill's fear of governmental regulation of the minutiae of life has been echoed by any number of twentieth-century libertarian thinkers, and has been elaborated in the novels of E.I. Zamyatin, George Orwell, Anthony Burgess, and others intent on dramatizing the dangers of Big Brother. Mill's arguments have also had a restraining influence on police-power legislation, at least in the United States; legislators have been reluctant to pass, and judges on occasion reluctant to uphold, blatant interference with individual activities when no clear injury to others has been demonstrated (*University of Chicago Law Review*, 1970).

Yet the unpleasant fact remains that millions of Americans are smoking, eating, drinking, and drugging themselves to an early death, and that significant improvement in the nation's health awaits eradication or at least reduction of such unhealthy practices. Confronted with premature and preventable disease, but aware of the political unacceptability of neocameralist arguments, public health advocates have had to turn elsewhere for justification of restrictions on unhealthy individual activities. Increasingly they have turned to an analysis of social costs.

The idea of social costs is not new; it can be traced back at least as far as Jeremy Bentham, who stressed the need for a hedonic calculus. One of Bentham's disciples, the great English sanitarian Edwin Chadwick, made repeated use of social costs, and in 1842 even performed a rudimentary cost-benefit calculation in his *Report on the Sanitary Condition of the Labouring Population of Great Britain* (Chadwick, 1965). In

1850 an American physician, J.C. Simonds, computed the net cost of preventable disease for the city of New Orleans, and in 1873 Max von Pettenkofer made a similar estimate for the city of Munich (Sigerist, 1944). Social costs were also an important part of the celebrated brief of Louis Brandeis and Felix Frankfurter in *Bunting v. Oregon* (Frankfurter and Goldmark, 1915), the Supreme Court case testing the constitutionality of the ten-hour work day. What is new about the social-costs argument is its increasing application to issues of individual unhealthiness. Basically, it is an attempt to revive the harm-to-others doctrine, with an important and strategic twist: indirect monetary effects are substituted for direct health effects. Tobacco smoking, for example, is harmful not only to the smoker, but also to those who must defray the costs of tobacco-related illness. The smoker who develops emphysema or lung cancer accumulates large medical bills, most of which are covered by private or government insurance. We all pay. As John Knowles (1977:59) put it, "One man's freedom in health is another man's shackle in taxes and insurance premiums." Additional costs may be generated by disability payments or widows' pensions. There are also losses of productivity if, as is likely, the illness results in increased absenteeism or premature death (Cooper and Rice, 1976). A similar case can be made for stricter control of alcohol, mandatory use of seat belts, life jackets, and motorcycle helmets, or banning consumer products linked to cancer. In the end, all such arguments come down to this: since your unhealthy acts hit the rest of us in our pocketbooks, we have a right to pressure you to change. The appeal is ultimately to utility; bad habits are penalized in the name of the greatest (economic) good for the greatest number—although, ironically, Mill would have denied the validity of this type of analysis on the ground that there are other, unaffordable costs associated with enforced conformity.

The social-costs argument is thus a convenient way of retaining the harm-to-others doctrine while attacking activities that involve individual risk to health. This is not to imply that the traditional disease-prevention argument has been abandoned; indeed, both rationales often surface in the same controversy. Antismoking forces, when advocating no smoking in public places, talk about the harm to the other person but, when discussing proposals such as drastically increased cigarette taxes, shift to the social-costs argument. Similarly, antialcohol forces point to the dangers posed by drunk drivers, as well as to the costs of treating heart disease, cancer of the esophagus, cirrhosis, and other alcohol-related disorders. But in other cases, such as the use of seat belts, saccharin, or even skateboards, the argument for regulation is generally made on the basis of social costs alone.

Problems with the Social-Costs Argument

I offer the foregoing as a historical commentary, a description of the way those who formulate and enforce public health policies have sought to justify their actions. In the remainder of this essay, however, I am concerned with critically evaluating the social-costs argument. Although the argument has its merits, particularly at a time when medical costs are rapidly increasing, there are several potential problems to which attention should be drawn. These may be summarized as the need to determine net social costs, the difficulty of determining net social costs, and the obligation to reduce social costs in the manner entailing the least coercion.

The Need to Determine Net Social Costs

A common rebuttal to the social-costs argument is that some allegedly unhealthy activities also generate economic benefits: tobacco is a cash crop, the tobacco industry employs thousands of persons, magazines depend heavily on revenues from cigarette advertising, and so forth. Moreover, there are certain opportunity costs associated with restrictive policies; tobacco farmers, for example, might derive substantially less income if they were forced to switch to corn or wheat. These are not necessarily fatal objections, but they do suggest that advocates of restrictive policies must be able to show that they will reduce the net social costs. In the case of tobacco, it must be shown that the savings resulting from the contemplated action (irrespective of distributional effects) outweigh the economic losses; otherwise, no appeal can be made to the principle of the greatest good for the greatest number. In practice, one finds some cases built on a careful weighing of costs and benefits, and others built only on a recital of social costs (cf. Atkinson and Townsend, 1977; Wolfe, 1977). Cases of the second type are incomplete and inadequate bases for coercive legislation, insofar as they have failed to establish that net harm will result to others.

The Difficulty of Determining Net Social Costs

In theory, the computation of net social costs is easy enough; one totals up costs and savings and then subtracts one sum from the other. In reality, however, such analyses are complex, expensive, and often incomplete. Two factors complicate the task: the difficulty of accurately assessing health costs, and the near impossibility of quantifying the intangible benefits individuals derive from unhealthy activities.

Evaluation of the dangers posed by consumer carcinogens furnishes an example of the first type of difficulty. Chemicals such as cyclamates or food and hair dyes are typically declared carcinogenic on the basis of rodent bioassay; that is, if an unusually large number of rats or mice develop cancer when fed a steady diet of these substances, the substances are considered likely human carcinogens. The problem is that the rodents receive relatively high doses, and it is difficult to calculate exactly what effect prolonged exposure to low doses will have on human populations. The task is not impossible; dose-response extrapolation models have been proposed, but these are still controversial (Jones and Grendon, 1975; Albert, Train, and Anderson, 1977; National Academy of Sciences, 1979). Epidemiologic studies can sometimes supplement bioassays, but these are not foolproof, as it is difficult to isolate and quantify all relevant variables. Moreover, as the saccharin controversy illustrates, epidemiologic findings sometimes conflict with the rodent studies (Armstrong et al., 1976; National Academy of Sciences, 1979). In short, whenever a case is made that we can save a certain number of lives by banning or restricting a given carcinogen, the figures presented must be understood as approximations, whose accuracy depends on the quantity and quality of the data available, as well as on the sophistication of the mathematical models used to analyze the data. Finally, even if the exact levels of morbidity and mortality associated with a particular carcinogen were known, the computation of social costs would still be difficult, since the calculation of the value of lost livelihood requires certain tricky assumptions about average earnings and the prevailing interest rate (Acton, 1975).

No existing mathematical model, however, can quantify the satisfaction that people derive from risky activities. Tackle football is a good example. Of the 1,200,000 persons who participate in organized tackle football each fall in the United States, between 50 and 86 percent sustain time loss injuries, a remarkable rate that would be intolerable in virtually any occupation other than sports. Some of the injuries are so serious that the young players are rendered quadriplegic; 3 of every 100,000 die (Torg et al., 1977). It might also be argued that the economic losses (in equipment sales, stadium receipts, television royalties) resulting from a ban on contact football would in the long run be made up by the increased popularity of less dangerous sports, such as soccer. Thus, on strict social-cost grounds, contact football should be forbidden. This argument, of course, neglects the whole range of emotional values that players and spectators attach to the game. How much is a traditional rivalry worth, or the disappointment of a fan who has followed a team for years? Every risky activity produces some satisfaction: the smoker relaxes after lighting up, the drinker experiences heightened confidence, the saccharin user satisfies his sweet tooth while congratulating himself for avoiding sugar and cutting calories. Are these real and substantial benefits, or are they passing sensations, which should be sacrificed in the name of social savings?

Reducing Social Costs while Minimizing Coercion

There are many different actions or combinations of actions that can bring about a reduction of net social costs, but often these actions involve a varying degree of curtailment of individual liberty. Of the array of proposals to minimize the costs of smoking, there are at least three—government-sponsored development of safer cigarettes; voluntary, government-subsidized smoking cessation clinics; and the education of school children—that involve no appreciable coercion. On the next level are policies that restrict the promotion and merchandising of tobacco: banning advertising, forbidding cigarette vending machines, and sale by prescription only. These proposals are coercive in the sense that they curtail corporate marketing options, even, in the case of advertising, options that are arguably protected by the First Amendment. But, from the consumer's point of view, relatively little coercion is involved, since purchase is still possible, though on less convenient terms. This is not necessarily true of sharply increased taxes on tobacco products, a policy that would seriously affect both manufacturers and consumers. Many smokers, especially the poorer ones, would be forced to restrict consumption or to sacrifice other commodities. As Mill (1977:298) succinctly put it, "Every increase of cost is a prohibition, to those whose means do not come up to the augmented price; and to those who do, it is a penalty laid on them for gratifying a particular taste." The most drastic measure of all would be total prohibition, the state in effect saying that the risks of smoking are so great that no one should legally be allowed to take them. The point to be made about such policy alternatives is that the least coercive combination, consistent with the maximum reduction of net social costs, is the most desirable. If, for example, it were to be determined that the introduction of safer cigarettes, coupled with intensive propaganda in schools and a ban on cigarette vending machines, would effect approximately the same savings as a near-prohibitive tax on tobacco, then the former combination of policies would be preferred because it is the least destructive of individual liberty.

Unfortunately, there are statutory mandates in the United States that push regulatory agencies toward the more drastic alternatives. A prime example of this is the Delaney Clause of the 1958 Food Additives Amendment to the Pure Food, Drug and Cosmetic Act. The clause, sponsored by Representative James J. Delaney of New York, states that ". . . no additive shall be deemed to be safe if it is found to induce cancer when ingested by man or animal, or if it is found, after tests which are appropriate for the evaluation of the safety of food additives, to induce cancer in man or animal" (U.S. House Committee on Interstate and Foreign Commerce, 1974:13; Kleinfeld, 1973). Unsafe additives, of course, are not allowed on the market, so that human or animal studies linking an additive to cancer theoretically trigger an automatic ban. In some cases this may be the appropriate action, but in others less drastic measures may be in order. As mentioned earlier, the evidence that saccharin causes cancer is contradictory; moreover, some groups, such as the obese and the diabetic, may derive benefits from its use—although the amount of benefit derived is controversial (cf. Cohen, 1978; Rosenman, 1978; National Academy of Sciences, 1979). This would seem to suggest a compromise measure, such as sale by prescription only, but the clause admits of only one action (proscription) and does not permit the assessment of net social costs. By contrast, some laws bearing on toxic substances, such as the Clean Air Act, Water Pollution Control Act, Safe Drinking Water Act, and Federal Insecticide, Fungicide and Rodenticide Act, permit social-costs analyses; other statutes, such as the Toxic Substances Control Act, require them as a matter of course (Eskridge, 1978). Whether or not proposed restrictions on a toxic substance are evaluated in terms of net social costs is often a matter of chance, depending on the language of the law under which the substance happens to fall. Reform may be on the way; a recent report by the National Academy of Sciences (1979), *Food Safety Policy: Scientific and Societal Considerations*, criticizes the existing law as complicated, inflexible, and inconsistent, and calls for the weighing of health and other benefits as well as the marketing of high-risk additives to selected subpopulations, such as diabetics, if circumstances warrant.

Conclusion

The harm-to-others doctrine, which has served for centuries as the basis for coercive public health measures, has become increasingly outmoded as the pattern of disease has shifted in developed countries. Today the leading causes of morbidity and mortality—accidents and noncommunicable diseases—are related intimately (though by no means exclusively) to individual irresponsibility and excess; yet grounds for state action are problematic, since, in many cases, only the individual's immediate health and well-being are at stake. Some public health officials, especially those in totalitarian societies, have responded by appealing to an abstract doctrine of organic national health, in effect reviving the main lines of the cameralist position. In Western democracies, however, the tendency has been to fashion a utilitarian rationale based on an analysis of social costs. This approach is, I believe, necessary and appropriate, especially in view of the enormous financial burden imposed on others by the costs of treating chronic disease in the modern welfare state. The problem is that such calculations are inherently difficult, and there is always the danger that we will be forced to take or to refrain from some action for no appreciable benefit. This danger can be minimized, however, if we insist that any given social-costs argument must be measured against three basic standards. First, does the analysis weigh concomitant economic losses? That is, does it compute net social costs? Second, is the assessment of risk based on substantial and consistent data, and are the models used to calculate reduced mortality and morbidity plausible ones? Third, has thought been given to selecting the policy or policies that entail the least coercion? Unless a social-costs argument meets these criteria, it must be considered incomplete, as there is no way of determining whether it is consistent with its implicit maxim, the greatest good for the greatest number.

References

Acton, J.P. 1975. *Measuring the Social Impact of Heart and Circulatory Disease Programs: Preliminary Framework and Estimates.* Santa Monica: Rand Corporation.

Albert, R.E., Train, R.E., and Anderson, E. 1977. Rationale Developed by the Environmental Protection Agency for the Assessment of Carcinogenic Risks. *Journal of the National Cancer Institute* 58:1537–1541.

Armstrong, B., et al. 1976. Cancer Mortality and Saccharin Consumption in Diabetics. *British Journal of Preventive and Social Medicine* 30:151–157.

Atkinson, A.B., and Townsend, J.L. 1977. Economic Aspects of Reduced Smoking. *Lancet* 2:492–494.

Chadwick, E. 1965. *The Sanitary Condition of the Labouring Population of Great Britain,* Flinn, M.W., ed. Edinburgh: Edinburgh University Press.

Cohen, B. 1978. Relative Risks of Saccharin and Calorie Ingestion. *Science* 199:983.

Cooper, B.S., and Rice, D.P. 1976. The Economic Cost of Illness Revisited. *Social Security Bulletin* 39:21–36.

D'Entrèves, A.P., ed. 1974. *Aquinas: Selected Political Writings,* trans. J.G. Dawson. Oxford: Basil Blackwell.

Department of Health, Education, and Welfare, Public Health Service, National Center for Health Statistics. 1978. *Facts of Life and Death.* Washington, D.C.: Government Printing Office.

Eskridge, N.K. 1978. Conflicting Academy Reports Leave EPA Bewildered. *BioScience* 28:309–311.

Frank, J.P. 1976. *A System of Complete Medical Police,* Levsky, E., ed. Baltimore: Johns Hopkins University Press.

Frankfurter, F., and Goldmark, J. 1915. *The Case for the Shorter Work Day, . . . Franklin O. Bunting vs. the State of Oregon, Brief for the Defendant in Error,* vol. 1, 428–451. New York: National Consumers' League.

Hesse, E. 1946. *Narcotics and Drug Addiction,* trans. F. Gaynor. New York: Philosophical Library.

Jones, H.B., and Grendon, A. 1975. Environmental Factors in the Origin of Cancer and Estimation of the Possible Hazard to Man. *Food and Cosmetics Toxicology* 13:251–268.

Kleinfeld, V.A. 1973. The Delaney Proviso: Its History and Prospects. *Food Drug Cosmetic Journal* 28:556–566.

Knowles, J.H. 1977. The Responsibility of the Individual. In Knowles, J.H., ed., *Doing Better and Feeling Worse: Health in the United States,* 57–80. New York: Norton.

Mill, J.S. 1977. On Liberty. In Robson, J.M., ed., *Collected Works of John Stuart Mill,* 18:213–310. Toronto: University of Toronto Press.

National Academy of Sciences. 1979. *Food Safety Policy: Scientific and Societal Considerations,* part 2. Springfield, Va.: National Technical Information Service.

New York City, Metropolitan Board of Health. 1866. *Annual Report.* New York: Wescott, Union Printing House.

Nohl, J. 1961. *The Black Death: A Chronicle of the Plague Compiled from Contemporary Sources,* trans. C.H. Clarke. London: Unwin.

Rosenman, K. 1978. Benefits of Saccharin: A Review. *Environmental Research* 15:70–81.

Sigerist, H.E. 1944. The Cost of Illness to the City of New Orleans in 1850. *Bulletin of the History of Medicine* 15:498–507.

Torg, J.S., Quedenfeld, T.C., Moyer, R.A., Truex, R., Jr., Spealman, A.D., Nichols, C.E., III. 1977. Severe and Catastrophic Neck

Injuries Resulting from Tackle Football. *Journal of the American College Health Association* 25:224–226.

University of Chicago Law Review. 1970. Limiting the State's Police Power: Judicial Reaction to John Stuart Mill. *University of Chicago Law Review* 37:605–627.

U.S. House Committee on Interstate and Foreign Commerce. 1974. *A Brief Legislative History of the Food, Drug, and Cosmetic Act.* Washington, D.C.: Government Printing Office.

Wolfe, S.M. 1977. Economic Costs of Smoking (mimeo). Washington, D.C.: Public Citizens' Health Research Group.

Research for this article was supported by the Samuel E. Ziegler Educational Foundation.

Address correspondence to: David T. Courtwright, Chairman, Department of History, University of Hartford, West Hartford, Connecticut 06117.

II Some Aspects of National Policy

Perspectives on Government Policy in the Health Sector

JAMES F. BLUMSTEIN

MICHAEL ZUBKOFF

Health expenditures and prices have accelerated markedly in recent years, both in absolute and relative terms. The pressures for some form of governmental intervention have generated widespread debate about national health policy. Determinants of health are complex, and policy development must follow the identification of issues and review of theoretical policy analysis. Formation of a theoretical basis will have a significant impact on substantive policy outcomes. Unfortunately, past and current proposals and policies have given insufficient attention to the traditional public finance criteria for government intervention; as a result, the importance of market forces has frequently been overlooked. Before wholesale rejection of the market as a means of promoting rationality, government should examine alternatives that foster increased effectiveness of the market mechanism. Even within this context, however, some forms of regulation will be necessary; also, traditional public finance norms would allow certain kinds of expanded government intervention. Market-perfecting policy instruments would result in different kinds of government programs, and much of future policy will be shaped by political decisions about substantive health policy issues.

The debate over a national health strategy is likely to continue as an important political issue for some time. The issues must be dealt with in broad terms in recognition of the wide variety of components that enter into the "production" of good health. Moreover, the theoretical foundation on which governmental action can be justified must be clearly identified and articulated because the policy consequences of choosing a theory of intervention are significant. The options available for governmental intervention are numerous, but before moving to an exclusively regulatory approach, government should attempt to reinvigorate the market as a device of social ordering in the health sector. This strategy would call for increased governmental regulation in areas where the market cannot reasonably be expected to function (for example, where a natural monopoly exists), but it would emphasize use of policy tools that retained the decentralized market system of decision making where possible and feasible. Government policy would then be aimed at restoring the ground rules and promoting the conditions that are prerequisites for an effective market. Consistent with this orientation, government could rationally justify support of compulsory insurance programs for emergency care and functional dislocation (or catastrophe). In addition, government could reasonably act to reduce the incidence of such illnesses through preventive measures. Although presentation of these areas of additional governmental intervention is not intended to be exhaustive, the discussion serves to illustrate the kinds of programs that could be justified under traditional public finance criteria for intervention.

Background

National health outlays have expanded both in absolute and relative terms at a staggering pace in recent years (Cooper and Worthington, 1973). For example, in fiscal 1972, national health expenditures amounted to $83.4 billion, an increase of $7.8 billion above the previous year and a rise of 10.3 percent, yet the rate of increase in health expenditures in fiscal 1972 was the lowest incremental rise since fiscal 1966.[1]

The enactment of Medicare and Medicaid in 1965 is in large part responsible for the recent spurt of growth of the health sector. The Medicare and Medicaid approach expanded the effective demand for medical services but did not simultaneously spur short-run increases in supply. Over the past seven years, the predictable has occurred: The substantial increase in demand, unmet by any similar short-run increase in supply, has resulted in acute stress on the system. As would be expected by conventional theory, the system has reacted to this imbalance by generating higher prices. Between 1965 and 1970, as measured by the Consumer Price Index of the Bureau of Labor Statistics, consumer prices in the medical

[1] Over the years 1940–1970, the percentage of Gross National Product (GNP) spent in the health sector went from 4.0 percent to 7.1 percent, and in fiscal 1971 and 1972 the health component of GNP rose to 7.6 percent. Thus, in the 25-year period 1940–1965, the percentage increased from 4.0 percent to 5.9 percent, while in the seven-year period 1965–1972 the percentage jumped almost as much as in that entire period (5.9 percent to 7.6 percent).

care sector skyrocketed, rising at a rate of 6 percent, compared to a similar overall price increase in the economy of 4.2 percent (Rice and Cooper, 1972). Some subsectors within the medical sector have experienced even greater price inflation, with prices in the hospital subsector rising by 10.6 percent in 1972, for example (Cooper and Worthington, 1973).

To a significant extent, the current emphasis on health care issues results from the runaway cost of medical services to consumers. This striking increase in costs has dramatized, in a politically potent way, the importance people have placed on medical care. As a result, great political pressure has arisen for the federal government to intervene to remedy the situation it helped create (U.S. Congress, 1971).

With full recognition of the extraordinary cost of this inflation, there is still an argument that the unbalanced strategy adopted in the mid-sixties succeeded in compelling full-scale, comprehensive consideration of basic issues in the health field much sooner than would otherwise have been the case. Some have argued that the inability to make important decisions is a major governmental shortcoming. Induced official decision making, in response to shortages and bottlenecks, may therefore prove beneficial in the long run. The stress on the medical sector brought about by the unbalanced strategy of demand stimulation has dramatized the weaknesses in the system, making the consuming public acutely aware of the system's inadequacies. In just seven years it has not only become apparent but also widely accepted that there are serious problems which necessitate some form of significant governmental response.

The impact of the "unbalanced strategy" of Medicare and Medicaid has led to federal efforts to develop a coordinated health program. Typically, federal intervention in the health area has been on an ad hoc basis without any overall plan, formulation of objectives, or theoretical underpinning. In 1969, Robert Finch, then-Secretary of the Department of Health, Education, and Welfare, candidly acknowledged (U.S. Congress, 1970: 224) that:

> . . . up to and including the present there has never been a formulation of national health policy, as such. In addition, no specific mechanism has been set up to carry out this function. As a consequence the national health policy is a more or less amorphous set of health goals, which are derived by various means and groups within the Federal structure.

In February, 1971, and April, 1972, President Nixon sent messages to Congress in which he outlined the need for developing a national health strategy, and in May, 1971, the Administration issued a detailed position paper. The liveliness of the ongoing debate seems largely attributable to the stresses resulting from the one-sided reliance on demand stimulation of Medicare and Medicaid. Whether the costs will have been worth bearing is uncertain and depends in part on successful identification of federal health objectives, formulation of federal health policy, and implementation of a federal health strategy.

The Basis for Government Involvement in the Health Sector

Public policy considerations regarding an appopriate federal role in health must not be restricted to a medical services orientation. To be sure, most of our discussion will focus on the medical care sector, but the complexity of the concept of health and the varied factors that contribute to its "production" must constantly be borne in mind.

The Concept of Health

The concept of health has a large social component. Illness may to a large degree be conditioned by culture, and its definition may be the product of a social bargaining process.[2] There is a second important social consideration which must enter into health policy formulation. A biological systems approach to illness, of course, is a critical aspect of defining the scope of the policy problem. Nevertheless, it is insufficient for policy purposes unless the functional elements of illness are incorporated into the analysis.

---

[2] An illustration of this social factor arises from the women's rights movement. By custom, working women in many occupations have been required to take a maternity leave after the fifth or sometimes the sixth month of pregnancy. An example of this bargaining process is the effort of the women's rights movement to eliminate automatic, mandatory maternity leave provisions, claiming, in effect, that this definition of "illness" imposed on women by society is illegal discrimination on the basis of sex. (See Wilson, 1970:3–12.) The United States Supreme Court has agreed to decide whether the claimed discrimination is unconstitutional (Cleveland Board of Education v. La Fleur, 1973:3565).

Health is not an ultimate but an instrumental value—an enabling condition, which helps lead to what is now typically labeled an improved "quality of life." Consequently, from a policy perspective, it may be important to look at the impact of an illness in determining what the appropriate governmental response should be. In this regard, it might be helpful to shift our emphasis from health or illness to disability and dislocation.

The "Production" of Health

Physicians are trained to look at the human being primarily as a physical specimen—a functioning biological organism. Coincident with this orientation, it is no wonder that they are likely to view the question of health from a biological systems approach. The biological orientation is understandable for those who are engaged in the delivery of medical care and may be serviceable for the medical practitioner, but it is not adequate as a basis for public decision making since the provision of medical care is not the only input in the "production process" of health. Normally, one thinks of going to the doctor because of an ailment and having the physician prescribe a cure. Except for certain fields like public health, which emphasizes preventive medicine, the medical profession in the United States has been remarkably cure-oriented. Only recently has the notion of health maintenance received the public prominence that it should have. But still, we tend to think of health largely as the result of a successful visit to a physician for a remedial service.

However, if greater attention is to be given health maintenance, with functional dislocation the major concern of policy, then serious questions of resource allocation arise within the health sector. Rational allocation of health dollars may require heavy investment in nonmedical items. In some societies, for instance, emphasis on such things as improving the quality of the community water supply or spraying against disease-carrying insects might result in the greatest overall increase in the community's health (Zubkoff and Dunlop, 1973).

As we have noted, health maintenance has begun to receive attention among health professionals, but the concept still carries with it a top-heavy medical service orientation. Most significant for our society, there are a considerable number of environmental factors which contribute substantially to our health problems; any governmental decision to become involved in the health sector must consider possible allocation alternatives in personal and nonpersonal environmental areas as a means of promoting health.

Three families of environmental problems which contribute to poor health are especially worthy of note. First are what might be called technological factors resulting from industrialization. The most common example of this type is air pollution. Unsafe working conditions and accidents resulting from defective equipment are other examples within this category of environmental factors which contribute to health risk.

A second category of environmental considerations might be called personal health maintenance. Under this heading are such things as overeating and failure to exercise. Health experts now believe that personal lifestyle habits have an important bearing on the incidence of disease. Also in this category are accidents of another type—those which result not from defective machinery (which of course might also arise from careless workmanship) but from personal carelessness or negligence. Accidents, caused both by defect and by human failure, account for a substantial amount of the cost associated with the health sector (U.S. Department of Health, Education, and Welfare, 1971:28-30).

The third category of environmental considerations is socio-economic status. It seems that the poor experience greater incidences of illness and shorter life expectancy; however, this is only partly the result of inadequate medical services (Antonovsky, 1967). A significant factor is poverty itself because it is accompanied by such things as inadequate sanitation, overcrowded housing, and bad nutrition (Lave and Lave, 1970: 255; Kadushin, 1964). In this regard, governmental programs which seek to alleviate specific conditions related to poverty have a significant health component; in determining an appropriate governmental response to health problems, the alternative allocation possibilities and their potential effect on improving health must be considered. It may be, for example, that emphasis on personal medical services may be an uneconomic allocation of health dollars unless a certain minimum standard of environmental quality is established (McDermott, 1969).

The Rationale for Government Action

In developing a federal health strategy, the government must identify its objectives. And implicit in this process of problem identification and goal formulation is an adoption of some theoretical basis on which to center governmental intervention.

The principles that have evolved in the field of public finance are founded on some normative judgments. Public finance norms assume that the market is the best means for allocating scarce resources. There is also an implicit assumption that the government in a democratic society promotes the welfare of individual citizens and does not necessarily act for the welfare of an organic society. This basically individualistic ethic is not limited to public finance theory but is reflected in other fields such as law.

A major policy question is thus whether to accept the public finance criteria for determining an appropriate federal role. Before addressing that issue, though, the traditional criteria for intervention will be discussed.

The basic economic justification for governmental intervention is as a remedy for some market failure. In essence, the traditional basis for governmental involvement has been remedial, when the market, for one reason or other, does not achieve an efficient allocation of resources. When traditional criteria serve as the basis of governmental action, substantive policy outcomes are left to the decentralized, impersonal marketplace; government's role, in this traditional regime, is primarily procedural, restoring the process of the market (or if necessary approximating the results which would have been achieved by a functioning market).

Traditional Criteria. Four traditional public finance criteria for government intervention are (1) externalities, (2) public goods, (3) monopoly, and (4) other market imperfections.

Externalities. Where there is a divergence between private and public costs and benefit, the competitive market system will not automatically achieve the social optimum. In these circumstances, some form of governmental action may be justified—either regulation, taxation or subsidy.

An externality is a direct influence of a producer's or a consumer's activity on the activities of other producers and consumers that is not evaluated or accounted for by the market. The market system is characterized by general interdependence and interaction among producers and consumers, but their interacting influences are exerted "indirectly" via relative prices within the market mechanism. Externality-generating influences, however, are exerted on producers and consumers "directly," outside the market mechanism (Mishan, 1971:2). They are not the deliberate outcome of a market relationship but rather an unintended or incidental result of legitimate but unrelated activity.

In the health field, national efforts historically have been directed primarily toward disease control and prevention in the area of public health (Chapman and Talmadge, 1970). From the outset, there has been little controversy about the propriety of some governmental role in combating epidemics; the government initiatives involved both prevention of communicable disease through immunization and control of epidemics through such measures as quarantines. The mandate for governmental intervention in public health, in traditional terms, arose from the very clearcut externalities involved in the spread of communicable disease. Understandably, and predictably, governmental initiatives in public health came early and drew widespread support.

The early federal emphasis on public health conforms to the traditional public finance criteria for government involvement since the private decision about prevention or cure does not reflect the total societal cost calculation. The United States Supreme Court has recognized the importance and constitutional legitimacy of governmental action, for example, in compelling smallpox vaccinations, even when the person involved claimed that his religion forbade the use of medicinal aids (Jacobson v. Massachusetts, 1905). Thus, governmental initiatives in public health have widely been recognized as justified in order to overcome the inadequacy of private decision making; this intervention, even by compulsion, has been sustained in the face of a constitutional challenge which pitted against governmental intervention the rights of free exercise of religion, a value whose special status is guaranteed by the First Amendment.

Public Goods. A second traditional basis for governmental involvement is the so-called public or social good. A public good is really an extreme example of an externality, a case in which benefits are entirely external (Musgrave, 1971:306). The decisive characteristic of a public good is that one individual's consumption does not interfere with anyone else's. In this sense, then, consumption of a public good is nonrival and contrasts with a pure private good from whose consumption the particular consumer derives the entire benefit.

Frequently, public goods are characterized by an inability to exclude people from the benefits that accrue. For example, national defense is often used as the typical illustration of a public good; theoretically, all citizens alike benefit from construction, say, of an aircraft carrier, and it is impossible (or at least extremely difficult) to exclude people from benefiting. As a consequence, no individual has an incentive to reveal the true value of the benefit because he will gain regardless of how much he contributes. This is commonly referred to as the "free-rider" problem. Private choice, in the aggregate, may not be a satisfactory process of decision making for achieving a socially desired outcome because of the difficulties of accurately determining true values in the market.

In the health field, the results of a successful immunization program may be characterized as a public good. Consumption is nonrival, and all members of the community share in its benefits without exception. The individual decision about treatment for a communicable disease is an example of a private decision that has external effects, but the "production" of epidemic control warrants governmental intervention because it is a public good of which consumption is nonrival.

Monopoly. A third traditional basis for governmental involvement is the monopoly case, of which there are two forms. The first occurs when cost structure and market size make competition inefficient and unfeasible. If market size and production technology allow a single firm to operate in the decreasing cost portion of its long-run cost curve, with any additional output at lower marginal cost, then the economies of scale cannot be exhausted at any given level of market demand. This form of monopoly is called a "natural monopoly." The utility companies are often cited as the example of this form of monopoly. In the utility case, the economies of scale in production and distribution are so marked that if several companies were in competition, costs would be substantially higher and significant inconvenience and misallocation of resources would occur.

The second type of monopoly is an "unnatural monopoly." An unnatural monopoly has been able to create an artificial situation, in which a producer is supplying its market with a good for which there are no close substitutes. The monopolist, in order to maximize profits, will restrict output and charge higher prices.

The presence of a monopoly indicates a breakdown in the perfectly competitive market and therefore justifies governmental intervention. With respect to "unnatural monopoly," regulation is aimed at restoring the conditions of competition in the marketplace, thus assuring that the economic game is played according to the rules of the market. Antitrust is a policy tool designed to promote competition and to prevent monopolization. With respect to "natural monopolies," however, the maintenance or reestablishment of competitive conditions is not a desirable policy response. The public utility model has been used in these cases. Returns on capital are permitted, but, through price regulation, these returns are supposedly kept as close as possible to those earned in the competitive market.

Characteristics of both the "natural" and "unnatural" monopolistic situations exist in the hospital subsector. The hospital is apparently subject to significant economies of scale in its production process (Hefty, 1969). As a result, hospitals in many communities probably operate in the decreasing cost portion of their long-run cost curve, and many small communities cannot hope to have more than one hospital. These isolated rural hospitals are essentially natural monopolies in that they are providing a service for which there is no close substitute and in which additional entry is not economically feasible because of the high capital cost and economies of scale.

Some observers report that hospitals are also monopolies in terms of patient access. In general, patients do not have a free choice concerning the hospital to which they are admitted because certain traditional characteristics of the physician-hospital relationship and the physician-patient relationship have limited access. Since the patient's lack of knowledge forces him to rely upon the physician's decision whether or not to hospitalize, and since the physician in turn is limited to those hospitals in which he has privileges, patient choice is curtailed not only by the number and location of hospitals but also by the institutional relationships between doctor and patient and doctor and hospital. This form of institutional constraint can be addressed by government policy that promotes access; it is not a "natural" monopoly, and policy tools aimed at opening up the system would be appropriate under the traditional criteria.

Monopoly elements also exist in the physician market through restriction on entry. The artificial shortage of physicians has resulted primarily from federal and state legislation concerning licensure requirements and from the educational requirements established by the American Medical Association. It has been argued that supply has been limited in order to restrict competition and thus allow physicians to set their own (higher) prices (Kessel, 1970; Kessel, 1958; Friedman and Kuznets, 1954:137); thus, the physician's monopolistic position must be classified as an "unnatural monopoly." This implies that government should modify those regulations restricting supply or impeding factor substitution.

Other Market Imperfections. There are situations in which the conditions of the competitive system do not obtain but which do not conform to the specific criteria for intervention already discussed. One of the foremost assumptions of the competitive model is that there is perfect knowledge in the market. The concept of "consumer sovereignty" cannot operate when the consumer is unable to make an informed choice. In the medical sector, consumers often lack the expertise required to make informed judgments. Because of this, the patient must delegate to the physician much of his freedom of choice. Consequently, although the traditional competitive model assumes that demand and supply are independent, demand in the medical sector depends largely on the judgment of the physician-suppliers (the "dependence effect"). The number of visits to the physician, the kinds of laboratory tests called for, the decision to hospitalize or not and for how long, and even the need for surgical operations are normally based on the judgment of the physician-supplier (Feldstein, 1968).

The perfect knowledge assumption of the competitive model also implies that there is no uncertainty within the market concerning future events. The unpredictable incidence of illness and accidents creates difficulties for the individual. Statistical indices can be worked out for large groups, but the incidence of sickness for an individual is largely random. Moreover, it is unlikely that a consumer is able to assess accurately the probability of illness and the costs involved should disability or catastrophe strike (Calabresi, 1970). In addition, dislocation may result from catastrophic or debilitating illness or accidents; this often means prolonged recuperation and absence from work. Consequently, exacerbating the unpredictability of illness are the severe consequences of dislocation.

Another problem in analyzing the medical sector is the undefinable nature of the output produced. Since each medical service is difficult to define or standardize, the medical sector does not produce a clearly defined unit. But until a single definition of health has been accepted, the concept of output cannot be clarified, and even if "health" could be defined precisely, it would still be difficult to measure. Researchers have suggested the use of proxy variables to represent the product. Some of these are the number of patient visits, the number of patients for outpatient services, the number of cases, patient days, bed days, or gross measures such as morbidity or mortality rates. These measures have proved useful in the development of certain internal management control procedures, but, in the context of a broader conceptual perspective, the measures lack both comprehensive and adequate focus on the rationale behind the provision of medical services. Consequently, changes in the medical delivery system which increase the number of hospital days or patient visits may or may not result in an improvement in the population's health. The problems associated with defining output and measuring productivity simply emphasize the nonhomogeneous nature of the product involved. Without a measure for productivity, comparisons between programs or the evaluation of a single program in terms of quality of care and the efficiency of production are difficult. What is needed is an evaluation methodology which, instead of focusing separately on inputs or proxy output measures, would combine both the input and output concepts into one methodology.

The process of defining output for the health sector is made even more difficult because most health services represent a combination of both consumption and investment aspects which are difficult to separate.[3] Many services are considered investments because they increase the productivity and extend the working life of the employed members of society. Other services provide temporary relief from pain and suffering and yield immediate benefits to the individual only in the current time period. Since outlays for medical services have both consumption and investment components, and

[3] This same problem exists in measuring the output of education (Becker, 1964; Schultz, 1963, 1970). The problem of identifying output is further complicated because medical services are often produced jointly with medical education.

since such classification is difficult and imprecise, output measures for the health industry are speculative at best.

The important role played by the nonprofit institutions in the medical care sector poses more difficulties in relation to the workings of the competitive model. The profit motive encourages technical efficiency and low-cost production. The marketplace disciplines firms that become overly inefficient. Nonprofit producers do not have the same pressures for efficient production nor the same incentive to adjust output in order to achieve higher profit (Newhouse, 1970; Lee, 1971). This problem is exacerbated by the form of third-party cost-plus payment that characterizes existing medical insurance plans (Pauly and Drake, 1970; Havighurst, 1970). Such a system of reimbursement provides few incentives for either the hospital or the physician to achieve greater efficiency, and leads to higher consumer costs.

In short, many of the distinctive characteristics of health and medical services satisfy the traditional grounds for government intervention. The irregular, uncertain, and sometimes communicable nature of illness, the unusual characteristics of the inputs and outputs, and the unusual forms of organization utilized to deliver health and medical care indicate that some form of government involvement is called for.

Merit Goods. Traditional public finance criteria for governmental intervention do not challenge the underlying assumption of consumer sovereignty. Governmental action is necessary to achieve the result that, but for various imperfections, would have been achieved through operation of the market. But the objectives of government policy in the traditional scheme of things must be quite limited, paralleling as closely as possible the outcome of the market and deviating from the market system itself as little as feasible.

In recognition of the fact that government often acts in ways which do not conform to the traditional public finance criteria, economists have developed a concept of a "merit good" as a basis for governmental involvement. The satisfaction of merit wants is provided for through the public budget, apart from what is purchased by private consumers. "The satisfaction of merit wants, by its very nature, involves interference with consumer preferences" (Musgrave, 1959:13; Musgrave, 1971:312–313).

The theoretical underpinning for the merit good concept, however, is rather flabby at this point. Clearly there are very significant
redistributional aspects to the substitution of collective consumer
decision making for the market. But more is at stake than redistribution. Since the provision of services is defined categorically, as in
some of the proposed compulsory national health insurance programs, the eligibility criteria may not impose any means test.

At least two explanations are offered for the presence of merit
goods. The first is a basic rejection, for a spectrum of items, of the
notion that people know what is in their own best interests. No matter how this argument is sliced it is paternalistic. Basically, the
rationale is that in certain cases there is inadequate consumer information or insufficient consumer expertise to evaluate options. Either through misleading advertising or through lack of expertise,
consumers may not have sufficient information or competence to
make intelligent consumer purchases. Some see this as a justification for governmental imposition of collective consumer choice
through the political system.

But another link in the analytical chain is necessary before this
conclusion is warranted. Lack of information can be remedied by
governmental regulation which requires producers to make available accurate data on their products. The "Truth in Lending" statute
and the various labeling statutes are attempts to improve the information at the disposal of the consumer so as to approach the competitive ideal of perfect knowledge. Only if providing this information
is unacceptably expensive is the alternative of collective purchase justified. It is, of course, possible that in some cases information costs are so prohibitive that other action is necessary. But imposition of collective consumer choice in such a situation would,
presumably, still attempt to mirror the outcome of the marketplace
as closely as possible. Consequently, this basis for intervention does
not explain why provision of a "merit good" rests on a different
theoretical foundation from more traditional forms of intervention,
such as labeling. Nor does it explain why, if the redistribution element is put aside, medical care should be supplied through the federal budget. Provision of medical services through the federal budget will not enhance the ability of the average citizen to understand
the factors involved. If an explanation is to be found for the political mood that medical services should be provided to all as a right,
we must look elsewhere than the lack of information or expertise.

A second explanation of the merit good phenomenon is that it is a case of disguised (or at least controlled) redistribution (Musgrave, 1971:315): "What seems to be a case of merit goods may, in fact, reflect interdependence of utilities and their provision may be an instrument of redistribution." Seen this way, the merit good label turns out to be applicable to any categorical program of assistance. These programs have been roundly criticized by many welfare economists who claim that transferring nonnegotiable commodities is a less efficient method of redistribution than substituting money for in-kind transfers. In effect, the market economists argue that transfers in kind deprive the recipients of the right to choose freely their own marketbasket of goods, and that this creates waste at a net cost in welfare.

The merit good construct seems like an attempt to explain why, despite constant academic criticism, politicians continue to advocate categorical assistance programs. Redistribution may be in the nature of a social good with interdependent utilities so that A derives satisfaction from B's consumption, especially if B's income is low relative to that of A. From this perspective, a merit good may be an example of a voluntary redistribution, and the donor may gain more satisfaction if the donee consumes medical care rather than whisky. For this reason, it may be easier to muster a political consensus for provision of medical care as a right than for a redistribution of a similar amount of income through a direct grant.

The public reaction of alarm and indignation to the demogrant proposal of Senator McGovern in the 1972 presidential campaign is evidence that the political phenomenon exists. The explanation may be that the price exacted by these voluntary donors is control of the way the redistributed funds are spent. Thus, we come full circle. Again, we have a paternalistic reason for this type of control, although with a different motivation for the paternalism. The condition on which the redistribution is given is the loss of consumer sovereignty for the donee.

One further word for the theoretical discussion in the medical care context is now appropriate. The political decision to provide categorical assistance through the federal budget for personal medical services was made in 1965 with the enactment of Medicare and Medicaid. From a pragmatic point of view, therefore, it is only reasonable to acknowledge that medical services have been defined as a merit good, at least for the medically indigent and the aged. This poses a troublesome conceptual question about the current debate over compulsory national health insurance for everyone. Since the medically indigent already are the beneficiaries of Medicaid assistance, what is the argument for compulsory universal national health insurance? If the redistribution goal is largely inconsequential, we are left with the information-competence argument. But those who are not medically indigent could assume the burden voluntarily of insuring against the risks of illness. Moreover, if government took steps to assure a competitive market for insurance, consumers would be able to choose from among a variety of packages instead of being confined to a single, govenment-imposed medical market-basket.

An argument can be made that individuals rationally might vote to tax themselves for medical insurance as a means of forced savings. This would apply especially to those unable to discipline themselves to invest in medical insurance if left with money which could be spent on more immediate pleasures. The argument has some superficial appeal: let the weak-willed, who recognize their own infirmity, pull the magic political lever once and assure themselves of adequate savings to purchase medical insurance. But why should the political system be used by a majority (by assumption) to impose on an unwilling minority a consumer good which (by hypothesis and by definition) the minority chooses not to consume (at least not in the form presented in the compulsory system)? As long as the only actor involved is the individual voter who is in the majority, there is no problem. But when the minority voters are brought in, the issue of an imposed choice must be faced. In some cases, failure to impose the majority will could result in deprivation for the majority because the good cannot reasonably be purchased or produced in any other way. But in the case of medical insurance, a private market exists. If a consumer is afraid of himself, there is a means of privately forcing saving—through contractual arrangement in which an individual can bind himself to save by creating legally enforceable obligations. Through this system of private ordering with the force of law, individuals can effectively limit their own freedom but at the same time not impose their consumer choices on an unwilling minority because of their own frailties. So long as adequate alternatives exist—e.g., private ordering through contract and governmental action to promote greater consumer choice among insurance packages—it is difficult to justify compulsory medical insurance on the basis of the forced-saving argument.

One might also argue that without compulsory national health insurance a dual system of medical services will be perpetuated, one for the relatively affluent and one for the poor. The argument proceeds as follows: because of its importance, nonindigents have a duty to supply adequate medical care to indigents; but a system that does not include governmental financing for the nonpoor may allow for inferior care for the poor, and so equality demands that universal government financing be made compulsory so as to eliminate a dual system. This argument is weak on at least two grounds. First, conceptually, the merit good approach would seem to warrant redistribution in kind of medical services that could be characterized as basic or necessary (Michelman, 1969). Once the duty of society to provide adequate care is met, however, inequality in provision of additional services is no more (and no less) of a societal problem than any other inequality in access to goods or services. The "specialness" of medical care exists only up to a certain threshold; beyond that it becomes just another consumer item. Implicit in the argument that nonindigents have a duty to provide access to care to those who could not otherwise afford such access is an understanding that inequalities in total consumption may continue to exist as they do in other sectors of the economy. Indeed, it is unlikely that any system of compulsory national health insurance would bar consumers from spending supplementary private funds for additional medical care, and if this option is left open, a "dual" system will develop in any case.

Second, even if unequal consumption of medical services is admitted, a proponent of compulsory national health insurance could point to the access to quality-care problems that have faced Medicaid patients. But if indigents have command of sufficient resources to purchase an adequate level or package of care in the marketplace, only imperfections in the market would inhibit their purchase of mainstream medicine. This is not to deny the problems the poor have had in gaining access to first-rate physician services or in having as broad a scope of choice as those who pay fees out of their own pockets (and who are likely to have socioeconomic, cultural, or racial backgrounds more akin to a physician's other patients) (Zubkoff, 1973). It is to state that a remedy for that problem could and should be fashioned that more precisely deals with the access-to-quality-care problem. The imposition of a compulsory, universal national health insurance program is not a policy instrument tailored to deal with the problem identified and may not even contribute to its amelioration.

It could also be argued that compulsory health insurance—that is, health insurance as a universal merit good—is necessary because individuals cannot assess correctly the probability of incidence of debilitating illness (Calabresi, 1970:55–58). The information cost associated with fully educating consumers of the dangers of disability might well be exorbitant. Moreover, as with Social Security, there may be serious secondary effects upon third parties when a person is disabled and, in the case of medical care, society (either through government or charitable agency) would likely come to the aid of an unfortunate disabled person. In such a case, a consumer might be likely to purchase less disability insurance than he might otherwise, relying on society to bail him out if something goes wrong. For this reason, the political process might be the only way to achieve an optimal solution. However, the lack-of-knowledge–extreme-side-effects argument can be stretched only so far; it does not cover nondisability or nonemergency situations and, moreover, conforms to the traditional criteria for intervention. The merit good theory is not needed to deal with this situation.

The political decision about the scope of the merit good in medical services is important for policy determination. If the merit good concept is applied, then policy makers must think in terms of substantive policy objectives and priorities, not only of remedial procedural tinkering. The result of such a governmental decision is increased governmental (and most likely centralized) control over the allocation process in the health field, and the types of policies formulated and programs developed would have markedly different objectives.

The Range of Choice for Governmental Intervention

Any discussion of the strategy for governmental intervention in the health field must first take stock of the tools available to the government. The selection of tools will depend in large measure upon what resolution the political process reaches on the merit good issue. If government continues to treat medical services as a federal program of categorical assistance for the poor and the aged, an assumption made here, then such issues as adequate access (both financial and geographical), determining the precise scope of the benefit package, and defining the class of people to whom the package will be provided will receive highest priority. If government intervention is based more on the criteria reflected in the traditional model, then the primary focus of policy will be restoration of the market as a functioning institution.

Determination of the breadth and depth of the benefit package is the major demand–side issue, and the problem arises once the decision is made to provide medical care through the budget to categorically defined groups. On the supply side, various tools are available both in cases where traditional criteria govern and where the merit good concept prevails. At one extreme, government could do nothing at all if the market mechanism is functioning well. At the other extreme, government could supply directly all medical services, in effect expanding the VA hospitals to provide care to the entire civilian population. In between these extremes are the following forms of intervention: (1) piecemeal dynamic intervention aimed at restoring the market mechanism; for example, reducing the barriers to entry by modifying licensure requirements and reducing the monopoly power of voluntary medical associations; (2) ad hoc static regulation aimed at short-run symptomatic remedies; for example, utilization review and wage and price controls; (3) regulation of output by a regulatory body such as a public utility commission with control of such things as product, pricing, investment, and cost standards (Posner, 1971).

At present, government policy primarily reflects a heavy reliance on such short-run symptomatic remedies as price controls. The outcome of the political debate about the basis for involvement will largely determine the shape of future federal programs in the health field.

Two illustrations will help indicate the differences in concern that can arise from differences in the orientation of federal policy. The supply of providers has not kept pace with the rapid increase in demand for medical services. There may be many reasons for this gap, but the longer the lag time between increased demand and ultimate supply response, the greater the impact of increased demand on the economy. Diminishing the length of the supply-response lag is an example of a market-perfecting policy for government. Consistent with such a goal would be encouraging medical schools to increase their output of new physicians by reducing the required training from four to three years. Similarly, government could reduce the institutional barriers to entry (as reflected in the various licensure laws) by relaxing the formal educational requirements for medical manpower. Again, by altering the institutional requirements, government would be fostering increased supply by "dynamic" regulation.[4]

Intervention on the supply side through subsidy would have to be justified by the presence, say, of externalities. Otherwise, government policy based on traditional criteria must be limited to the function of facilitating market accommodation, without regard to substantive outcome. Along these lines, if the outcome of the market's functioning were to mean that certain geographic areas would not have sufficient medical care, then the traditional model would adopt a "so be it" response. However, it is now clear that the political judgment has been made that adequate access to medical services is a major policy objective of the federal government (U.S. Congress, 1971).

A second illustration of the influence on policy orientation of one's theory of intervention arises in the context of hospitals. There have been some suggestions that increased emphasis be placed on hospitals which operate on a for-profit basis. Proponents of this approach argue that proprietary hospitals have financial incentives to keep costs in line and that efficiency has been better in the for-profit

[4] The approaches to supply shortages mentioned above assume that the market adequately performs the allocative function but that structural and institutional rigidities operate so as to impede its proper performance. In such situations, government action, under traditional theory, must strive to restore competitive conditions. It is important, however, to underscore what assumptions underlie the traditional response. As prices in the health sector rise in response to the excess demand, the expectation is that increased incomes to health professionals will induce more people to become members of the health professions. As these new workers take their place in the profession, one would expect the imbalance of demand and supply to disappear and the extranormal increase in prices to dissipate. Therefore, it is appropriate within the traditional framework to smooth the path of supply response or to act affirmatively to shorten the period of lag. It would be inappropriate, however, for government through subsidy to induce more people to pursue careers in the health professions in the absence of externalities or other public finance justifications. This allocation function is one for the market; if its functioning is restored, the results would follow rationally without explicit governmental inducement.

hospitals. But one of the strongest counterarguments is that reliance on for-profit hospitals would mean that certain kinds of less profitable medical services would either be less available or would strain the financial resources of the voluntary hospitals. In essence, the critics of the for-profit hospitals argue that the hospital is a major focus of modern medical service delivery and that it must continue to afford comprehensive treatment for reasons of health policy. If a hospital were to cut back in areas in which profit levels were not high, there might be a concomitant deterioration in the quality of overall medical service. The solution to this problem adopted by the voluntary hospitals is that profitable medical services subsidize the less profitable.

Those with a market orientation would rebut the critics of the proprietary hospitals by arguing that since a subsidy is being paid for reasons of health policy, a more rational approach would be to determine on whose shoulders the subsidy should fall and then to subsidize openly either the voluntaries or the proprietaries on that basis. It may be difficult to justify a system which covertly taxes patients with profitable illnesses to support those with less profitable ones. So long as health policy dictates that less profitable illnesses need to be treated, these same policy considerations should be brought out into the open to determine who should pay for this subsidy and at what level. It seems doubtful that one class of the sick should support another class without regard to such factors as income. Nevertheless, the less affluent afflicted with profitable diseases now subsidize the more affluent with unprofitable illnesses. The market-oriented would argue that health policy goals should be subsidized through the budget, and that the rest of the hospital's operations should face market competition.

The purpose of the discussion of manpower and hospitals has not been to advocate one approach over another but rather to illustrate the consequences for policy of adopting one orientation or another toward the appropriate basis of governmental action. The next sections address the question of whether the market mechanism or the regulatory mechanism should serve as the basis for future governmental involvement in certain areas of the health field.

Modes of Intervention: The Utility Approach

Since much of the impetus for review of the governmental role in medical care derives from the recent increases in costs to consumers, it might seem logical for the government to grab the bull by the horns and focus policy directly on the stabilization of prices. The outcome of such a policy determination would be to choose the regulatory model as the best means of keeping down prices in the medical care sector. There have been some suggestions, for example, that a public utility approach be used for regulation of hospitals. The American Hospital Association embraced this concept in February, 1972 (Priest, 1970; American Hospital Association, 1972).

Adoption of the utility concept amounts to a wholesale recognition that competition and the marketplace cannot function effectively in the medical sector. For two reasons, we reject the avenue of total regulation, at least at this time. First, the history of utility-style regulation in this country has been anything but encouraging; any argument for complete rejection of the market must bear a heavy burden in showing that the proposed solution is desirable and workable, and also that the alternatives are doomed to failure. We believe this showing has not been made. Second, a good case can be made that the market system itself has not been given a chance to operate in the medical sector in light of the special restrictions which have been imposed by government. For this reason, further reliance on the market as a mechanism for social ordering may still be an available option.

Recent criticism of public utility regulation has focused on three points (Donahue, Jr., 1971; Posner, 1971). First is the difficulty that a regulatory agency inevitably has in determining the legitimate costs of the regulated firms. The agency cannot rely on the regulated firm's own calculations but must attempt to determine acceptable costs independently. This is an extremely difficult task involving highly complex accounting, and the consequence of error may be either inadequate capital for the regulated industry or excess monopoly profits. The stakes are high whereas the mechanism is rather imprecise.

Second, price regulation may distort the incentives of the regulated firm. For example, a firm that sells both regulated and unregulated products may seek to subsidize the competitive enterprise by allocating costs to the unregulated portion of its business. Also a regulated firm may attempt to take out nonmonetary profits in the way of prestige items like thicker carpets, bigger offices, a shorter work week, etc. The result of this is higher but less visible costs not easily susceptible to regulatory control.

Third, public utility regulation is a political as well as an economic process. Experience with regulatory agencies since the New Deal Era indicates that the regulated industries frequently exercise a great deal of control over their own regulation. This phenomenon is often more acute at the state level, and much of the regulatory activity in the medical care sector would most likely occur at this level. The proposal by the American Hospital Association for utility regulation by a state body is evidence that the industry feels that its interests will be well protected through state utility-type regulation.

Given the track record of utility regulation, government should hesitate to commit itself wholesale to the regulatory path in the medical sector. A much heavier burden of justification would be necessary before commitment to such a total system could be justified. Not only is the history of public utility regulation undistinguished, but, in the context of the medical care field, special considerations suggest that its extension would be unwise (Posner, 1971:8–10).

One special problem is product specification. If a regulatory commission were to attempt to establish appropriate rates for physician's services, the problem would arise as to define what the good or service involved was. Unless this was defined with precision, a regulated firm could substitute an inferior product for the one which was the basis of the rate established by the regulatory commission. Both the physician's and the hospital's service are much more amorphous products than typical products of regulated firms like electrical energy or telephone service. The technology of measuring output in health is in its infancy right now, and there is widespread disagreement about what output measures are appropriate. The real difficulty here is that the ultimate product—good health—is very difficult to measure of itself. Consequently, surrogate measures such as days off the job or days in the hospital are used, but these are at best only inadequate measures of output.

Another special concern in the medical care sector is cost control, but utility regulation is extremely weak in imposing cost consciousness. Regulated prices are derived after determination by the regulatory body of a fair and reasonable rate of return. This procedure provides an incentive for padding expenses on which a return can be earned and has the defects that inhere in cost-plus pricing. Consequently, utility regulation might very well exacerbate the inflationary pressures that already exist within the medical care sector.

Finally, organized medicine has time and time again shown its political clout.[5] Since the history of utility regulation shows that the regulated often control the regulators, the prognosis in the medical sector is not good. If anything, the extraordinary political influence of organized medicine should signal a pause before acceptance of a wholesale regulatory takeover.

Modes of Intervention: Countervailing Market-Oriented Mechanisms

This discussion suggests, then, that in the medical care sector a dose of competition might be what the doctor ordered (Havighurst, 1970). For example, the introduction of health maintenance organizations (HMOs) may encourage greater cost consciousness in the hospital sector. At present, third-party reimbursement on a cost-plus basis is the general rule for hospitals. Moreover, most of the third-party payment schemes do not reimburse patients for ambulatory care but require hospitalization before reimbursement is permitted. This structural bias toward hospitalization increases the cost of medical care because hospital care is the most expensive form of medical treatment. The HMO, through the prepayment device, will have an incentive to keep hospital costs down since incomes come from capitation fee, not fee for service. Reduced expenditures will result in increased income, so the prepaid HMOs will have an interest both in bargaining with hospitals to keep costs down and in emphasizing ambulatory and other less expensive forms of care.

Furthermore, the HMOs will be in a position to deal effectively in the marketplace. While consumers may not have the expertise to make medical decisions, and physicians may now have no incentive to serve the role of intermediary on behalf of the patient, the reward system for the HMO will encourage it to act on the consum-

---

[5] One must wonder why there is much a push for regulation *now* on the part of hospitals. Possibly this desire to be regulated is a response to the increased public pressure on hospitals to contain costs and at the same time meet community needs. A regulatory commission may serve the hospitals—e.g., by keeping out low-service competition, or by protecting the hospitals from the public—but it seems unlikely to serve the public (Chapman and Talmadge, 1970).

er's behalf in keeping costs down. Moreover, because of its professional expertise, it will be better able to deal effectively with hospitals and other providers (Wolfe and Zubkoff, 1973).

Of course, the introduction of HMOs will be no panacea for the problem of consumer ignorance or hospital inefficiency. Especially in areas where there may be inadequate choice among health maintenance organizations, there may be a similar problem with respect to fees set or quality of services offered by the HMO itself. We do not suggest that regulation has no place but rather that competition does have an important role to play. The introduction of new institutions and new devices for consumer participation might well make the market a more viable institution for social ordering in the medical context than anyone has thought.

In the past, government has responded to the distinctive traits of the medical sector by imposing restrictions on the providers. The detailed licensure statutes, the comprehensive regulation and planning of facilities construction, and medical education are examples of the minute piece-meal manner in which the medical sector is now regulated. It might be time, however, to look toward the more traditional role of government in attempting to make the market work. If consumer ignorance is a major problem—and it is—then government could become involved in more intensive health education programs.

One approach might be to establish roles such as health advocates to whom consumers could turn for advice and who could serve as intermediaries on behalf of consumers in dealing with providers. Moreover, greater responsibility could be imposed on doctors to disclose the mysteries of their practice. Too many doctors assume a role of aloofness so that patients feel inhibited from inquiring about what is going on. It is possible that legal institutions could have an effect "so as to compel the doctor to share critical decision-making power with the patient and to encourage the development of a partnership mode in doctor-patient relations to replace the prevalent authoritarian pattern" (Yale Law Journal, 1970:1534).

In addition to helping foster a more open doctor-patient relationship, the legal system can limit the extraordinary dominance by the physician of the entire health profession. Current statutes frequently preclude anyone but licensed physicians from providing certain care, even though there is far from clear evidence that such a requirement is necessary for quality care (Carlson, 1970). Modifications in licensure laws could therefore permit other health professionals to assume broader responsibility[6] and could perhaps reduce the individual's medical care bill by allowing for a different, less expensive "production technology" for good health. Many states have recently liberalized their licensure laws in recognition of the expanded roles that can be played by allied health professionals.

Other Modes of Consumer Influence

There are other mechanisms which can also be used to foster more effective use of the market. To the extent that health maintenance organizations themselves suffer from lack of effective competition, consumer participation in the organization and management of the group could help alleviate some of the consumer complaints that currently exist while affording the providers insight into consumer attitudes and desires.

In an engaging recent book, Professor Hirschman (1970) discusses the problems associated with the deterioration of the quality of output of an organization. His discussion and analysis have relevance for our discussion of nonregulatory mechanisms for promoting operating efficiency and responsiveness in the medical sector. Hirschman notes that competition is a mechanism for restoring organizational efficiency and, in his terms, promoting recuperation. Hirschman points out that the process of recovery can be spurred by two different though interrelated phenomena which he calls exit and voice.

In response to an absolute or comparative decline in quality, some customers stop purchasing a firm's product or some members leave an organization. "[T]his is the exit option. As a result, revenues drop, membership declines, and management is impelled to search for ways and means to correct whatever faults have led to exit" (Hirschman, 1970:4). This process of exit is the one normally associated with the competitive market system; the discipline of the marketplace is imposed on a firm through the opportunity of consumers to go elsewhere.

However, there is another way in which consumers can seek improvement in the functioning of a firm or an organization. They

---

[6] See, e.g., New York's new definition of nursing, Education Law §§6901, 6902, McKinney's Consolidated Laws of N.Y. (1972 supp.).

can express their dissatisfaction directly to its management or through general protest. This is what Hirschman calls the voice option. This also causes management to seek possible remedies for the expressed dissatisfaction. Hirschman's work offers a theoretical basis for such things as consumer activities which focus on corporate responsibility.[7]

In terms of the medical care sector, Hirschman's analysis suggests another private mechanism by which consumers can attempt to exercise a greater measure of influence, if not sovereignty. Without resorting to the traditional regulatory framework, government can foster private institutions and mechanisms through which consumers can enhance their ability to deal effectively in the marketplace. If HMOs prove to be monopolistic, for example, then government can institutionalize voice by consumers as a means of promoting continued operational vitality. In any case, the possibility of influencing organizational effectiveness in situations in which traditional modes of competition may be inadequate offers an alternative that should be explored further before wholesale regulatory takeover is pressed.

Illustrative Programmatic Intervention

To say that nongovernmental institutions that retain private ordering should be promoted is not to deny that some governmental intervention in the health field may be warranted, even under the traditional criteria. Of course, market-perfecting policies are appropriate under the traditional criteria; so are such activities as public health and biomedical research, the first areas of comprehensive federal involvement. But persuasive argument can be made that the traditional criteria justify government involvement in at least three other areas. The types of intervention discussed in this section are illustrative of the kinds of programs that can be supported on the traditional theoretical foundation.

Emergency

The market for medical services is actually composed of several submarkets; an important submarket is that for emergency care.

[7] For a discussion of a specific attempt to influence the corporate management of General Motors, see Donald E. Schwartz (1971).

Defining the precise boundaries of what constitutes emergency care surely is an uncertain venture, but hospital emergency rooms now typically break down their visits according to emergency and non-emergency classifications (Zubkoff, 1971:120–134). Similarly, under Medicare, hospitals that are not eligible for federal reimbursement for general patient services are eligible for payment for emergency services. The Medicare regulations establish guidelines describing the kinds of services and the circumstances that qualify as emergencies within the Medicare statute. Questions of definition and categorization still persist and sometimes necessitate adjudication (Carey v. Finch, 1970), but, nevertheless, it does make sense to think of emergency care as a somewhat distinct submarket of the medical services market.

The market for emergency care is characterized by highly inelastic demand elasticity so that an increase in price has only a minimal effect in reducing demand (Campbell, 1971:53–54). In the normal nonemergency case, a patient may rely heavily on the physician's judgment to determine the quantity of medical services consumed, but a patient can shop around for several opinions and even compare prices. As the Medicare legislation acknowledges, a patient confronted with a medical emergency faces a situation of nonchoice where even the limited options open to a patient with a nonemergency medical problem are not available. The free choice of the marketplace does not realistically exist for a person with a medical emergency.

Recognizing the distinctive characteristics of medical emergencies, some courts have imposed a requirement on hospital emergency rooms to treat all comers without respect to ability to pay, even though those same hospitals may have no duty to provide nonemergency care to indigents (Stanturf v. Sipes, 1969). This approach reflects the attitudes with which medical providers and society at large respond to medical emergencies. Providers historically have given free emergency care more readily than nonemergency care. Also, society is more likely to respond charitably to an emergency than to a nonemergency situation.

On the one hand, emergencies are highly unpredictable, and services must be purchased as an indivisible package with the concomitant discontinuities of supply. On the other hand, providers and society are likely to feel an obligation to treat a patient in an emergency situation. In such a case, a strong analogy exists to Social Security, in which compulsory insurance is justified on the ground that if an individual chooses not to insure himself privately, society will bear the onus of any mistaken private decision out of a sense that the elderly should not be permitted to go destitute.

In any case of emergency medical care, there is a strong argument that consumers will undervalue this insurance because of a calculation that if things get really bad, someone will bail them out. In this way, private decision making would permit a beggar-thy-neighbor private choice. Thus, this is a case in which an externality may be involved, since the detriment resulting from a poor private choice does not fall on the individual himself but on others (society at large or at least on the providers of care). Such an analysis makes it possible to draw a parallel with the compulsory liability insurance that many states impose on automobile drivers. Since the burden of harm wrought by a reckless and impecunious driver falls not on that driver but on his victims, government can justifiably impose mandatory insurance on the driver as a cost of operating his automobile. From the perspective outlined here, government financing of emergency medical care may be warranted on similar grounds. In those areas where competition among providers of emergency services is nonexistent or infeasible, some form of regulation could also be supported under the traditional criterion of natural monopoly.

Dislocation

A second area in which government involvement may be appropriate is dislocation—that is, illness or accidents that result in catastrophe or disability and therefore substantially disrupt the functioning of a person as a social and economic being. Like emergency, dislocation may elicit charity from society; individuals' perception of this likelihood might result in an understated revealed preference by consumers for insurance to deal with emergency situations.

The concern with dislocation reflects the functional approach to health discussed at the outset (Mechanic, 1968; Wilson, 1970). People unable to work may face a loss of income at the same time that medical bills impose a direct financial burden. To be sure, individuals can insure privately against many forms of dislocation, but the impact of a mistaken choice by a head of a household can have

133333

major secondary effects on others who are dependent. It is unrealistic, for example, to expect children, given their subordinate role within the family unit, their lack of independent funds, and their limited access to information and limited experience, to make an informed private choice weighing risks about catastrophe or disability. Similarly, there is little reason to impose parental risk preferences on children, especially since society normally assumes a special responsibility to care for children whose parents are incapacitated.

Of course, the protection-of-children argument runs the danger of proving too much, justifying potentially disruptive governmental intrusion into the constitutionally protected realm of family rearing (Pierce v. Society of Sisters, 1925; Meyer v. Nebraska, 1923). But the decision of a parent to forgo dislocation insurance in favor of some other form of consumption significantly affects those members of the family unit whom society frequently feels obliged in other contexts to protect, even against their own parents. Compulsory education laws and prohibitions on child labor are illustrations of governmental intervention to safeguard the interests of children. Since the burden of private error in the instance of dislocation falls on others besides the chooser, traditional criteria for government intervention would permit compulsory insurance. Whether this type of program would unduly interfere with countervailing values of family control of child rearing is the kind of analysis that goes into constitutional decision making; suffice it to say that taxation of this type has not typically been considered a significant infringement of parental prerogatives nor a substantial intrusion of government into intrafamily life.

By government action, losses that result from dislocation can be spread among many people (interpersonal loss spreading) and over time (intertemporal loss spreading) (Calabresi, 1970:39–42). In this way, the impact of functional dislocation on any individual or family would be reduced. The question then must be faced of why a system of total compensation for dislocation should not be established in the form of a comprehensive social insurance scheme. It is true that the current health policy debate has largely taken place in isolation from the simultaneous controversy over the no-fault concept of automobile insurance, yet the issues that arise in determining the scope of governmental involvement in the health field must also be addressed in policy terms in the accident law field. One of the difficulties with adopting a governmental system of total insurance for dislocation is that it would very likely lead to an increase in disbursements for at least two reasons. First is that without strict administrative limitations, such a reimbursement system would attract attempted freeloaders and promote overuse. Second, provision for comprehensive coverage for dislocation might reduce the incentives for people to exercise caution in their daily lives. To be sure, the problem of reducing the incidence of dislocation is more acute in the context of accidents than in the context of disease; nevertheless, the complexity of the "production function" of health does indicate that there may be significant ways to reduce the incidence of illness which causes dislocation. Thus, any system devised must balance the need for encouraging personal health maintenance with the need to ameliorate the problems brought on by dislocation.

Prevention

This leads to a third area of government involvement: prevention. To the extent that some form of social insurance for dislocation is implemented, an obligation falls on government to minimize, to the degree feasible, the incidence of dislocation. In the accident law field, reduction in the incidence and severity of accidents—primary cost avoidance in the parlance of Professor Calabresi—is achieved in part through rules of legal liability. From a health perspective, government can move broadly to help cut down on dislocation. Examples of government movement in this direction are such measures as mine safety and general occupational health legislation. Similarly, environmental programs that lower the incidence of debilitating respiratory illness also fall within this category, as do such social programs as sanitation, food inspection, and nutrition which help lower risks of serious disease. The government initiative in broad prevention programs is essentially a form of technological intervention so as to minimize the amount of dislocation with which it must cope. If a governmental response in cases of dislocation is warranted, an aggressive governmental role in preventive measures is also justified to keep the costs down—the counterpart of the objective of accident law to keep the primary costs of accidents down.

In addition, government emphasis on preventive measures may

often be justified on the basis of the public-good features of many preventive programs and the externalities associated with such measures. For example, an improved water supply or cleaner air will benefit members of the community without consumption being rival (at least to the point of overutilization). Similarly, public health measures that seek to eradicate communicable diseases benefit those who are not directly immunized. Consequently, government support of preventive measures can be justified under the traditional criteria both because they may contribute to a lower incidence of dislocation and also because delivery of preventive services is often characterized by public-good and externality-generating features (Zubkoff and Dunlop, 1973).

Conclusion

The dialogue about national health policy is bound to continue into the foreseeable future. In this paper, we have attempted to put the issues of health policy into an analytical framework that will be useful for those involved in policy formulation and implementation. It is our belief that insufficient attention has been paid to first principles of policy analysis; as a consequence, some previous and proposed policy instruments have not and would not successfully address the problems identified. More particularly, it is our view that policy must accommodate itself to the realities of the economic market and that additional attention should be given to governmental initiatives that promote increased effectiveness of the market as a device of social ordering. Of course, regulation will have a place in any comprehensive national health strategy, but intervention should follow from theoretical analysis and should encourage market perfection wherever feasible and appropriate.

James F. Blumstein
Associate Professor of Law
Vanderbilt Law School
and
Acting Director
Urban and Regional Development Center
Vanderbilt University
Nashville, Tennessee 37235

Michael Zubkoff, PH.D.
Associate Professor of Health Economics
Mehary Medical College and Vanderbilt University
and
Associate Chairman, Department of Family and Community Health
Meharry Medical College
Nashville, Tennessee 37208

An earlier version of this paper was presented at a Seminar on Problems of Regulation and Public Utilities at the Amos Tuck School of Business Administration, Dartmouth College, August 23, 1972. The authors wish to express appreciation to Soo-Keun Kim for his research assistance, and to the Department of Family and Community Health of Meharry Medical College, the Vanderbilt Urban and Regional Development Center, the Ford Foundation, the Vanderbilt University Research Council, and the Amos Tuck School for support.

References

American Hospital Association
  1972 Guidelines for Review and Approval of Rates for Health Care Institutions and Services by a State Commission, accepted by Board of Trustees on February 9, 1972. Chicago: American Hospital Association.

Antonovsky, Aaron
  1967 "Social class, life expectancy and overall mortality." Milbank Memorial Fund Quarterly 45 (April):31–74.

Becker, Gary S.
  1964 Human Capital. New York and London: Columbia University Press.

Calabresi, Guido
  1970 The Costs of Accidents: A Legal and Economic Analysis. New Haven and London: Yale University Press.

Campbell, Rita R.
  1971 Economics of Health and Public Policy. Washington, D. C.: American Enterprise Institute.

Carey v. Finch
  1970 316 F. Supp. 1263 (E. D. La.).

Carlson, Rick J.
1970 "Health manpower licensing and emerging institutional responsibility for the quality of care." Law and Contemporary Problems 35 (Autumn): 849–878.

Chapman, Carleton B., and John M. Talmadge
1970 "Historical and political background of federal health care legislation." Law and Contemporary Problems 35 (Spring):334–347.

Cleveland Board of Education v. LaFleur
1973 U. S. Law Week 41 (April 24): 3565.

Cohen v. Chesterfield
1973 U. S. Law Week 41 (April 24): 3565.

Cooper, Barbara, and Nancy Worthington
1973 "National health expenditures, 1929–72." Social Security Bulletin 36 (January): 3–40.

Donahue, Charles, Jr.
1971 "Lawyers, economists, and the regulated industries: thoughts on professional roles inspired by some recent economic literature." Michigan Law Review 70 (November): 195–220.

Feldstein, Martin S.
1968 Economic Analysis for Health Service Efficiency. Chicago: Markham Publishing Company.

Friedman, Milton, and Simon Kuznets
1954 Income from Independent Professional Practice. New York: National Bureau of Economic Research.

Havighurst, Clark C.
1970 "Health maintenance organizations and the market for health services." Law and Contemporary Problems 35 (Autumn): 716–795.

Hefty, Thomas R.
1969 "Returns to scale in hospitals: a critical review of recent research." Health Services Research 4 (Winter): 267–280.

Hirschman, Albert O.
1958 The Strategy of Economic Development. New Haven: Yale University Press.
1970 Exit, Voice and Loyalty. Cambridge: Harvard University Press.

Jacobson v. Massachusetts
1905   197 U. S. 11.

Kadushin, Charles
1964   "Social class and the experience of ill health." Sociological Inquiry
       24 (Winter) : 67–80.

Kessel, Reuben A.
1958   "Price discrimination in medicine." Journal of Law and Economics
       1 (October) : 20–53.
1970   "The AMA and the supply of physicians." Law and Contemporary
       Problems 35 (Spring) : 267–283.

Lave, Judith R., and Lester B. Lave
1970   "Medical care and its delivery: an economic appraisal." Law and
       Contemporary Problems 35 (Spring): 252–266.

Lee, Maw-Lin
1971   "A conspicuous production theory of hospital behavior." Southern
       Economic Journal 35 (July) : 48–58.

McDermott, Walsh
1969   "Demography, culture, and economics and the evolutionary stages
       of medicine." Pp. 7–28 in Kilbourne, Edwin D., and Wilson G.
       Smillie (eds.), Human Ecology and Public Health. London: Collier
       and MacMillan Co., Ltd.

McKinney's Consolidated Laws of N.Y.
1972   Education Law §§6901, 6902. McKinney's Consolidated Laws
supp. of N. Y.

Mechanic, David
1968   Medical Sociology. New York: Free Press.

Meyer v. Nebraska
1923   262 U. S. 390.

Michelman, Frank
1969   "On protecting the poor through the fourteenth amendment." Har-
       vard Law Review 83 (November) : 7–59.

Mishan, E. J.
1971   "The postwar literature on externalities: an interpretative essay."
       Journal of Economic Literature 9 (March): 1–28.

Musgrave, Richard A.
  1959 Theory of Public Finance. New York: McGraw-Hill.
  1971 "Provision for social goods in the market system." Public Finance 26: 306–320.

Newhouse, Joseph P.
  1970 "Toward a theory of nonprofit institutions: an economist's model of a hospital." American Economic Review 60 (March): 64–74.

Pauly, Mark V., and David F. Drake
  1970 "Effects of third-party methods of reimbursement on hospital performance." Pp. 297–314 in Klarman, Herbert E. (ed.), Empirical Studies in Health Economics. Baltimore: Johns Hopkins Press.

Pierce v. Society of Sisters
  1925 268 U. S. 510.

Posner, Richard
  1971 "Regulatory aspects of national health insurance plans." University of Chicago Law Review 39 (Fall): 1–29.

Priest, A. J. G.
  1970 "Possible adaptation of public utility concepts in the health care field." Law and Contemporary Problems 35 (Autumn): 839–848.

Rice, Dorothy P., and Barbara S. Cooper
  1972 "National health expenditures, 1929–71." Social Security Bulletin 35 (January): 3–19.

Schultz, Theodore W.
  1963 The Economic Value of Education. New York: Columbia University Press.
  1970 Investment in Human Capital: The Role of Education and of Research. New York: Free Press.

Schwartz, Donald E.
  1971 "Towards new corporate goals: co-existence with society." Georgetown Law Journal 60 (October): 57–109.

Stanturf v. Sipes
  1969 447 S. W. 2d 558 (Mo.).

U. S. Congress
1971   The President's Message to the Congress Proposing a Comprehensive Health Policy for the Seventies. Weekly Compilation of Presidential Documents, vol. 7, no. 8: 244–260. Washington, D. C.: Office of the Federal Register.

U.S. Congress, Senate Committee on Government Operations
1970   The Federal Role in Health (Ribicoff report). Senate Report 809, 91st Cong., 2d sess. Washington, D. C.: U. S. Government Printing Office.

U. S. Department of Health, Education, and Welfare
1971   Towards a Comprehensive Health Policy for the 1970's: A White Paper. Washington, D. C.: Government Printing Office.

Wilson, Robert N.
1970   Sociology of Health. New York: Random House.

Wolfe, Samuel, and Michael Zubkoff
1973   "Problems of financing prepaid group practice in the university." Journal of Medical Education 48 (April, P. 2): 93–98.

Yale Law Journal
1970   Note, "Restructuring informed consent: legal therapy for the doctor-patient relationship." Yale Law Journal 79: 1533–1576.

Zubkoff, Michael
1971   "Emergency room services." Pp. 120–134 in Ginzberg, Eli, and Conservation of Human Resources Project Staff, Urban Health Services: The Case of New York. New York: Columbia University Press.
1973   "The troubled transition: from 'for free' to 'purchase'." Hospital Administration (Winter, in press).

Zubkoff, Michael, and David Dunlop
1973   "Consumer behavior in preventive health services." In Mushkin, Selma (ed.), Proceedings of Round Table on Consumer Incentives for Health Care. New York: Milbank Memorial Fund (Fall, in press).

The Marriage of National Health Insurance and *La Médecine Libérale* in France: A Costly Union

VICTOR G. RODWIN

University of California,
Berkeley

I F ONE WERE TO ASK, AS AN INTELLECTUAL EXERCISE, how to design a cost-maximizing health care system, a likely response might be to cite at least three conditions: 1) national health insurance (NHI); 2) private fee-for-service medical practice and professional autonomy—what the French call *la médecine libérale;* and 3) minimal state intervention to regulate physician fees, monitor the volume of medical services rendered, and more generally influence the social organization of medicine. The first two conditions are distinguishing features of the French health care system. The third condition does not hold; quite the contrary, since World War II the French State has actively intervened in the health sector. It has established a negotiating system to set physician fees and a system of physician "profiles" to monitor the volume of care; it has examined the criteria by which health resources should be allocated; and it has tightened control over hospital reimbursement rates, hospital investments, and capital expenditures for medical technology. Since 1960, however, the average rate of increase of French health expenditures has exceeded that of the United States (see Table 1), and the trend appears likely to continue (Sandier, 1979).

Clearly, French policy makers have failed to contain rising health care costs. They have pursued contradictory policies. On the one hand, they have protected the right of access to medical care by extending

Milbank Memorial Fund Quarterly/*Health and Society*, Vol. 59, No. 1, 1981
© 1981 Milbank Memorial Fund and Massachusetts Institute of Technology
0160/1997/81/010016-28 $01.00/0

TABLE 1

Health Care Expenditures and Related Variables: Average Annual Rate of Change (%), 1960–1973

Types of Services	Expenditures at Current Prices				Expenditures Deflated by CPI				Volume Expenditure Deflated by Price Index				Price Index			
	Total		Per capita		Total		Per capita		Total		Per capita		Current		Deflated by CPI	
	U.S.	France	U.S.	France	U.S.	France	U.S.	France	U.S.	France	U.S.	France	U.S.	France	U.S.	France
Physicians' services	9.4	12.7	8.1	11.5	6.0	7.8	4.8	6.6	4.6	5.8	3.3	4.7	4.6	6.5	1.4	1.9
Laboratory tests	—	17.8	—	16.5	—	12.6	—	11.4	—	13.7	—	12.5	1.6	3.6	-1.5	-0.9
Other professional services	6.3	20.2	5.0	18.9	3.0	15.0	1.8	13.8	1.6	15.7	0.4	14.5	4.6	3.9	1.4	-0.6
Dentists' services	8.9	13.2	7.6	12.0	5.5	8.2	4.3	7.1	4.7	7.9	3.5	6.8	4.0	4.9	0.8	0.3
Ambulatory care services	9.0	13.6	7.7	12.4	5.6	8.7	4.4	7.5	4.3	7.6	3.1	6.4	4.5	5.6	1.3	1.0
Drugs and drug sundries	7.4	13.5	6.2	12.3	4.1	8.6	2.9	7.4	7.8	12.6	6.5	11.4	-0.3	0.8	-3.4	-3.6
Eyeglasses and appliances	7.9	9.1	6.7	7.9	4.6	4.3	3.4	3.2	4.5	5.8	3.3	4.7	3.3	3.1	0.1	-1.4
Hospital care	11.7	14.7	10.4	13.6	8.3	9.6	7.0	8.5	6.6	8.1	5.3	7.0	4.8	6.1	1.6	1.4
Personal health care	10.5	14.2	9.2	12.9	7.1	9.2	5.9	8.0	6.3	9.1	5.0	7.9	4.0	4.6	0.8	0.1

Source: Adapted from Rösch, G., and Sandier, S. 1975. A Comparison of the Health Care Systems of France and the United States. In Teh-wei Hu, *International Health Costs and Expenditures*. Proceedings of an International Conference on Health Costs and Expenditures. Sponsored by the John Fogarty International Center for Advanced Study in the Health Sciences, National Institute of Health, Bethesda, Maryland, U.S.A., June 2–4, 1975. DHEW Publication No. (NIH) 76-1067.

health insurance coverage; on the other, they have protected the prerogatives of *la médecine libérale.* The simultaneous pursuit of these policies has been costly, both economically and politically, and for that reason the combination of French NHI and *la médecine libérale* is not likely to endure.

To explain this view, I will examine 1) the ideological and institutional roots of the French health care system, 2) the evolution of French health policy, 3) the effect of reimbursement incentives on physicians and hospitals, and 4) the politics of cost control.

Ideological and Institutional Roots of the French Health System

Two conflicting ideas underlie the French health care system: liberal-pluralism and solidarity. "Liberal" refers not to the twentieth-century American sense of social reform and government intervention, but rather to the nineteenth-century European sense of laisser faire, individualism, and free choice. "Pluralism" refers to the existence of organizational diversity and dispersed centers for making decisions. In the health sector, the term liberal invokes a set of principles: selection of the physician by the patient and vice versa, freedom of prescription by the doctor, and professional confidentiality. These characteristics presumably ensure a personal, symbiotic doctor-patient relationship. The term pluralism justifies a variety of health-insurance funds offering a range of benefits and a diversity of health care delivery modes such that physicians can preserve their autonomy as individual professionals in their work and maintain control, as a group, over the structure of medical care organization. Together, these components of liberal-pluralism have cemented the French State's commitment to *la médecine libérale* (Caro, 1969).

The idea of solidarity—*solidarité*—is a peculiarly French concept that refers not to the American trade-union sense of "solidarity forever," but rather to the belief in mutual aid and *national* cooperation (Hayward, 1959). It conflicts with the idea of liberal-pluralism because it questions the virtues of laisser faire and professional autonomy in the name of a higher ideal: collective action to serve a concept of social justice. In the health sector, the idea of solidarity has provided the ideological foundation for the French NHI program and the social security system of which it is a part (Schorr, 1965). It suggests that health insurance is a right for all—sick and well, high and low income, active and inactive—and that premiums ought therefore to be calculated on the basis of ability to pay, not anticipated risk.

After World War II, in the spirit of solidarity, the Social Security Ordinance of 1945 was passed, calling for NHI under one unitary fund (Bridgman, 1971). Virtually the entire French population (99 percent) is now covered. The majority (75 percent) are covered by the *Caisse Nationale d'Assurance Maladie des Travailleurs Salariés* (CNAMTS)—the national health insurance fund for salaried workers.* Although the CNAMTS is only one of several NHI funds within the French social security system, it finances the bulk of health services— roughly 70 percent of total health expenditures and 30 percent of the capital for hospital construction and modernization. In French administrative law, the CNAMTS is a private organization charged with managing a public service. But in reality it is quasi-public since it falls under close ministerial supervision; and it is parafiscal since it is financed not directly from government revenues but almost entirely by employer and employee payroll taxes. As of August, 1979, employees contributed 4.5 percent of their total salary and 1 percent of their salary below a ceiling of 4,470 francs ($1,200) per month. Employers contributed 4.5 percent of the total wage and 8.95 percent of the wage below the ceiling (*Le Monde*, 1979).

Established in 1967 as part of De Gaulle's administrative reform of the entire social security system, the CNAMTS was designed to exercise greater authority over the previously independent regional and departmental sick funds and to ensure financial balance over the entire system's receipts and expenditures. Representatives of the state, of management (employer associations), and of employees (trade unions) were appointed to a national board of directors and the entire institution was placed under stricter supervision by the Ministry of Labor and Social Security. Despite De Gaulle's reform, the social security system is one of those rare French administrative structures in which a tradition of accountability, decentralization, and regional autonomy is strong (Catrice-Lorrey, 1979). Indeed, before the centralization achieved under the 1967 reform, members of the regional and local sick funds were elected (Galant, 1955). It is surely for this

---

* A key to the acronyms used in this paper appears on page 43.

reason that the CNAMTS has always been more concerned with assuring its subscriber population of access to medical services than with pursuing explicit policies to control rising health care costs.

In spite of attempts by French legislators to devise a unitary NHI fund under the banner of solidarity with equal benefits for all, the commitment to liberal-pluralism exacted compromises. To begin with, in addition to the CNAMTS, agricultural workers (8 percent), the self-employed (7 percent), and a set of special interest groups (9 percent) have their own health insurance funds. Also, flagrant disparities persist in levels of health insurance benefits and copayments between and even within health insurance funds. For example, the self-employed are eligible for fewer benefits and required to pay higher copayments than salaried workers and numerous special interest groups such as miners, merchant seamen, subway workers, railway workers, veterans, and public employees, all of whom still maintain their right to more favorable benefits. What is more, the process of extending health insurance coverage has taken almost thirty years and is still not complete. As late as 1970, a national survey (Guibert, 1973:46) indicated that more than 1.6 percent of the population—over 800,000 residents of France—were not eligible for benefits under NHI. At the present time, roughly 1 percent of the population remain ineligible for NHI benefits but are covered by welfare programs administered by the Ministry of Health.

It should not be surprising that the idea of liberal-pluralism exacted compromises. Organizational arrangements for the delivery of medical care in France are supported by strong physician and hospital associations. Efforts at health care reform have provoked conflicts between the medical profession and the state, between representatives of public and private sectors, and more generally between the ideas of liberal-pluralism and solidarity. Indeed, these conflicts have shaped the evolution of French health policy.

Evolution of French Health Policy

Since World War II, as in other industrially advanced nations, the French medical profession has practiced in a socioeconomic context whose growth and changing patterns have transformed the health sector from a *gemütlich* "cottage industry," composed of entrepreneurial physicians providing most of their services in the patient's home, to a major industrial complex organized around hospitals that support highly specialized staff and affiliated activities such as the pharmaceutical industry, biomedical laboratories, and firms producing and marketing medical technology. In the presence of such change, the French State has wavered between protecting the interests of *la médecine libérale* and adapting the health sector to the demands of a modern economy.

The Medical Profession and the State

General practitioners and specialists in France are free to set up practice wherever they like.[1] And consumers are free to choose among physicians in private practice, in public hospital outpatient departments, or in any one of 592 health centers (CNAMTS, 1977:47) established and managed by municipalities, trade unions, and nonprofit associations. In addition, local health insurance funds also manage dispensaries that provide preventive services such as checkups, screening, and laboratory tests to roughly 1.2 percent of the total population (IGAS, 1974). But diversity notwithstanding, under the banner of free choice the bulk of ambulatory care is provided by physicians in private practice.

Upon visiting their physicians, consumers pay the full charge of their visit, as set by a negotiated fee schedule. In return, the physician gives them a receipt to present to their local health insurance fund, either by mail or in person. The fund then reimburses the consumer 75 percent of the charge as set in a national fee schedule. The remaining 25 percent represents a consumer copayment. In general, the size of the copayment depends on the kind of medical service consumed. For most laboratory tests, dental care, and drug prescriptions, the copayment is 30 percent; for specially designated or particularly

---

[1] In modern France, as in ancient Rome, not only do all roads lead to the capital city but consumption of goods and services is concentrated there as well. In addition to its other attributes, Paris is renowned for its high density of physicians. Lyon, too, as well as the Riviera, are centers around which *la médecine libérale* has thrived. More precisely, the geographic distribution of physicians ranges from 59.1 per 10,000 population in Paris to 9.6 in Haute-Saône (in the west of France between Alsace and the Alps) (Ministry of Health, 1978).

expensive drugs it is 20 percent; and for hospital services it is 20 percent unless the hospital stay exceeds thirty days or requires costly therapy for prolonged illness such as diabetes, polio, and cancer, in which case medical care is free of charge to the consumer. To be insured against the copayment, French consumers may join any one of 7,840 mutual aid societies (Ministry of Health, 1979:56) or purchase commercial insurance. Some mutual aid societies, e.g., the *Mutuelle Générale de l'Education Nationale (MGEN)*, provides comprehensive health care services, in kind, thus supplementing the normal range of benefits provided under the NHI program. Estimates indicate that in 1974, roughly 32 million (over 60 percent of the French population) subscribed to some form of supplementary insurance (IGAS, 1975:218).

Since 1928, when the first French health insurance bill was passed, there have been periodic conflicts within the medical profession and between medical trade unions and the state over the conditions of medical practice under health insurance. Henri Hatzfeld (1963) argues that these conflicts have resulted in the taming of the French medical profession. Others, including physicians, even speak of proletarianization insofar as conditions of medical practice have been substantially altered (Steudler, 1973). Still another point of view, albeit in the minority, is that the medical fraternity continues to dominate health policy, but that physician trade unions, themselves, will soon demand a shift from fee-for-service to salary reimbursement (Stephan, 1978). These issues are explosive. But there is a growing consensus on one point (Hatzfeld, 1963:297), that "the physician appears condemned to lose a part of his professional autonomy: his activities and income will no longer be determined by his freedom to set charges and by his success; he will become a man employed on a salary based on status or a man hired on contract; his place in social organization will become more precise, more established."

The growth of biomedical knowledge and technology has changed the employment structure in the health sector by increasing the division of labor and hierarchy and reinforcing technician-type services performed by paraprofessionals. *La médecine libérale* is gradually receding behind new forms of collective and often salaried practice. Group practice has emerged over the last fifteen years to include roughly 30 percent of all physicians in private practice (*Le Monde*, 1974:24). Other forms of ambulatory care are also growing: hospital outpatient departments, home care programs, and day-long hospital procedures, e.g., ambulatory surgery.

As early as 1929, in a letter to the minister of labor, Paul Cibrie, the secretary general of the first medical trade union, *Confédération des Syndicats Médicaux Français* (CSMF), expressed concern over the emergence of third-party payment (Cibrie, 1954:68):

> The medical profession is under no illusions about the consequences of the contractual liberty allowed for under the law. We understand administrative procedure well enough to know that the [health insurance] funds will want to impose allowable charges and third-party payment. And we have great difficulty identifying an impartial institution capable of arbitrating between the opposing positions of the medical profession and that of the health insurance funds.

Until 1960, French physicians in private practice remained free to set their own fees. With the Ministerial Decree of May 12, 1960, de Gaulle expanded the regulatory power of the state and, to qualify for reimbursement under NHI, the medical profession was forced to accept a national negotiating system of annual contracts with price ceilings on uniform fees (Steudler, 1977). This system not only ended the traditional freedom of physicians to set their own fees; it also destroyed the unity of medical trade unions, for strong partisans of *la médecine libérale* opted out of the NHI system and formed a rival trade union—the *Fédération des Médecins de France* (FMF). But by 1964, 85 percent of French physicians, including most members of the FMF, were participating in the NHI program.

In 1971, when the present negotiating structure was devised, the CSMF struck a new agreement with representatives of the NHI funds and the state (Glaser, 1978:39–50). Once again, the FMF demanded the freedom for doctors to determine their own fees; once again, they ended up participating in the NHI program. At present, 98 percent of French physicians have agreed, in principle, to accept the national fee schedule. If consumers choose to seek medical care from doctors who are not participating in the NHI program, they will be reimbursed roughly 25 percent of the rate established by the fee schedule; thus their copayment will be significantly higher. In return, physicians are covered under NHI and the health insurance funds have agreed not to compete directly with *la médecine libérale* by establishing new primary care dispensaries. In addition, physicians are granted the right to exceed the uniform fees under two conditions: 1) when the patient presents unusually high demands, and 2) when the doctor is considered prestigious. As of 1977, 28 percent of specialists and 5 percent of general practitioners in France were considered prestigious, on the basis of criteria such as university degrees and honors conferred (CNAMTS, 1977:31).

Thus, despite concessions by physicians in private practice, *la médecine libérale*—at least through 1971—not only survived but prospered.

Hospitals and the State

Hospital care in France is provided in public hospitals, in proprietary hospitals known as *cliniques,* and in private nonprofit hospitals that are a cross between the public hospital and the *clinique.* Roughly one-third of acute hospital beds are in the private sector; over one-half of private-sector beds are in *cliniques.*

In 1977, there were 10.8 hospital beds per 1,000 population in France as compared with 6.5 in the United States. This difference may well be due to the fact that, since France has no nursing home industry comparable to that in the United States, French hospital data reflect beds that are used in a nursing-home capacity. If one includes nursing home beds in the United States data, there are 12.0 hospital beds per 1,000 population in the United States (Sandier, 1979:62).

Whether an individual is referred to a public or a private hospital for inpatient care, payment is not required upon admission. Instead, 80 percent of the charges are billed to the patient's health insurance fund and the other 20 percent directly to the patient. This same procedure is used for diagnostic hospital services provided on an outpatient basis and for costly drugs and laboratory tests. Moreover, after three days of hospitalization, as part of an incomes policy, French patients are eligible for a supplementary sickness benefit. Beginning on the fourth day, the health insurance fund will pay cash benefits for up to a year, and in some cases for up to three years.

French hospitals have not escaped the changes occurring in the health sector; indeed, they have led the way. As the public hospital has shed its former image of a philanthropic warehouse caring for (and sometimes experimenting on) the indigent sick, it has become the medical specialist's workshop, an institution where the most prestigious functions of the health care system are performed: teaching, basic research, and diagnosis and therapy for complex illnesses. In 1958, with the passage of the Hospital Reform Act, university medical schools were merged with the best-equipped public hospital facilities (Jamous, 1969). The new institution, called a *Centre Hospitalier Universitaire* (CHU), was assigned the responsibility for providing high technology medicine and superspecialty services to regions with populations of over a million.

One of the principal provisions of the Hospital Reform Act was to initiate a shift in the reimbursement of hospital-based physicians from fee-for-service toward salary payment. During the legislative debate on the proposed reform, the medical profession opposed the bill on the grounds that the shift in reimbursement mechanisms would gradually turn all physicians into civil servants. Some of the younger physicians, however, supported the reform as an attack on the feudal hierarchy of the university, and on the values of *la médecine libérale* as well. The highest ranking clinical professors, *les grands patrons,* resisted vigorously, and succeeded in conserving that part of *la médecine libérale* that they considered most dear—the right to hospitalize their private paying patients in "private" beds within their *service* at the public hospital. Nevertheless, 30 percent of French physicians are now fully salaried and roughly one-half of the remaining 70 percent are employed part time on a salaried basis, largely in public administration and public hospitals.

Like the Flexner Report and Regional Medical Programs in the United States, the Hospital Reform Act had important effects: to consolidate and control the diffusion of high-technology medicine and to reduce the gap between biomedical knowledge and its application. During the first fifteen years of the Fifth Republic (1958–1973), health planners in the Ministry of Health embarked on a major hospital construction program. In addition to the institutional reform, they pursued a policy of hospital modernization, including conversion of communal wards into private rooms. This was known as *l'humanisation des hôpitaux.* However, as late as 1970, almost 15 percent (80,000) of public hospital beds were still in bleak communal wards (Castaing, 1975). Despite efforts to "humanize" the public hospital and provide it with the most up-to-date medical equipment and specialty services, in the late sixties, even the most prestigious public hospitals, such as those of *l'Assistance Publique* (AP) in Paris, were losing patients to the *cliniques*, largely because material conditions there were far superior to those in the public sector, but also because part-time salaried physicians often referred their patients to *cliniques* to avoid queuing.[2] Moreover, in the private sector, the patient ostensibly chooses his doctor whereas in the public sector he does not have the prerogative of exercising free choice.

Cliniques have been the strongest refuge for *la médecine libérale* in the hospital sector. They differ from public hospitals in terms of size, case mix, and occupancy rates. The average *clinique* has 38 beds (Ministry of Health, 1973a); the average public hospital has 240 (Ministry of Health, 1973b). *Cliniques* have only 10 percent of all medical beds and almost half of all surgical and obstetric beds. They tend to avoid emergency care and specialize in routine cases, especially maternity care and noncomplicated surgery. Also, they tend to have higher occupancy rates than public hospitals. In terms of organizational strategy, *cliniques* have served as an institution within which the medical profession has retained control over its own work outside the bureaucratic structures of the public sector.

Throughout the sixties and early seventies, hospital capacity in the *cliniques* grew at an even faster rate than in public hospitals. In 1963, *cliniques* represented 26.4 percent of all acute hospital beds; in 1978, they had grown to include 34.8 percent (de Kervasdoué, 1980). This growth in number of beds was accompanied by increasing ideological conflicts between public and private sectors and growing polarization between a new "medical technostructure" (Steudler, 1974) of salaried physicians in public hospitals and physicians practicing in the *cliniques*. Ideological debates on the relative virtues of the private and public sectors have frequently been published in the press (*Le Monde*, 1976a). Associations of private *cliniques* have released studies showing that *cliniques* are managed more efficiently than hospitals, and have argued that the state should consequently encourage their growth. Representatives of the public sector have pointed out the limitations of such analyses and reminded their private sector colleagues of the burdens

---

[2] In 1973, the public image of *l'Assistance Publique* in Paris sank so low that the central administration ran spots on television, in movie theaters, and in the daily press to sensitize public opinion. On April 8, a publicity campaign was launched, bringing 70,000 to 80,000 Parisians to 28 of AP's 37 hospitals (AP, 1973).

of teaching, research, and high-cost illness, all of which must be borne by the public hospital (FHF, 1976). The state's ambivalent response to these debates has led simultaneously to frequent denunciation and to rapid growth of the private sector at public expense.

In 1970, the Hospital Law was passed in an effort to control rising health care costs. This legislation sought to improve management in public hospitals and regulate the private sector so as to promote a "harmonious" distribution of hospital beds. To do this, an elaborate planning and regulatory machinery was established (Brumter, 1979). Also, the hospital law called for reform of provider reimbursement mechanisms to create financial incentives for redistributing health resources in conformance with national and regional hospital plans.

The effect of this legislation has been to move French hospitals toward a public utility model of organization. Local hospitals are losing their autonomy as they become consolidated within broader administrative structures. Hospital planning is growing more important as investment decisions are increasingly scrutinized by regional commissions as well as the Ministry of Finance. However, the state has not yet developed provider reimbursement incentives for implementing the bold aims of the hospital law (Rodwin, 1978a; 1981).

Provider Reimbursement Incentives

The structure of the French health care system and the failure to contain rising costs cannot be explained by considering only explicit state policies. We must also examine the provider reimbursement incentives under French NHI to discern the implicit policies that underlie the health system.

On Paying the Doctor

Fuchs (1974) has observed that physicians are the most important determinant of both the level and the configuration of health resources: they decide who shall be hospitalized and they prescribe medical procedures, laboratory tests, and drugs. There is a wide range of methods of physician remuneration ranging from fee-for-service to capitation or salary payment, or some combination of these. Since there is much evidence that reimbursement incentives affect physician behavior at the margin (Contandriopoulos, 1979; Monsma, 1970), it is important to devise reimbursement systems to encourage good medicine, prevent abuse, and discourage neglect (Glaser, 1970).

In the French fee-for-service system, the fee schedule, or relative value scale, is known as the *Nomenclature Générale des Actes Professionnels.*[3] Originally written by the CSMF in 1930, it classifies medical procedures by so-called key letters. For example, C signifies a consultation with a general practitioner; B signifies laboratory tests; Z signifies all radiological procedures; and K signifies surgical and specialty procedures. The Bs, Zs, and Ks are always followed by a coefficient that is supposed to reflect their relative value on an elaborate scale of medical procedures. For example, an appendectomy or simple hernia operation is coded as K-50, whereas the surgical removal of an ingrown toenail is coded as K-10. Physician fees are equal to the coefficient times the value of the key letters that serve as the explicit object of bargaining during the national fee negotiations.

Relative value scales such as the *Nomenclature* are based on an implicit concept of medical practice that assumes that physician activities can be disaggregated into a precisely defined hierarchy of medical procedures. Such a concept fits comfortably the notion of *la médecine libérale,* for it calls attention to the choice and diversity of medical procedures. Moreover, it fits well within a system of strong state intervention and tightly controlled prices, for every effort made by physicians may be called a "procedure" and assigned a price. Unlike England, where the combination of capitation and salary reimbursement of physicians provides virtually no routine data collection on the volume of physician activity, in France it is impossible to engage in health services research without encountering utilization data (based on billings) classified by key letters and coefficients of medical procedures.

Economists suggest that fee schedules be designed so that relative value points reflect relative costs (Reinhardt, 1975:167). By this criterion, the *Nomenclature* is a crude instrument. For example, the value of a particular K procedure is constant, regardless of whether it is performed by a general practitioner, a certified surgeon, or a car-

---

[3] The most recent version of the *Nomenclature* is published in *La Revue du Practicien* (1979:1–154). As of February, 1979, the C was equal to 40 francs ($10.00); the V was equal to 53 francs ($12); the K was equal to 8.30 francs ($2); and the Z to 5.20 francs ($1.25).

diologist, and regardless of the presence and degree of pre- or post-operative complications. In contrast, pricing rules for the Z category of procedures are more refined. They not only distinguish between reimbursement rates for radiologists versus gastroenterologists but also include amortization and operating charges based on the capital value of the technology and equipment required by the procedure. As for consultations and home visits (C and V), their rate of reimbursement is constant, regardless of whether the doctor spends five minutes or an hour, thus encouraging "fast medicine." There is an additional problem with the French *Nomenclature:* the relative values are not annually readjusted to account for changes in technology—for example, economies of scale in the production of laboratory tests or the introduction of microprocessors that reduce the unit cost of radiological equipment. Thus, there are built-in price distortions in the physician fee schedule that do not encourage good medicine, prevent abuse, or discourage neglect.

Since changes in both the relative value scale and the value of the multiplier are the result of a bargaining process between a monopoly (the medical profession) and a monopsony (the NHI funds), fee-setting in this context leads to a classic bilateral monopoly situation that, in economic theory, is "indeterminate." The resulting fees are largely determined by ability to bluff, skill in bargaining, and, above all, power, all of which fall outside the economist's preoccupations (Ruderman, 1976). In France, as Jean-Claude Stephan (1978:130) argues, the medical profession—at least until 1976—succeeded in maintaining its accustomed level of income, "thanks to a multiplication of procedures."

In the United States, studies have demonstrated how the existing reimbursement structure encourages costly institutional care, specialized services, and excessive use of technology (Blumberg, 1978; Schroeder and Showstack, 1978). In France, there are no equivalent studies. However, the average annual rate of increase in the volume of radiological procedures and laboratory tests has been respectively two and three times that of physician consultations (Lecomte and Sandier, 1976:218). As a percent of the total volume of services in the private sector, radiological procedures increased from 17.2 in 1968 to 23.4 in 1977 (Sandier and Tonnelier, 1978:19). Surely this may be a sign of technological "progress," but it is also the result of favorable reimbursement incentives.

A comparative study of France and the United States (Lenoir and Sandier, 1976) concludes that the volume of per capita drug consumption in France is even higher than that in the United States, where pharmaceutical consumption is often considered excessive (Silverman and Lee, 1974). Anecdotal evidence reported in France's leading consumer advocacy magazine suggests that French physicians have a tendency to err on the side of "overprescription" (*Que Choisir,* 1978). Whether such overprescription of laboratory tests, diagnostic procedures, and drugs would occur under a different reimbursement structure is hard to say. What is clear is that the volume of medical care and ancillary services in France is high. During the 1971 negotiations between physician trade unions and the state, French policy makers acknowledged this problem and made regulation of the volume of medical services a central issue.

Since 1971, the French health insurance funds have established a system of "profiles" on the procedures performed by each physician. The objective of this style of regulation is symbolic: to sensitize physicians to the financial implications of their activities. The system is based on finding irregularities in medical practice and issuing sanctions to doctors who overprescribe tests and drugs. But this is exceedingly difficult because criteria on proper work loads have not yet been agreed on. If the entire medical profession is influenced by reimbursement incentives to increase medical procedures, particularly specialty services and high-technology medicine, the effect of the profiles will be negligible.

Since the 1976 negotiations, the system of physician profiles has been computerized. Enormous amounts of data have been collected on patterns of physician activity. After several years of sorting out technical problems, the system is now operational and is most often described as a first step in implementing a system of quality control, similar to professional standards review organizations (PSROs) in the United States. However, in France medical confidentiality is a sacrosanct principle, and physicians have tenaciously refused to divulge data on patient diagnoses, even under anonymous statistical codes. As a result, it is virtually impossible to judge the validity of most medical decisions and, consequently, the quality of medical care. Thus, the physician profiles are not likely to control the volume of medical services.

On Paying the Hospital

From 1950 to 1978, expenditures, in current prices, on hospital care in France have increased at an average annual rate of 15.1 percent as compared with 10.4 percent in the United States (Sandier, 1979:83). Hospital expenditures now represent almost 50 percent of total health expenditures. Just as the financial incentives built into the *Nomenclature* have contributed to the growing volume of medical services, so methods of hospital reimbursement have favored the growth of inpatient hospital care and affected the structure of the hospital sector.

As in the United States, hospitals in France are paid largely on the basis of costs incurred. In public hospitals, although certain nonmedical specialties such as laboratory and radiological departments bill NHI funds on a fee-for-service basis, the principal unit of reimbursement is the patient day. Its value is calculated by dividing total operating expenses, including teaching, research, and administrative costs, and a range of ancillary services, by the total number of patient days. In the private proprietary sector, the patient day is less of a catchall category for, in contrast to the public hospital, operating-room costs, expensive drugs, laboratory costs, blood transfusions, and prostheses are all billed separately on a fee-for-service basis.

Until 1968, the NHI funds negotiated the rate of a patient day for *cliniques* on the basis of the daily fee of the closest public hospital. Since the public hospital must, by law, keep its occupancy rate under 95 percent, be equipped to handle all emergencies, and be open twenty-four hours a day, the average costs of public hospitals tend to be significantly higher than those of *cliniques*. This system of hospital reimbursement enabled the medical entrepreneur to skim the cream off the market. Since 1968, the NHI funds have allowed increases in patient-day rates for *cliniques* only when authorized by the Ministry of Finance. Such price control has restricted the windfall profits of the sixties. But the *cliniques* responded by removing as many procedures as possible from inclusion in the patient-day rate. This practice explains the finding of Lévy et al. (1977:108) that the activity of *cliniques* is best characterized by the quest for both high revenues and long lengths of stay during which a large number of medical procedures are performed.

Aside from favoring the private sector through reimbursement of patient-day costs, the NHI funds have systematically underestimated the amortization rate for capital expenditures in public hospitals as compared with *cliniques* (Ministry of Health, 1970; Brunet-Jailly, 1976). There is a justification. Representatives of the NHI funds argue that they already overpay the public sector by subsidizing teaching and research expenses through reimbursement of the patient-day fee. Despite these subsidies, however, and their impressive hospital construction and modernization program throughout the sixties and early seventies, public hospitals have been chronically short of investment funds.

Beginning in 1973—three years after the passage of the Hospital Law—increasing regulation of capital expenditures in the private sector constrained the development of *cliniques* to the point where certain banks no longer consider them a good investment opportunity (Beau, 1979). This situation is probably more an indication of the present containment phase of health sector development than an anti-*clinique* policy on the part of the state. The Ministry of Finance has also pressured public hospitals to tighten regulation over patient-day rates and to improve hospital management.

It is unlikely, however, that managerial and administrative technologies can be adapted to the practice of medicine, for there is consensus neither about what outputs are being produced, nor about how one might measure them (de Kervasdoué, 1979). In addition, hospital managers are bound by rigid regulations (e.g., those governing civil service employees) that restrict their capacity to innovate and to be flexible. Since they work within a system of cost-based hospital reimbursement, hospital managers have a financial incentive to maintain high hospital occupancy rates in order to increase revenues. Despite symbolic efforts to initiate home-care programs and day-long hospital procedures, financial incentives discourage the development of ambulatory surgery (Stein, 1979) and extensive outpatient departments.

Since the passage of the Hospital Law, there have been efforts to devise new payment incentives such as prospective budgets for public hospitals. As for the private sector, since 1968 policy makers have classified *cliniques* in various ways in order to devise more sophisticated methods for calculating the patient-day rate. But despite exhortation in the public sector and elaboration of new payment rules in the private sector, the basic principles of hospital reimbursement remain unchanged. Financial incentives in France tend to encourage hospital-based care and generous provision of medical procedures. In short, in France as in the United States, controlling health care costs is a perpetual uphill battle.

The Politics of Cost Control

Health expenditures of the CNAMTS are big and growing bigger. Eighty-one percent of total health expenditures in France are financed by third-party payers—71.1 percent by the NHI funds, 3.2 percent by welfare, 3.7 percent by mutual aid societies, and roughly 3 percent by private insurance (CREDOC, 1979). This leaves 19 percent that are financed directly by the consumer, compared with 30 percent in the United States (Sandier, 1979). In addition to health expenditures, pensions and family allowances contribute to the vast income and expenditure flows administered by the social security system. After 1971, the "social budget"—all state welfare expenditures and social security transfer payments—exceeded the state budget as a whole (Ministry of Health, 1974:474), and at present it equals one-fourth of the French gross domestic product (GDP) (Ministry of Health, 1979b).

The Ministry of Finance has not ignored the growth of such expenditures and indirect taxes, for they lead to social security deficits, increase fiscal and parafiscal pressures (from income and payroll taxes), and affect both disposable income and the production costs of industry. Increasing costs of production get passed on to consumers either through real wage losses or price increases, and this runs counter to the Ministry of Finance's goal of promoting industrial development and international competitiveness. Continued growth of health expenditures has forced consideration of two central economic questions for national health policy: 1) Should the rate of increase of the social budget be permitted to exceed the rate of increase of GDP? 2) Are the marginal benefits worth the rising costs to patients and taxpayers? In a section entitled "The Limits of Solidarity," the Finance Committee of the Sixth Plan (NPC, 1971) answered both questions with a categorical no; so did the 1976 economic plan of Prime Minister Raymond Barre (*Le Monde,* 1976b). However, translating economic decisions into palatable political programs is no easy task.

Political Stalemate

In their paper on "permacrisis" in French social security, Cohen and Goldfinger (1975:66) argue that "the lack of smooth fit between the imperatives of the economic system and the necessities of the political system is the key to understanding the contradictions of social security." In the health sector, the contradiction is expressed by economic pressures to keep rising deficits under control in a political environment of increasing social demands on the NHI funds.

Proposed stopgap measures to increase the CNAMTS' revenues have included providing state subsidies, increasing health insurance premiums (payroll taxes), and raising the wage ceilings to which these payroll taxes are applied. However, such measures provoke political resistance. The Finance Ministry wants to reduce state expenditures in order to keep a more balanced budget. Employers resist increased payroll taxes, for such taxes increase wage costs, leading to higher production costs and prices, and thereby hurt their competitive position. Wage earners fight increased payroll taxes through trade unions; upper-level executives refuse to consider elimination of the wage ceilings; and special beneficiaries such as miners, merchant seamen, and railway workers do not merely oppose increasing the rate of payroll taxes; they also fight to protect their own particular and often advantageous insurance benefits. Beneficiaries of health insurance agree on only one point—that their premiums not be increased.

Despite these pressure groups, the state has taken a judicious combination of all of the proposed stopgap measures in order to raise the revenues to finance rising health care costs. The result has been to leave the delicate balance between interest groups unaffected. A political stalemate has emerged whereby short-term financial deficits are reduced while the basic structure of French health insurance stays the same.

In November, 1976, a blunt internal memorandum from the Finance Ministry (1976) advised the following cost control measures: 1) reduce the growth of medical personnel, especially physicians; 2) stabilize the aggregate number of hospital beds; 3) review and strengthen the system of physician profiles; and 4) limit the allowable number of medical procedures performed per physician. The Council of Ministers announced their support for these measures in April, 1977. In addition, they established several experiments with alternative modes of hospital reimbursement, proposed a copayment fee for each day spent in the hospital, froze patient-day rates for hospitals and *cliniques,* and reduced reimbursement rates for certain "nonessential" drugs from 70 to 40 percent of the controlled prices.

Subsequently, in the last days of July, 1979, the Council of Ministers announced a new plan for salvaging the NHI funds as well as the entire social security system. Launched while physicians and labor leaders were on vacation, this plan raised health insurance premiums, imposed a cap on public hospital expenditures, and froze the patient-day rates of *cliniques* (*Le Monde,* 1979). In addition, the Council of Ministers broke the government's agreement with physician trade unions by denying a previously scheduled fee increase for October, 1979, and January, 1980, and by refusing both to raise fees and to sign a new agreement (scheduled for 1980) until physicians and hospitals agreed to work in a closed budget system within which the volume of prescribed procedures would be more tightly controlled.

These measures provoked prompt and vitriolic response from the medical profession. The association of public hospitals (*Fédération Hospitalière de France*) condemned the concept of closed budgets for hospitals (Raynaud, 1979). The CSMF protested against this "threat to the quality of care, to professional autonomy and to free choice" (Bles, 1979). Such reactions are predictable. What is more difficult to predict, however, is whether *la médecine libérale* will continue to prosper in the face of serious government efforts to control health care costs.

Concluding Observations

The Business of Medicine

Medicine in France has been not only big business but also good business. The level of physicians' income is a good indicator of the medical profession's strength and the returns to *la médecine libérale.* Brunet-Jailly's (1976) analysis indicates that the average net income of physicians reimbursed by the CNAMTS was approximately twice as large as the average salary of top-level executives in the sixties. According to a study by CREDOC (Glarmet-Lenoir, 1979:26), the average income of physicians was 51 percent higher than that of top-level executives and 114 percent higher than that of engineers in 1975. More recently, a study by the Organization for Economic Co-operation and Development (OECD) (1976:24), using 1974 data, indicated that the ratio of an average doctor's income to that of an average production worker's was higher in France than in all other OECD countries—7.0 compared with 5.6 in the United States and a low of 2.7 in the United Kingdom. Data from the French equivalent of the Internal Revenue Service (*Direction Générale des Impôts,* 1978) reveal that, from 1973 to 1976, physicians' income increased faster than that of other professions such as lawyers and engineers. Finally, the CERC study (1976) estimates the average net income of the French general practitioner at 200,000 francs ($50,000) and the average net income of the French specialist at 225,000 francs ($56,000) in 1976.

Cost Control Policies

In a system characterized by fee-for-service payment under NHI, to control costs it may be necessary, as Thorsen (1974) suggests, to devise a mechanism for controlling physicians' fees. However, there is no evidence that such a strategy is sufficient. On the contrary, the French experience suggests that the success of cost control policies is likely to depend both on the outcome of the fee negotiations and on the extent to which the volume of medical procedures can be restrained. Thus far, the system of physician profiles has not reduced the proliferation of medical procedures. And proposed changes in hospital reimbursement incentives have yet to be enacted, let alone alter the configuration of health resources.

In 1979, as part of a long-run cost-containment strategy, the French government passed legislation reducing the number of physicians trained by cutting enrollments in medical school (*Le Monde,* 1979). At the present time, two other legislative bills are pending. One bill proposes to grant the Ministry of Health authority not merely to authorize new hospital beds but also to close "unneeded" ones. The other proposes to change, once and for all, hospital reimbursement incentives by introducing prospective budgeting for all public hospitals.

Effective control of health costs depends on the state's ability to control the many factors that account for mounting costs (Lévy et al., 1978). In addition, it depends on the extent to which the state is able to link its explicit policies to the implicit incentives that govern provider reimbursement. This, in turn, depends on political forces, for manipulation of financial incentives at the national level is constrained by pressures to which the state and the entire social security system, including the CNAMTS, must respond (Rodwin, 1978b). For the time being, the politics of cost control is in limbo.

NHI: Cui Bono?

The introduction of NHI in France was no doubt a progressive contribution to social policy for it eliminated financial barriers to medical care. It did not, however, reduce social class disparities in medical care consumption; in fact, it made them worse. Between 1965 and 1972 the social class disparities in per capita consumption of all goods and services stayed roughly the same, whereas the disparities in per capita medical care consumption increased. Per capita medical consumption varies by a factor of 50 percent between income levels; it varies by twice that amount between occupational groups (Brunet-Jailly, 1976). This variation is largely explained by the propensity of higher occupational groups to use proportionately higher volumes of specialized medical services (Lecomte and Sandier, 1976).

As we have seen, provider reimbursement incentives under French NHI have reinforced existing patterns of medical care organization by benefiting *la médecine libérale.* Moreover, the growth of NHI appears to have been more successful in enriching the CNAMTS' most powerful beneficiary—the medical profession—than in assuring the CNAMTS' subscriber population equal access to medical care. Under the pressure of rising costs, however, the Ministry of Finance may soon persuade the CNAMTS to reduce the level of health insurance benefits, impose a closed budget on all hospitals and participating physicians, and allow dissenting physicians to opt out of the NHI program while recovering reimbursement for allowable charges. This policy option would encourage the growth of a two-tiered medical system in France; yet it is receiving serious consideration as a strategy for preserving *la médecine libérale.* Indeed, the critical question for the future is whether *la médecine libérale* can survive at all as a distinguishing feature of the French health system.

Victor G. Rodwin

The Prospects for la Médecine Libérale

As the French State attempts to break the stalemate over cost control, it is likely to reconsider its commitment to *la médecine libérale*. Once this happens, the business of medicine may turn bad. In spite of the new legislation reducing enrollments in French medical schools, projections indicate that the rapid influx of new medical school graduates will double the number of physicians between 1970 and 1985 (CES, 1979). Together with tougher cost containment policies and growing efforts to control the volume of medical services rendered, more physicians may contribute to lowering average physician income. Indeed, there is evidence that this is already beginning to occur (Glarmet-Lenoir, 1979:41).

In France, the idea of solidarity has justified NHI as well as increasing state intervention to rationalize the organization, centralize the financing, and preside over the transformation of the health sector. The idea of liberal-pluralism has not only restricted state efforts to create a unitary NHI fund with equal benefits for all; it has also restricted efforts to control costs by forcing accommodation to the demands of powerful interests in the health sector. As we have seen, the conflict between these ideas has supported contradictory policies. But the situation is now at a turning point.

In the future, *la médecine libérale* in France is likely to erode and, within the health sector, the notion of liberal-pluralism will wane. Whether or not this is a change for the better depends on how social choices about the allocation of health resources will be made. As for the past, it seems safe to conclude that the marriage of NHI and *la médecine libérale* thwarts efforts to control rising health care costs. Costly unions—at least in the present era—do not tend to be eternal.

References

AP (*Assistance Publique*). 1973. *Rapport d'Activité des Hôpitaux de Paris*.
Beau, N. 1979. *Le Monde,* January 10.
Bles, G. 1979. Cited in Le Film des Evénements, *Médecin de France,* No. 143, August 9.
Blumberg, M. 1978. Rational Provider Prices: An Incentive for Improved Health Delivery. In Chacko, C.K., ed., *Health Handbook, 1978*. Amsterdam: North Holland.

Bridgman, R.F. 1971. Medical Care under Social Security in France. *International Journal of Health Services* (4):331–341.

Brumter, C. 1979. *La Planification Sanitaire.* Strasbourg: Université des Sciences Juridiques, Politiques, Sociales et de Technologie, Faculté de Droit et de Sciences Politiques. February.

Brunet-Jailly, J. 1976. Quelques Evidences sur l'Evolution du Système de Santé. *Revue Economique,* No. 3.

Caro, G. 1969. *La Médecine en Question.* Paris: Maspero.

Castaing, M. 1975. L'Hôpital, Ce Malade Chronique. *Le Monde,* February 21.

Catrice-Lorrey, A. 1979. *Dynamique Interne de la Sécurité Sociale et Service Publique.* Paris: Université Paris-Sud, Centre de Recherches en Sciences Sociales du Travail.

CERC (*Centre d'Etude des Revenus et des Coûts*). 1976. *Les Revenus des Médecins Libéraux Conventionnés.*

CES (*Conseil Economique et Social*). 1979. *L'Adaptation des Professions Médicales et Paramédicales aux Besoins de Santé de la Population Française.* March.

Cibrie, P. 1954. *Syndicalisme Médical.* Paris: Confédération des Syndicats Médicaux Français.

CNAMTS. 1977. *Démographie des Professions de Santé en 1977.*

Cohen, S., and Goldfinger, C. 1975. From Real Crisis to Permacrisis in French Social Security. In Lindberg, L., Alford, R., Crouch, C., and Offe, C., eds., *Stress and Contradiction in Modern Capitalism.* Lexington, Mass.: D.C. Heath.

Contandriopoulos, A.P. 1979. Evolution du Profil de Pratique des Médecins du Québec de 1971 à 1973. Paper presented to the meeting of the Canadian Society for Economic Sciences, May 9–11.

CREDOC (*Centre de Recherche pour l'Etude et l'Observation des Conditions de Vie*). 1979. *Comptes Nationaux de la Santé.*

de Kervasdoué, J. 1979. Les Politiques de Santé Sont-Elles Adaptées à la Pratique Médicale? *Sociologie du Travail,* Vol. 3.

————. 1981. La Politique de l'Etat en Matière d'Hospitalisation Privée. *1962–1978.* Analyse des Conséquences de Mesures Contradictoires. *Annals Economiques de Clermond-Ferrand,* 1980, No. 16.

Direction Générale des Impôts. 1978. *Etudes et Bilans. Les Notes Blues du Service de l'Information du Ministère du Budget.* October.

FHF (*Fédération Hospitalière de France*). 1976. *L'Hôpital Public Coûte-t-il Plus Cher que les Cliniques Privées?*

Finance Ministry. 1976. Internal Memorandum No. B-6B-8157 from the Office of the Budget to the Minister of Finance, December 13.

Fuchs, V. 1974. *Who Shall Live? Health, Economics, and Social Choice.* New York: Basic Books.

Galant, H. 1955. *Histoire Politique de la Sécurité Sociale Française*. Paris: Armand Colin.

Glarmet-Lenoir, Ch. 1979. *Les Revenus avant Impôt et les Tarifs des Médecins Conventionnés en 1977. Evaluation 1962–1977*. Paris: CREDOC.

Glaser, W. 1970. *Paying the Doctor: Systems of Remuneration and Their Effects*. Baltimore: Johns Hopkins University Press.

————. 1978. *Health Insurance Bargaining*. New York: Gardner Press.

Guibert, B. 1973. *Les Modes de Protection de la Population par les Systèmes Sociaux en 1970*. Paris: CREDOC.

Hayward, J.E.S. 1959. Solidarity: The Social History of an Idea in Nineteenth-Century France. *International Journal of Social History* 4(2):261–284.

Hatzfeld, H. 1963. *Le Grand Tournant de la Médecine Libérale*. Paris: Editions Ouvrières.

IGAS *(Inspection Générale des Affaires Sociales)*. *Rapports Annuels*. Paris: Ministère de la Santé Publique et de la Sécurité Sociale.

————. *1974. La Prévention.*

————. *1975. Les Formes Complémentaires de Protection.*

Jamous, H. 1969. *Sociologie de la Décision: La Réforme des Etudes Médicales et des Structures Hospitalières*. Paris: Centre National de la Recherche Scientifique.

Lecomte, T., and Sandier, S. 1976. Les Médecins Producteurs et Prescripteurs de Soins. *Droit Sanitaire et Sociale*, No. 46.

Le Monde. 1974. December 18.

————. 1976a. June 12, August 25, and October 15.

————. 1976b. September 23.

————. 1979. Le Redressement de la Sécurité Sociale, July 26.

Lenoir, Ch., and Sandier, S. 1976. *La Consommation Pharmaceutique en France et aux U.S.A.* Paris: CREDOC, June.

Lévy, E., et al. 1977. *Hospitalisation Publique, Hospitalisation Privée*. Paris: CNRS, A.T.P. No. 22.

————. 1978. *La Croissance Des Dépenses de Santé*. L.E.G.O.S. Université de Paris, IX. Dauphine.

Ministry of Health. 1970. Les Conditions Actuelles du Financement. In *Pour Une Politique de la Santé. Rapports Présentés à Robert Boulin*, Vol. 3.

————. 1973a. *Recensement des Establissements d'Hospitalisation Privés: Activité et Personnel*. Division d'Etudes et du Plan.

————. 1973b. *Bulletin de Statistiques*, No. 6, tome B.

————. 1974. *Santé et Sécurité Sociale, Tableaux*. Paris: Documentation Française.

————. 1978. *Santé, Sécurité Sociale: Statistiques et Commentaires.* Paris: No. 6, tome B, November-December.

————. 1979a. *Annuaire des Statistiques Sanitaires et Sociales.* Paris.

————. 1979b. *Chiffres Repères de la Santé.* Note d'Information No. 141. Service de Presse.

Monsma, G. 1970. Marginal Revenue and the Demand for Physicians' Services. In Klarman, H., ed., *Empirical Studies in Health Economics. Proceedings.* Baltimore: Johns Hopkins University Press.

NPC (National Planning Commission). 1971. Sixth Plan: *Economie Générale et Financement.* Paris: Documentation Française.

OECD (Organization for Economic Co-operation and Development). 1976. *Public Expenditure on Health.* Studies in Resource Allocation, No. 4, Paris.

Que Choisir? 1978. No. 126, February.

Raynaud, P. 1979. Réflexions sur la Réforme Budgétaire et de la Tarification Hospitalière: Réforme pour la Forme? Réforme de la Forme? Ou Réforme de Fond? *Revue Hospitalière de France.*

Reinhardt, U. 1975. Alternative Methods of Reimbursing Non-institutional Providers of Health Services. In *Controls on Health Care, Papers of the Conference on Regulation in the Health Industry,* January 9, 1974. Washington, D.C.: National Academy of Sciences.

Revue du Praticien. 1979. Volume 29, No. 17, March.

Rodwin, V. 1978a. Health Planning and Provider Reimbursement in France: Lessons for the United States. Paper presented to the Community Health Planning Section at the 106th APHA Meeting, October 16, 1978, Los Angeles. Available through NTIS, Washington, D.C.

————. 1978b. The Politics of Keeping Politics out of Health: French Health Policy and Planning Under the Fifth Republic. Paper presented to Conference on "The Impact of the Fifth Republic on France." New York: State University College, SUNY, June 9–11, at Brockport.

————. 1981. Health Planning in International Perspective. Chapter 13, Section II, "France: Health Planning under NHI." In Blum, H., *Planning for Health: Development and Application of Social Change Theory.* New York: Human Sciences Press, 2d edition (in press).

Ruderman, P. 1976. The Political Economy of Fee-Setting and the Future of Fee-for-Service. In Fraser, R.D., ed., *Health Economics Symposium. Proceedings of the First Canadian Conference, September 4–6, 1974.* Kingston, Canada: Industrial Relations Center, Queens University.

Sandier, S. 1979. *Comparaison des Dépenses de Santé en France et aux*

U.S.A. 1950–1978 (Rapport Préliminaire). Study commissioned by USDHEW, NCHSR. Paris: CREDOC.

———, and Tonnelier, F. 1978. *La Consommation de Soins Médicaux dans le Cadre de l'Assurance Maladie du Régime Générale de Sécurité Sociale*. Paris: CREDOC.

Schorr, A. 1965. *Social Security and Social Services in France*. Washington, D.C.: Social Security Administration, Division of Research and Statistics, Research Report No. 7.

Schroeder, S., and Showstack, J. 1978. Financial Incentives to Perform Medical Procedures and Laboratory Tests: Illustrative Models of Office Practice. *Medical Care* 16:289–298.

Silverman, M., and Lee, P. 1974. *Pills, Profits and Politics*. Berkeley: University of California Press.

Stephan, J.C. 1978. *Economie et Pouvoir Médical*. Paris: Economica.

Stein, S.L. 1979. *Ambulatory Surgery in the Public Hospital System of Paris*. Paris: Assistance Publique, Direction du Plan.

Steudler, F. 1973. L'Evolution de la Profession Médicale: Essai d'Analyse Sociologique. *Cahiers de Sociologie et de Démographie Medicales*, No. 2.

———. 1974. *L'Hôpital en Observation*. Paris: Armand Colin.

———. 1977. Médecine Libérale et Conventionnement. *Sociologie du Travail*, Vol. 2.

Thorsen, L. 1974. How Can the U.S. Government Control Physicians' Fees Under National Health Insurance? A Lesson from the French System. *International Journal of Health Services* 4(1):49–57.

Acknowledgments: This paper grew out of a broader project on health planning efforts in industrially advanced nations. For further detail, see my *Health Planning and Implementation: France, Québec and England* (Doctoral dissertation, Department of City and Regional Planning, University of California, Berkeley, 1980). The research has been supported by the National Institute of Mental Health; the Institute of International Studies, University of California, Berkeley; and the Council for European Studies, Columbia University, New York.

I am grateful to H.L. Blum, S.S. Cohen, P.R. Lee, S.L. Stein, M.M. Weber, and H.L. Wilensky for their help in the course of this research, and to J. de Kervasdoué and G. Pallez for providing irresistible incentives for me to spend 1979 in Paris. *Address correspondence to:* Dr. Victor Rodwin, Lecturer, Health Arts and Sciences Programs, Building T-7, University of California, Berkeley, CA 94720.

	Key to Acronyms
AP	*Assistance Publique*
CERC	*Centre d'Etude des Revenus et des Coûts*
CES	*Counseil Economique et Social*
CHU	*Centre Hospitalier Universitaire*
CNAMTS	*Caisse Nationale d'Assurance Maladie des Travailleurs Salariés*
CREDOC	*Centre de Recherche pour l'Etude et l'Observation des Conditions de Vie*
CSMF	*Confédération des Syndicats Médicaux Français*
FHF	*Fédération Hospitalière de France*
FMF	*Fédération des Médecins de France*
GDP	Gross Domestic Product
IGAS	*Inspection Générale des Affaires Sociales*
MGEN	*Mutuelle Générale de l'Education Nationale*
NHI	National Health Insurance
NPC	National Planning Commission
OECD	Organization for Economic Co-operation and Development
PSRO	Professional Standards Review Organization

Inflation and the
Federal Role in Health

LOUISE B. RUSSELL

Introduction

The health sector bears the dubious distinction of having suffered from intractable inflation for years, long before the rest of the economy discovered it. Price increases in health have been particularly rapid since the middle 1960s. Over the period 1965 to 1974, physicians' fees rose 5.7 percent per year on the average. Cost per hospital day climbed at an annual 12.1 percent; about half of the increase was due to higher levels of inputs per hospital day, putting the rate of pure price inflation at just over 6 percent per year (Waldman, 1972). During the same years the Consumer Price Index rose at a more modest 4.5 percent annually. [1]

This rapid inflation has paralleled an enormous expansion in the federal role in health. In 1965 federal health outlays amounted to $5.2 billion (Office of Management and Budget, 1974). By 1969, a swarm of new programs, of which Medicare and Medicaid are the largest, had brought the total to $16.7 billion. And by 1974 that amount had nearly doubled again, to about $32 billion (Table 1).

Understandably then, the problem of inflation has been intertwined with every aspect of the federal government's health programs. Rising prices have absorbed a large part of the billions of

---

[1] Unless otherwise noted, all data given in this paper are for fiscal years. Average annual rates of inflation are based on fiscal year data supplied by the Office of Research and Statistics, Social Security Administration.

In *Health: A Victim or Cause of Inflation?*, edited by Michael Zubkoff. New York, PRODIST, 1976.

Note: References for this paper begin on p. 349.

**TABLE 1   Total Federal Health Outlays
in Current and Constant Dollars,
Fiscal Years 1969–1974
($ millions)**

	1969	1970	1971	1972	1973	1974 [b]
Current dollars	$16,708	$18,345	$20,682	$24,147	$26,130	$31,942
Constant dollars [a]	16,708	17,137	18,092	19,968	20,724	24,072

[a] 1969 = 100
[b] Estimates
Source: Russell *et al.* (1974).

dollars spent through these programs—straining budgets and making it difficult to tell when higher outlays spell real advances and when they are canceled out by price increases. Because of the government's newly dominant role in health, it has become the focus of demands that something be done to combat inflation. And the fact that health sector inflation worsened just as the federal government expanded its share so dramatically has raised questions about whether the parallel is accidental. Have federal programs been a major contributor to health sector inflation? With the passage of national health insurance imminent, the answer to this question is particularly crucial.

The Federal Role in Health: Trends in Program Outlays

As the introduction noted, federal health programs spent $32 billion in 1974, about twice as much as in 1969, and six times the total for 1965, only ten years earlier. In recent years the increases have been a nearly even mix of real growth and price inflation. Between 1969 and 1974, while current dollars rose from $16.7 billion to $31.9 billion, real outlays grew much less, although still substantially—from $16.7 billion to $24.1 billion (Table 1). Thus about $8 billion of the current dollar increase was absorbed by rising prices. (See Appendix for deflator sources.)

A wide range of activities and programs makes up the federal health outlays, and they have not, of course, suffered equally from inflation or shared equally in the real growth. Health research, health manpower training, and construction support for health facilities can all be viewed as investments in the health care system. Health care services, whether federally financed through the private sector or provided directly in federal facilities, are the most important product of that system. The two remaining categories are prevention and control programs, and programs aimed at improving the organization and delivery of care. The programs and trends in each of these categories are discussed in the following pages.

Research

As a rule, the federal government's involvement in the health sector was quite limited until the 1960s. Health research is the major exception to that rule. For a number of reasons the political climate after World War II favored research over other ways of promoting the national interest in health, and it was at this time that the government established itself as the major source of financing (Strickland, 1972). In 1950 the nation spent $161 million on health research, with the federal government contributing close to half. By 1973 the government accounted for almost two-thirds of a total $3.5 billion spent on health research (National Institutes of Health, 1973).

A number of federal agencies—including the Defense Department, the Veterans Administration, and the Atomic Energy Commission—report substantial outlays for health-related research, but the National Institutes of Health (NIH) are unquestionably the financial and scientific center of both the federal and the national research effort. NIH controls more than two-thirds of all federal funds for health research. Principally through the ten research institutes, each created to focus attention and money on a particular area of research, these funds are spent on intramural research and distributed as grants and contracts to outside investigators.

Table 2 traces the recent history of federal outlays for health research. The total reflects NIH's fortunes, which reached a low point in the late 1960s after years of steady growth in congressional appropriations. As the table shows, the institutes' outlays grew relatively little in current dollars between 1969 and 1971. Because of inflation, they actually declined in real terms—by about 3.5 percent.

TABLE 2   Federal Outlays for Health Research,
in Current and Constant Dollars,
Fiscal Years 1969–1974
($ millions)

	1969	1970	1971	1972	1973	1974c
TOTAL a						
Current dollars	$1,476	$1,531	$1,546	$1,713	$2,003	$2,400
Constant dollars b	1,476	1,452	1,388	1,463	1,631	1,839
National Institutes of Health:						
Current dollars	836	862	899	1,079	1,325	1,616
Constant dollars b	836	817	807	921	1,079	1,238
Cancer Institute:						
Current dollars	163	169	181	245	345	447
Constant dollars b	163	161	162	209	281	342
Heart and Lung Institute:						
Current dollars	129	135	141	172	218	291
Constant dollars b	129	128	127	147	178	223
Other National Institutes of Health						
Current dollars	543	558	577	662	762	879
Constant dollars b	543	530	518	565	621	673
All other federal programs						
Current dollars	640	669	647	634	677	784
Constant dollars b	640	634	581	541	552	601

a Detail may not add to totals because of rounding.
b 1969 = 100
c Estimates
Source: Russell *et al.* (1974).

This unaccustomed period of stagnation was followed by a
period of renewed growth. By 1974 total outlays stood 63 percent
higher than in 1969 and, in spite of higher prices, had produced a
25 percent increase in real terms. The National Institutes fared
better than the average since a near doubling in current dollars
between 1969 and 1974 sustained a gain in constant dollars of nearly
50 percent. As the table also shows, however, the growth has been
very much concentrated in two of the institutes—the National
Cancer Institute, and the National Heart and Lung Institute. In
response to the National Cancer Act of 1971 and similar legislation
for heart diseases, the combined current dollar outlays of these two
institutes spurted to $738 million in 1974, and accounted for 46
percent of the funds allotted to all the Institutes, in contrast to the 35
percent allocated six years earlier.

Manpower Training

Until the 1960s, federal training outlays came primarily from the research training programs of the National Institutes of Health, and the programs of agencies, like the Defense Department and the Veterans Administration, that need staff for their own facilities. The 1960s brought the first legislation to finance generally the training of health care professionals as a contribution to the solution of several widely perceived national problems—actual or potential shortages of health manpower, the uneven geographic distribution of health manpower, and the decline of the general practice specialty in medicine. Under this legislation, DHEW's Bureau of Health Manpower Education was created and given responsibility for the new programs.

Table 3 shows the trends in federal training dollars over the years 1969-1974. The current dollar total doubled over the period, and training was a relative gainer in real, as well as current, dollars because inflation in training costs has apparently been more moderate than inflation in other health sectors—about 4.6 percent annually since 1965 (Russell, 1975). Less than half of the growth in current outlays was absorbed by inflation, putting real growth at 54 percent over the period.

The new programs are reflected in the trends for different types of health manpower. In 1969 funds for research personnel training still exceeded those for any other single category and accounted for more than a quarter of all federal training funds. But they declined in both current and constant dollars over the period, falling to 12 percent of the total by 1974. This trend should continue over the next few years—except for a temporary interruption due to the release, in fiscal 1974, of impounded 1973 funds—as current programs are phased out and a new and smaller program of research fellowships, proposed by the secretary of DHEW, is introduced.

By contrast the outlays for other categories of manpower have grown rapidly, reflecting the Bureau of Health Manpower's programs. The bulk of the bureau's funds—which, in 1974, accounted for about half the outlays for physicians' training, 70 percent of the funds for dentists, and 80 percent of the funds for nurses—is

TABLE 3   Federal Outlays for Health Manpower Training
in Current and Constant Dollars,
by Type of Training, Fiscal Years 1969–1974
($ millions)

	1969	1970	1971	1972	1973	1974 [c]
TOTAL [a]						
Current dollars	$805	$969	$1,120	$1,262	$1,416	$1,597
Constant dollars [b]	805	916	1,008	1,079	1,152	1,240
Research personnel training:						
Current dollars	210	221	215	219	164	185
Constant dollars [b]	210	209	195	190	136	147
Physicians' Training:						
Current dollars	170	185	225	269	318	407
Constant dollars [b]	170	175	204	233	264	324
Dentists' training:						
Current dollars	28	28	45	59	68	82
Constant dollars [b]	28	27	41	51	56	65
Nurses' training:						
Current dollars	61	72	80	95	129	127
Constant dollars [b]	61	68	73	83	107	101
All other training:						
Current dollars	249	361	444	461	536	584
Constant dollars [b]	249	342	402	400	446	464
Construction at Health Professions Schools:						
Current dollars	88	102	111	159	202	211
Constant dollars [b]	88	95	94	122	142	138

[a] Detail may not add to totals because of rounding.
[b] 1969 = 100
[c] Estimates
Source: Russell *et al.* (1974).

distributed as institutional grants to the schools in return for promised increases in enrollments. The remainder is spent for student loans and scholarships, and special programs. The outlays for 1974 also reflect new Defense Department programs to attract manpower, especially physicians, now that the draft is no longer applicable.

Construction Support

Along with health research, construction support is the oldest federal commitment to help the private sector meet national goals. The Hill-Burton program was established in 1946 to finance the construction of hospitals in rural areas. Since then, it has expanded to cover other types of health care facilities, although hospital construction and modernization have remained its major focus.

Louise B. Russell

With the arrival of the large federal programs of health care financing, the need for special programs of construction support has become a matter for debate. The Administration has argued that sufficient funds are provided through depreciation allowances included in the third-party payments of Medicare, Medicaid, and private insurers, and that construction support programs are redundant. It has regularly tried to kill the Hill-Burton program. Congress has, with equal regularity, revived it.

The outlays for recent years reflect these policy battles (Table 4). While outlays for research and environmental health facilities show relatively little change in current dollars, outlays for health care facilities dropped more than 20 percent between 1970 and 1974. Rising prices meant that, in real terms, these outlays were cut in half. Primarily because of this precipitous decline in outlays for health care facilities, total construction support lost ground in real terms over the entire period.

TABLE 4   Federal Outlays for Construction Support
in Current and Constant Dollars,
Fiscal Years 1969–1974
($ millions)

	1969	1970	1971	1972	1973	1974[c]
TOTAL [a]						
Current dollars	$634	$679	$663	$569	$554	$581
Constant dollars [b]	634	635	564	436	390	381
Health Care Facilities:						
Current dollars	340	387	360	300	253	265
Constant dollars [b]	340	362	306	230	178	174
Hill-Burton:						
Current dollars	264	284	266	244	167	190
Constant dollars [b]	264	265	226	187	117	125
Health Research Facilities:						
Current dollars	51	41	43	13	39	60
Constant dollars [b]	51	38	37	10	28	39
Environmental Health Facilities						
Current dollars	243	251	261	255	262	257
Constant dollars [b]	243	235	222	196	184	168

[a] Detail may not add to totals because of rounding.
[b] 1969 = 100
[c] Estimates
Source: Russell et al. (1974).

126

Health Services

Federal health services programs can be grouped into two subcategories—those that pay for care provided in the private sector, and those that provide care directly in federal facilities. Together these programs spent $13 billion in 1969 and more than $25 billion in 1974—about 80 percent of all federal expenditures for health (Table 5).

New programs of federal financing have been the source of the tremendous growth in federal health spending during the last decade. The largest, the Medicare program for the aged, did not exist in 1965; in 1974, when the disabled and those with chronic kidney disease were brought under the program, it spent more than $12 billion. Medicaid's predecessor accounted for $550 million in federal outlays in 1965 (Cooper et al., 1973); Medicaid spent nearly $6 billion of federal money on medical benefits for the welfare population in 1974. The Health Services Administration and the Alcohol, Drug Abuse, and Mental Health Administration added close to $1 billion more to the 1974 total.

Taken together, programs of federal financing have been among the relative gainers in the health budget. Their expenditures more than doubled between 1969 and 1974 and, in spite of inflation, supported an increase of 56 percent in real terms—compared to the real increase of 44 percent in the total health budget over the period.

The interesting thing about the growth in constant dollars for health services programs is the fact that a large chunk of it went, not to provide for larger beneficiary populations or for more hospital days and outpatient visits per capita, but for increased inputs per hospital day. Taking into account Medicare outlays for the aged, which amount to 86 percent of total 1974 outlays, we find that about $2.6 billion of the current dollar increase of $3.9 billion (1969-1974) was necessary to meet price increases, and another $1.1 billion was absorbed by increases in inputs per hospital day. If we limit our consideration to the program's expenditures for hospital care, it turns out that all of the real growth was funneled into increased inputs per day (Russell et al., 1974).

TABLE 5   Federal Outlays for Health Care Services in Current and Constant Dollars, Fiscal Years 1969–1974 ($ millions)

	1969	1970	1971	1972	1973	1974
PROGRAMS OF FEDERAL FINANCING, TOTAL [a]						
Current dollars	$9,988	$11,067	$12,835	$15,370	$16,287	$20,594
Constant dollars [b]	9,988	10,306	11,186	12,676	12,920	15,567
Medicare:						
Current dollars	6,598	7,149	7,875	8,819	9,479	12,180
Constant dollars [b]	6,598	6,658	6,865	7,273	7,513	9,195
Medicaid:						
Current dollars	2,285	2,727	3,362	4,426 [c]	4,600 [c]	5,827
Constant dollars [b]	2,285	2,539	2,930	3,651	3,649	4,405
Health Services Admin., and Alcohol, Drug Abuse, and Mental Health Administration: [d]						
Current dollars	378	423	554	799	720	909
Constant dollars [b]	378	395	481	659	579	701
Programs that supplement direct provision: [f] [e]						
Current dollars	300	375	492	583	669	726
Constant dollars [b]	300	349	429	481	530	548
All other programs:						
Current dollars	426	393	552	742	819	952
Constant dollars [b]	426	366	482	612	649	718

PROGRAMS OF DIRECT FEDERAL PROVISION, TOTAL[a,k]

Current dollars	3,045	3,231	3,550	4,108	4,535	5,099
Constant dollars [b]	3,045	3,009	3,090	3,375	3,575	3,816
Department of Defense: [k]						
Current dollars	1,485	1,466	1,558	1,773	1,923	2,085
Constant dollars [b]	1,485	1,366	1,355	1,457	1,519	1,567
Veterans Administration: [k]						
Current dollars	1,376	1,554	1,751	2,092	2,342	2,667
Constant dollars [b]	1,376	1,447	1,526	1,719	1,844	1,995
All other programs and construction of federal facilities: [k]						
Current dollars	184	211	241	242	271	347
Constant dollars [b]	184	196	210	198	212	254

[a] Detail may not add to totals because of rounding.
[b] 1969 = 100
[c] Outlays for 1972 include an advance grant made to the states for 1973 program expenses.
[d] Includes health programs of the Office of Economic Opportunity, which were transferred to HSA and ADAMHA in 1973 and 1974
[e] Estimates
[f] Includes Department of Defense and Veterans Administration programs
[k] Includes related construction

Source: Russell et al. (1974).

This point should be kept in mind whenever the outlays of health services programs are considered. For example, Medicare outlays per aged enrollee, in constant dollars, grew from $336 in 1969 to $368 in 1974 (Russell et al., 1974), a real increase of about 10 percent. But the growth in inputs per hospital day suggests that this real growth does not reflect additional hospital days or physician visits, two traditional measures of services. This view is supported by data on hospital days reimbursed, which show no trend between 1969 and 1974, and by the fact that Medicare's coverage of the medical bills of the aged fell from its 1969 high of 45.5 percent to 40.3 percent in 1973 (Cooper et al., 1974).

The federal share of Medicaid outlays per recipient (a less desirable base than the number eligible for Medicaid, which is virtually impossible to determine) has followed a choppy downward course, falling from $189 in constant dollars in 1969 to $162 in 1974 (Russell et al., 1974). Again if we refer to the role of inputs per hospital day in the constant dollar outlays, it seems reasonable to believe that hospital days and outpatient visits per Medicaid recipient have actually declined in recent years.

The outlays of the Health Services Administration (HSA) and the Alcohol, Drug Abuse, and Mental Health Administration (ADAMHA) have not been much affected by the phenomenon of rising hospital inputs. Virtually all of their funds, which dipped sharply in 1973 because of impoundments, are spent for outpatient services. HSA's major programs are the venerable Maternal and Child Health program and the much newer Community Health Centers; the latter offer comprehensive medical care to the poor. ADAMHA provides support for Community Mental Health Centers. Both agencies have been the recipients, in 1973 and 1974, of related health programs from the now dismantled Office of Economic Opportunity.

The Department of Defense and the Veterans Administration account for 90 percent of the outlays for the direct federal provision of health services. Through their own networks of hospitals and clinics, they serve two special beneficiary groups—active and retired servicemen and their dependents in the case of the Defense

Department, and veterans in the case of the VA. Their combined outlays grew by two-thirds in current dollars, to cover rising prices and sustain a real growth of 25 percent. Both agencies finance small insurance programs to supplement federal services with care in the private sector; the outlays for these programs grew much more rapidly, increasing by about 80 percent in real terms between 1969 and 1974.

Prevention and Control of Health Problems

The prevention and control category includes traditional public health programs like those of DHEW's Center for Disease Control, consumer protection activities, and programs to combat a variety of environmental hazards. As we expand our knowledge of the factors which are health related, so does the range of programs in this category. The new occupational safety agencies in the Departments of Labor and Health, Education, and Welfare are included in the outlays. By the same token, the Environmental Protection Agency should probably be represented, but only a small portion of its outlays is reported as health related at present. Still other programs have some claim to be considered. For example, given the importance of nutrition to health, one could argue that the food stamp program belongs here.

As presently defined, this category accounts for a small portion of the federal health budget—$1.1 billion in 1974 (Table 6), or about 3.5 percent. Within the total, consumer protection activities—the Food and Drug Administration, the inspection programs of the Agriculture Department, and the new Consumer Product Safety Commission—have increased their outlays rapidly. But on average, the category has grown at a somewhat slower rate than the health budget as a whole, with a 75 percent increase in current dollar outlays resulting in real growth of about 30 percent over the period.

Improving the Organization and Delivery of Care

This category is probably more important for its symbolic value than for anything else. It includes programs like the Comprehensive Health Planning and Regional Medical Programs, which focus on

TABLE 6   Federal Outlays for Other Health-Related Activities in
Current and Constant Dollars, Fiscal Years 1969–1974
($ millions)

	1969	1970	1971	1972	1973	1974 [b]
Prevention and control of health problems:						
Current dollars	$644	$699	$730	$814	$933	$1,129
Constant dollars [a]	644	659	645	679	739	830
Improving the organization and delivery of care						
Current dollars	117	168	238	312	401	542
Constant dollars [a]	117	158	210	260	317	399

[a] 1969 = 100
[b] Estimates
Source: Russell *et al.* (1974).

concerns that have grown along with the federal role in health—
concerns about the availability, quality, and cost of health care. The
difficulty is that these problems involve nearly every federal program to some degree. For example, one goal of federal training
programs is to improve the availability of care. Thus it misrepre-
sents the size of the federal effort to single out only those programs
as those whose primary focus is in this area. Even so these outlays
have soared in recent years and are an important indicator of federal
concern. Even after allowing for inflation, they have tripled—going
from $117 million in 1969 to $400 million in 1974 (Table 6).

Causes of Health Sector Inflation
and the Federal Role in Health

As Section II showed, the federal health budget has grown
substantially in real terms over the last decade. But inflation has
clearly taken a heavy toll as well—of the 91 percent increase in
current dollars between 1969 and 1974, just over half was absorbed
by rising price. While federal health programs have suffered from
inflation, the problem must be considered from another side. Might
they also have contributed to that inflation? How much can we say
about the part these programs play in health sector inflation?

The last decade has also seen a great deal of research into the problem of inflation in the health sector. Let us consider some of the evidence that has accumulated and, against this background, draw out some of the interesting implications of the federal outlays previously described. The discussion suggests possible answers to the questions asked in the first paragraph, but is not definitive. To begin then, we need to review what we now know, or think we know, about the causes of health sector inflation.

Most of the analysis of inflation has concentrated on the costs of health services, particularly hospital costs per day, which have been rising at the unprecedented rate of more than 12 percent per year since 1965. Different theories about the process emphasize different actors—the patient, the doctor, the hospital administrator, hospital labor unions—and different objects of expense—new technology, capital facilities, or even waste and inefficiency (Davis, 1973). But the theories return to one basic factor, which can be viewed as either permissive or motivating, that being health insurance—or, more broadly, third-party payments (Feldstein, 1971a; Salkever, 1972).

Third-party payments reduce the out-of-pocket cost of care to the patient. For example, under the high-option Aetna plan available to government employees, the patient pays only 20 percent of hospital costs after the deductible is met. The Medicare program pays virtually all hospital costs in full for the first 60 days, beyond a deductible of $84 (calendar 1974). All parties to the medical care process are aware of this and affected by it. The insured patient knows that he will have to pay only a small portion of the cost of services out-of-pocket, and is thus not greatly concerned about cost. The physician and the hospital administrator realize that, because their full costs (or charges) are not reflected in what the patient pays, those costs will not prevent him from seeking their services, and they will not have to worry about nonpayment of bills.

The Cost of Living Council has published some estimates that show how significant the effect of third-party coverage of hospital care has been. Using data from the American Hospital Association, the council reported that the cost of a day in the hospital rose from $16 in 1950 to $109 in 1973. But over the same period, the out-of-pocket cost to the patient fell from $10 per day to $9 (U.S. Congress,

1974). Clearly, third-party coverage provides very large subsidies for hospital care, relieving those who make decisions about hospital care of most of the financial costs and risks of those decisions.

This description applies directly to federal programs for health services. Like private health insurance, they reduce the cost of care to the patient. And the massive programs introduced during the last decade have vastly expanded the pool of third-party payments available to health service providers. The federal funds supplied by Medicare and Medicaid (remember that matching Medicaid funds from the states are not included) supplied about 22 percent of all the money spent on hospital care in 1973. All federal programs together paid for about one-third of the costs of the nation's hospital care (Russell et al., 1974).

There is no comparable work on the causes of inflation in other areas of the health sector, such as training or research. While it is beyond the scope of this paper to undertake such an analysis, one might begin by generalizing from the emphasis on subsidies in the theory developed for hospital costs. This suggests, by extension, that it is worthwhile to examine the size of the federal subsidy in these other areas.

It was noted in Section II that the federal government supplies almost two-thirds of all the money spent nationally on health research. Medical schools are the recipients of a major part of these funds—federal research grants and contracts have provided about a third of their financial support in recent years (Office of Management and Budget, 1973). The funds have had some noteworthy effects. For example, during the years 1951–1966, when NIH appropriations were growing steadily, the number of full-time medical faculty increased fivefold, while medical student enrollment increased about 30 percent (Strickland, 1972; National Center for Health Statistics, 1973).

Training programs are another major source of funds for medical schools. When institutional training grants are added to research monies, it turns out that the federal government has paid for about half the total cost of running medical schools in recent years (Office of Management and Budget, 1973). Yet another way to bring out the size of federal training subsidies is to relate them to the target groups of students. When institutional grants, student loans and scholarships, and special project funds—but not construction funds—are considered, the federal government paid out $5,042 per medical student, $4,280 per dental student, and $560 per nursing student in current dollars in 1974 (Russell et al., 1974). [2]

Federal subsidies are obviously quite large in a number of health areas. In the case of health services these subsidies are causally related to the high rates of cost inflation that have come to characterize health care. Argument by analogy suggests that they may be related to price inflation in other areas of the health sector. Does this mean that inflation is an unavoidable side effect of subsidies designed to promote other goals? What are the policy alternatives for combatting inflation? Again the discussion has developed to the furthest extent in health services. The solutions that have been proposed, not all of which are mutually exclusive, will be briefly discussed under two headings: regulation, and restructuring insurance.

Regulation

The kind of regulation most frequently proposed for the health sector is regulation of prices or costs. Sometimes particular subcategories of costs—for instance, payroll costs or facility acquisition costs—are suggested for special regulation. And there are, of course, many variations on any of the basic themes. For example, the basis for regulating hospital costs can be cost per day, cost per admission, or the entire annual budget of the hospital.

Regulation is a difficult and administratively complex process. It requires considerable knowledge of the industry on the part of the regulators. And almost by definition, it works against the incentives of the actors in the industry, thus making its own task more difficult. For example, attempts to regulate physicians' fees during the recent period of economy-wide regulation induced physicians to itemize

---

[2] The amount per medical student is based on DHEW funds only. Most of the outlays of the Defense Department and the Veterans Administration support internship and residency programs, rather than undergraduate medical training.

their bills, charging separately for items that had formerly been included in a single fee, and partially frustrating the purpose of the regulation. Similarly, it is difficult to control the provision of unnecessary services designed to increase provider revenues. Attempts to counter this sort of thing, such as physician profiles, add to the complexity of the regulatory process.

But the most important and difficult question to ask of any proposed solution to inflation, is: will it work? While there are no definitive answers, there are some pieces of evidence which deserve careful consideration.

The first is the experience with regulation of the health sector under Phases II, III, and IV. During the months covered by these phases, November 1971 to April 1974, hospital charges for a semiprivate room and for operating room services rose at rates well below those of the preregulation period (U.S. DHEW, 1974). The picture was blurred, however, by the fact that hospital costs continued to rise at rates close to those of the preregulation years (U.S. Congress, 1974), an important aberration since many insurance programs, public and private, reimburse on the basis of costs. And since the end of Phase IV, price increases have jumped to rates considerably higher than those obtained before regulation began.

But this regulation was short term, and during some of the period it was economy-wide. The proposal now is the permanent regulation of a single industry, health care. Other industries—such as the airlines and electric and gas utilities—have been under permanent regulation for many years, and social scientists have had time to study some of the effects of regulation on these industries. Their studies lead to a surprisingly unanimous conclusion: regulation of prices, or costs, has not been successful. Prices and costs appear to be at least as high, in some cases higher, than they would be in the absence of regulation (Noll, 1974).

Of course, the health sector differs from these regulated industries in many ways, and the level of subsidy—through private insurance and public programs—may be one of the most important. In the presence of these subsidies, few people see how some degree of regulation can be avoided. At the same time, there is no evidence to suggest how regulation can be made to work. The proposals made under the next heading deserve careful consideration for any help they can offer.

Restructuring Insurance

Proposals to restructure insurance are based on the principle that the problem of health sector inflation arises because decision makers are separated from the financial results of their decisions. The solution then is to reintroduce financial incentives in some fashion.

Most public and private insurance programs are currently designed to cover low and moderate levels of health care use quite well. They thus remove the financial incentives for cost control from the bulk of health care services—even though most people could handle most or all of these expenses without insurance. At the same time, they provide inadequate protection from truly "catastrophic" medical bills. The main proposal in this area, major risk insurance, would simply reverse this design, providing little or no coverage for moderate levels of use, and very high or even complete coverage for very large medical bills (Feldstein, 1971b).

Prepaid group practice, which has received considerable attention in recent years, is another way to restructure insurance. The argument for it is that doctors have the most to say about the use of medical services and that, if they are paid a flat annual fee per person, they will then be encouraged to provide only care that is needed, at the lowest possible cost.

Would major risk insurance help control inflation in the health sector? The answer is that no one knows, because it has never been tried. The studies showing that insurance is a major factor in rising hospital costs provide support for the presumption underlying the plan—that the process can be reversed, and inflation reduced, by the introduction of less extensive insurance. But until it is tried we cannot be sure it will be effective, nor can we dismiss it as ineffective. Since all participants in the health sector are involved in the inflationary process, any experiments with major risk insurance would have to include all of the population in a medical "market area." Physicians and hospital administrators would be little influenced if only a few of their patients were covered by it.

Summary and Conclusions

The role of the federal government in health has grown enormously in the last ten years. In 1965 federal outlays for health were $5.2 billion. The total jumped to $16.7 billion in 1969 and by 1974 it stood at $32 billion. These increases have meant substantial advances in real terms for most health programs, but the inflation in health sector prices that paralleled rising federal expenditures has taken a heavy toll as well—about half of the increase in current dollars between 1969 and 1974 was absorbed by rising prices.

Studies of rising hospital costs indicate that federal programs have contributed to this inflation. Together with private health insurance, they encourage inflation by separating those who make decisions in the health sector from the financial results of their decisions. Argument by analogy suggests that federal subsidies to other areas may contribute to inflation in those areas. In some cases the subsidies are quite large. As a prominent example, medical schools receive fully half their financial support from federal research and training programs.

Proposals for combatting health sector inflation can be grouped under two headings: regulation, and restructuring insurance. While few feel that increased regulation of the health sector can be avoided, past experience does not suggest any models for successful regulation of prices and costs. The principle behind proposals to change the structure of insurance is that some financial incentives must be built into the framework that shapes the decisions of participants in the health sector; these incentives may be able to substitute for regulation in some areas, and to serve as a way of reinforcing regulation in others.

Appendix: The Deflators

The deflators used to derive the constant dollar estimates are described in detail in Appendix A of Russell et al. (1974). Their sources will be indicated here. All deflators were adjusted to a base of 100 for fiscal 1969.

Research Deflator. Jaffe, S. A., *A Price Index for Deflation of Academic R & D Expenditures,* National Science Foundation Publication 72–310.

Training Deflator. Developed from faculty salary data published in various issues of the *Journal of Medical Education,* and the GNP deflator for nonfinancial corporations. Expenditure weights provided by the Association of American Medical Colleges.

Construction Deflator. Department of Commerce, *The Construction Review* (the American Appraisal Company index).

Health Services Deflator: Inpatient Services. Adjusted hospital cost per day in short-term community hospitals from the American Hospital Association. Further adjusted to correct for increases in inputs per day.

Health Services Deflator: Outpatient Services. Physicians' fees index from the Consumer Price Index, Bureau of Labor Statistics.

Deflator for Prevention and Control, and Improving the Organization and Delivery of Care. White-collar wages from various issues of the Bureau of Labor Statistics' national survey of professional, administrative, technical, and clerical pay.

Politics, Public Policy, and Medical Inflation

THEODORE R. MARMOR, DONALD A. WITTMAN, AND THOMAS C. HEAGY

The Problem of Inflation in Medical Care

Introduction

In the past twenty-four years the price of medical services has gone up 1.5 times as fast as the Consumer Price Index. The proportion of the Gross National Product devoted to health care increased by 71 percent from 4.6 percent to 7.8 percent.[1] Clearly, a continuation of these trends would have serious consequences. Moreover, many economists believe that the "continuing trend toward full or nearly full insurance coverage in the context of a nearly unregulated fee-for-service delivery system is likely to produce continued inflation in medical care" (Newhouse, 1976).

This paper dicusses the politics of anti-inflation policy in the health sector, and the determinants of governmental responses to problems known jointly as medical care inflation. The first section attempts to clarify the issue by distinguishing between four different concepts commonly used when discussing medical inflation. The

---

[1] For a discussion of these figures, see the next section, *Clarification of the Problem.*

In *Health: A Victim or Cause of Inflation?*, edited by Michael Zubkoff. New York, PRODIST, 1976.

Note: References for this paper begin on p. 351.

second section presents some of the standard solutions to these problems suggested by economists.

Of necessity, a discussion of how the political "market" works and the political attributes of the solutions proposed go hand in hand with a discussion of inflation. Our main conclusion is that the politics of medical inflation produces persistent expressions of concern about inflation rates, but actions which at worst exacerbate the problem or at best are weak. In addition, we find that the most decisive governmental reactions to medical inflation take the form of reducing medical care benefits in selected public programs rather than actions to reduce medical inflation generally. Finally, we suggest that this will continue to be the case until or unless the budget for health is centralized at one governmental level. We find, in general, that a decentralized payment structure reduces the government's interest in effective implementation of anti-inflationary policies.

Clarification of the Problem

Considerable confusion has arisen in the discussion of controlling medical inflation because commentators have discussed at least four different problems under the common rubric of "medical inflation."

Consider the problem of *absolute price inflation.* Absolute price inflation is measured by the medical services component of the CPI. According to this index, the annual rate of medical inflation has averaged 4.4 percent over the past twenty-four years (Bureau of Labor Statistics). This measure seems clearly inappropriate. What we are concerned with is medical price inflation only to the extent that it exceeds general inflation. If the inflation rates are identical, the problem is one of general inflation, not medical inflation.

Consider next the problem of *relative price inflation.* The difference between the annual rate of growth of the medical services component of the CPI and the total CPI measures relative price inflation. By this index, the rate of medical inflation has averaged 1.3 percent per year over the past twenty-four years (Bureau of Labor Statistics). This rate may appear small, but represents a total increase of 37 percent in the relative price of medical services over the period.

Next, *total real expenditures growth per capita* is measured by the percentage growth in expenditures per capita on medical services deflated by the total CPI. The annual rate of expenditure growth has averaged 4.8 percent (U.S. DHEW, 1974). This measure is inappropriate for reasons similar to that cited in regard to absolute price inflation: the measure incorporates the general growth of real GNP per capita. Only if the real expenditures on medical services grow at a faster rate than total real income, is its growth noteworthy.

With respect to *relative expenditure growth*, the increase of medical expenditures as a percent of GNP is an appropriate measure. The annual rate of growth has averaged 2.3 percent, from 4.6 percent of GNP to 7.8 percent of GNP, an increase of 71 percent. Relative expenditure growth can be divided into two components, relative price inflation (see above), and relative quantity growth. Relative quantity growth is that growth in medical services as a percent of GNP that would have occurred in the absence of any change in the relative price level of medical services. It includes both quantity changes (in the strict sense) and quality changes. Over the past twenty-four years, both have been major contributors to relative expenditure growth.

Neither relative price inflation nor relative quantity growth is a priori bad. People are concerned about relative price growth for at least two reasons. First, it represents a redistribution of income to the providers of health care services away from the providers of all other services in the economy. Second, lower income families spend a higher percent of their income on medical care. An increase in its relative price will have a disproportionate impact on the poor (Davis, 1976). Implicit in the concern about relative price growth is the assumption that relative prices are "too high." If they were "too low," an increase would be desirable. The role of unskilled hospital workers illustrates the ambiguity in arguing that the relative price growth experienced has been undesirable. A major part of the growth in the price of hospital services is explained by the increased wages of unskilled workers (Lave, 1976). But it can be argued that these workers were among the worst paid workers in the economy and that the relative increase in their wages was not only justified, but insufficient.

People are concerned with relative expenditure growth because, by definition, this growth reduces the share of GNP available to other sectors. But as in the case of relative prices, growth in relative expenditures is undesirable only if the level of relative expenditures is too high. Proponents of this position argue that for a variety of reasons (government subsidy, insurance, and so on) people consume more and better quality medical services than they really need; that expenditures for medical care are suffering from substantial diminishing marginal benefit; and that some of the money going to health care could be better used elsewhere in the economy (Newhouse, 1976). It can also be argued, however, that the increase in relative expenditures has been the desirable result of increased access for the poor and of better quality generally.

While there may be some disagreement concerning the optimal level of expenditures, it is unambiguous that if relative expenditures increase at current rates without limit, they will soon become intolerable.

For the remainder of this paper we will accept the arguments made earlier in the book that relative prices and expenditures in medical care are currently too high and that government action is justified to curtail further medical care inflation.

It is essential to note that limiting relative expenditures requires the simultaneous control of relative prices and relative quantity. However, some proposed policies would reduce relative price at the expense of increasing relative expenditures. If the goal is simply to control relative price, these policies are appropriate means. But, if the goal is to control relative expenditure, they are not. Ultimately, the choice of policy tools will depend on which of these two definitions of the medical inflation problem one is concerned about.

The appropriate response to the problem of medical inflation depends on its causes. Observers (Davis and Foster, 1972; Feldstein, 1971; Lave, 1976; Newhouse, 1976; Russell, 1976; etc.) have diagnosed six major causes of medical health inflation: (1) wealthier societies tend to spend a larger fraction of their resources on medical care; (2) cost-increasing technological developments in medical care in the postwar period, such as kidney machines and open heart surgery, have outweighed cost-decreasing developments, such as antibiotics; (3) doctors and hospitals have monopoly power; (4) the supply of doctors has been artificially limited, and substitutes are legally limited in scope; (5) greater use of medical insurance has reduced the marginal cost of medical care to the patients; and (6) the government substantially subsidizes health care. Of these causes, numbers 2 to 6 cause *high* relative prices (and/or expenditures), not *increasing* relative prices (and/or expenditures). For them to cause relative inflation they must increase in magnitude or effectiveness over time. Only to the extent that health inflation is caused by numbers 3 to 6 is it a "problem" requiring or responsive to government action.

Cures

There are three broad types of responses to the problem so diagnosed. One is to improve the market, that is, to make the market for medical care resemble efficient markets in other sectors where the interplay of people seeking private gain and paying out-of-pocket for their goods and services disciplines both the consumer and the provider. Such a strategy includes providing patients with more information about the market and likewise giving them greater financial stakes in acting on that information. Typically such remedies include the suggestion of patient financial participation through substantial co-insurance and deductibles. This type of remedy is exemplified by Martin Feldstein's major risk insurance proposal, whereby families would pay up to 10 percent of their income for medical care and anything above that would be paid for by the federal government in a catastrophic health insurance plan (Feldstein, 1971). The characteristic feature of that program is a deductible high in relation to average expenditure but low in relation to people's normal conception of what constitutes a financial catastrophe. The effect of doing so would mean that most people would be paying out-of-pocket for most medical care, but there would be deep coverage against those small number of instances where medical care disaster hits. Hence, according to Feldstein, the true purpose of insurance would be served: namely to protect people against the unbudgetable, unforeseen, and unpreventable disaster. One author estimates that each year catastrophic health expenses of $5,000 or more affect about 1.6 million Americans—or 0.8 percent of the population (Meyer, 1975). Other critics have argued for HMO expansion as part of the market improvement strategy (Newhouse, 1976).

A second answer to this set of problems is to compensate for the poor market structure which we have identified with public utility-type regulation (Sattler, 1975; Lewin, 1974; Lewin, Somers, and Somers, 1975). The standard site for such regulation is the states; an example of such regulation is electrical utilities. The standard subjects of such regulation are the number of health care facilities and the price they charge for their services. Many states are establishing commissions that deal with facility supply (certificate of need) and separate commissions that deal with pricing (primarily for hospitals). So-called rate commissions in Massachusetts, Maryland, Connecticut, and other states have been set up to regulate hospital prices (Sattler, 1975).

The third response is to replace the economic market with a political market by effectively nationalizing the industry. In this case there is a constraining bilateral relationship between buyers and providers: the buyer is the government and the providers are the industry's constituent parts. The government bargains with the providers on price, supply, and quality; and substitutes its concerns for the quality of the services and the level of expenditures for those of diffuse and decentralized consumers who are not well organized to influence health policy decisions. In effect, the government is dealing with the monopoly power of the providers by creating a monopsony for the consumers. The Kennedy-Corman bill (S3, HR 21) is an example of such an approach. It provides that the federal government pay for almost all medical care services and regulate the prices of those services by regional health boards in market areas throughout the country.

Theodore Marmor, Donald Wittman, and Thomas Heagy

The Response of Government

Solutions to medical care inflation have been supplied by economists for years, yet the government has not been "buying" their advice. In fact, past actions by the government, such as tax subsidies for medical insurance, have contributed to medical inflation. Let us see why this is so and why there is little reason to expect that the government will act boldly to reduce medical inflation (relative price or expenditure growth) in the future. The object of our analysis is to understand the political "market" in which decisions on controlling medical inflation are made.

The Theory of Imbalanced Political Interests: Concentrated versus Diffuse Benefits and Costs

The political "market" refers to institutional arrangements—the relationships among organized pressure groups, voters, authoritative governmental agencies, and affected citizens—that determine what governments do. As Stigler (1971) states in connection with governmental *regulation*, the theory of public policy ought to explain "who will receive the benefits and burdens of governmental [action]." Some characteristic features of the American political process will be discussed, and among the most important is the natural imbalance between the interests of mass publics and those of health care providers on issues like inflation.

By imbalanced political markets we mean a contrast to another model of the political system—the egalitarian theory of one man-one vote—implying equal power by all participants. There are many theories of imbalanced political markets. We would like to stress one—the notion of concentrated versus diffuse interests. By concentrated interests, we mean that the effects of the policy (whether subsidy or tax, compulsion or prohibition) are significant to the party. By diffuse interests we mean unimportant benefits or costs to individuals whatever the aggregate level of those costs or benefits. A $1.00 per capita tax is an illustration of a diffuse cost of substantial aggregate magnitude in the United States as a whole.

The incentives to press claims for concentrated interests are much greater than those for diffuse ones. The prospect of having one's well-being greatly affected creates substantial incentives to act to protect one's interest. An interest marginal to one's well-being—even though large when aggregated over the class of affected parties—provides weak incentives to act. This distribution of incentives results in a systematic imbalance of the probabilities of interest representation. It is not the case that the theory of imbalance in the political market explains the outcomes of political struggles by itself. For the outcomes are a product not simply of the representation of interests, but also of other political resources that fuel the representation of those interests. But the structure of interests does largely determine which groups play a role in the channels of policy action and whose preferences are likely to count most in that process (Allison, 1971; 1973). The theory of imbalanced interests holds that concentrated groups, other things being equal, will be more effective in the political process than diffuse ones (Stigler, 1971; Posner, 1974).

It is useful to compare the concentrated-diffuse market theory with other concepts of imbalanced political markets. One stresses that some voters are more informed than others about the political process. Clearly, if some voters are totally uninformed, their interests will be neglected by vote-maximizing candidates for political office (Wittman, 1975). Thus the political market is imbalanced toward the more informed voter.

Groups also differ in terms of wealth. It is obvious that, other things being equal, the rich can exert greater influence per capita on election results than the poor through donations; and similarly influence political decisions in between elections.

If a group has nonpolitical reasons for being well organized (for example, labor unions), it will have greater political capability, through simple economies of multiple functions, than a group whose sole purpose is political activity. The fixed organizational overhead is already paid in the former case; in the latter a larger fraction of the organization's resources go to organizational maintenance.

Since the results of most political activity constitute a collective good, the differential ability of various groups in overcoming the collective good problems of political activity creates an unbalanced power differential.

These theories are, it should be noted, partially overlapping and an exogenous variable in one may be endogenous in another. For example, having more concentrated benefits and costs gives members of a group greater incentives to be better informed.

In addition, there is usually a substantial correlation among the characteristics that lead to greater political influence. For example, doctors are better informed (on health issues), wealthier, better organized, and have more concentrated interests than do patients. This obviously makes it difficult to pinpoint the specific effect of their concentrated interests on public policy as opposed to the effect of the other characteristics. This is why the case of welfare mothers is enlightening. On the basis of every criterion of political power except concentrated interest, one would expect them to have virtually no success in the policy arena. The extent to which they have been successful in increasing benefits in the postwar period might be explained by the theory of concentrated interests.

Imbalanced Interests and Inflation

What is the connection between the theory of imbalanced political interests and the response to the problem of relative inflation generally? The theory predicts that excessive relative inflation in any sector will generate modest, usually ineffective, governmental policy responses to the problems. Consider, for example, the ways in which relative price inflation in the construction and medical care industries has worked out in the past half decade. Relative inflation has been a serious problem in both sectors—indeed, has produced double-digit inflation in the early 1970s—and constitutes a considerable problem in the aggregate, which makes up a very large component of the GNP. Substantial relative inflation imposes large opportunity costs on both national and individual expenditures.

The problem is that such inflation is an example of a public "bad," the solution of which mobilizes the resistance of concentrated interests in the affected industry. Governmental action to control relative inflation in construction costs would have a smaller percentage effect of the total expenses of the average household than on workers' income in construction unions. Medical care inflation likewise would affect providers (hospitals, nursing homes, physicians, nurses) much more than it would patients.

Application to Medical Care Inflation

Who are the people who will have the most say on health care? The answer is relatively clear-cut. Doctors, hospital administrators, unions, and insurance companies will have a relatively greater voice in the political process than their mere numbers would indicate; less represented than their numbers would indicate will be taxpayers in general and patients in particular. The reason is quite simple. The providers are very knowledgeable and concerned about health care policy since it is so important to their lives. On the other side, the expected benefits or costs of a health care policy are relatively unimportant to the consumer (except for the chronically ill). His interests are diffuse, being not only health, but also food, clothing, shelter, education, and recreation as well as employment. It does not pay the consumer to take strong action. This is not to say that consumers have no effect; they clearly do, but it must be emphasized that their voice is systematically underrepresented in the political process.

The theory suggests that political leaders have little incentive to follow politically controversial economic advice on how to combat relative inflation in the medical care market. If relative inflation in medical care is everybody's problem—that is, if the burdens are widely distributed among millions of health care purchasers—the benefits of improving that situation generally do not provide compelling political incentives to act. A 10 percent decrease in health expenditures—an average of reduction from $400 per capita per year to $360 per year—would reduce the total health bill of the United States by a striking $10 billion. But, while society would save that much, the efforts to produce such a reduction would mobilize the powerful countervailing efforts of providers. A 10 percent decrease in one's average health bill is of marginal concern to citizens, yet medical care pricing policy preoccupies providers. As a result, governments have greater pressure upon them to resist anti-inflationary policy than to act on it.

The main exception is that governments in their buying capacity have a substantial interest in reducing their own program costs. The various governmental departments act as if the total government expenditures are relatively inelastic, and therefore compete with each other and try to undermine excessive expenditure increases by other departments. There is, therefore, an internal government market which partially serves to put a brake on programmatic expenditure increases. This means that the form of financing is very important. For example, the government will not be internally as concerned about increases in costs if the revenues are derived from payroll deductions as it would be if the revenues came out of general revenues. Some support can be seen in the fact that the providers strongly prefer payroll deductions to financing from general revenue.

From another perspective, the more any particular level of government pays for medical care, the more it will be concerned about price and expenditure increases. Again, there is some evidence to support the theory. Great Britain, with a centralized public finance payment structure, has a significantly lower inflation rate and level of expenditure than the United States, Canada, and Sweden, which vary in their private versus public support mix (with Sweden being close to 100 percent government-supported), but all being financed at various levels (Anderson, 1972; Fraser, 1974; Marmor et al., 1975). Table 1 presents longitudinal data from several western industrial nations in terms of the changing proportion of resources spent on health care.

Medicare and Medicaid offer an example of the complex interplay of the forces we have been discussing. During the period 1966–1970 total government expenditures for both Medicare and Medicaid increased very rapidly; expanding beneficiary roles, increased utilization, and general medical inflation all contributed (Andersen et al., 1973; Anderson, 1972). By the 1970s, expenditures had grown enough that the Nixon Administration made serious efforts to hold down these program costs. Except for the brief period of price controls (Russell, 1976), which had no permanent

TABLE 1   Total Expenditures for Health Services
as a Percentage of the Gross National Product,
Seven Countries, Selected Periods,
1961–1969

	WHO Estimates [a]		SSA Estimates [b]		Average Annual Rate of Increase in Health Expenditures [c]	
Country	Year	Percentage of GNP	Year	Percentage of GNP	Year	Rate of Change (percentage)
Canada	1961	6.0	1969	7.3	1961–69	13.2
United States	1961–62	5.8	1969	6.8	1962–69	10.1
Sweden	1962	5.4	1969	6.7	1962–69	14.0
Netherlands	1963	4.8	1969	5.9	1963–69	16.1
Federal Republic of Germany	1961	4.5	1969	5.7	1961–69	10.3
France	1963	4.4	1969	5.7	1963–69	14.9
United Kingdom	1961–62	4.2	1969	4.8	1962–69	9.5

[a] Brian Abel-Smith, An International Study of Health Expenditure, WHO Public Paper No. 32 (Geneva: 1967).
[b] Joseph G. Simanis, "Medical Care Expenditures in Seven Countries," Social Security Bulletin (March 1973), p. 39.
[c] Office of Health Economics, London, "International Health Expenditure 11," Information Sheet No. 22 (May 1973), Table 2.
Source: The Report of the Health Planning Task Force prepared under the auspices of the Research and Analysis Division of the Ontario Ministry of Health.

effect, these efforts were aimed at reducing benefits in the Medicare and Medicaid programs rather than trying to deal with the general problem of medical inflation (Stevens and Stevens, 1974). The net result was to stop (but not reverse) the growth in Medicare payments per beneficiary; and to reverse the growth of Medicaid payments per beneficiary (both in terms of constant dollars). During the same period (the 1970s) the number of beneficiaries continued to rise (but at a slower rate) so that total expenditures (in constant dollars) continued to rise in both programs, but at much slower rates (see Davis, 1976, for a more detailed discussion in this volume).

The theory of concentrated costs and benefits appears to succeed in predicting the broad outline of past governmental responses to medical inflation and the impact on Medicare/Medicaid. It has more difficulty in predicting which of the two programs would be more affected by concern over its program costs. Since payment for Medicaid is more decentralized (by federal and state governments and including some cost-sharing by beneficiaries), we would expect less pressure to reduce its expenditures than Medicare's. On the other hand, since Medicare is financed by a payroll tax, we would expect the opposite. We would expect these two factors at least partially to offset each other so that the theory cannot make a prediction. It may be that the factor that tipped the scales against Medicaid has nothing to do with concentrated costs and benefits, but rather the greater political attractiveness of the old compared to the poor (Stevens and Stevens, 1974).

How then can we apply this theoretical approach to the politics of inflation control in medical care to the three classes of solutions cited earlier? The market improvement strategy discussed earlier is a classic example of a general anti-inflationary stance unlikely to be acted upon. Were the economic market to be improved and the relative rate of inflation reduced, the beneficiaries would be the diffuse public paying lower insurance premiums and lower medical prices than otherwise. But the resisters of such policy—resistant both to its enactent and to its successful implementation—are those very providers whose concentrated interests would be mobilized. The point about the market improvement proposals is not that they are all conceptually *ineffective*, but that the greater their likely effectiveness, if enacted, the greater the opposition of the concentrated interests and, therefore, the more *politically* unlikely their implementation.

The government—the set of institutions which would have to generate market improvements—would benefit from an anti-inflationary policy for medical care to the extent it pays now for medical care services. But note that while the federal government pays for approximately one-quarter of total medical care expenditures (Social Security Administration, 1974), a successful anti-inflationary policy through market improvement would impose on the federal government 100 percent of the political costs of such changes. This leads to the prediction that the greater the share of costs a single level of government has in the medical care market, the greater its potential interest in a general anti-inflationary strategy for medical care.

For regulation of the public utility type, the issue is the effectiveness of such policies, not the political feasibility of enactment. The demand for state regulation is partly a gesture toward controlling relative medical care inflation and partly an expression of the belief that direct controls of supply and price can, through state commissions, actually moderate inflation.

To the extent supply restrictions are demanded—as illustrated by certificate-of-need legislation—two points are relevant. First, supply restrictions will undoubtedly apply only to facility expansion and not to current hospital bed supply. This is protective legislation for present hospitals even if it can be shown that supply restraints affect total expenditure growth. Second, supply constraints may even exacerbate relative price inflation.

Those advocates of rate review—medical care price setting— typically argue that in the United States the rate-setting function should be separated from the governmental payment for medical care services in programs like Medicare and Medicaid. This separation of the payer from price regulator is likely, on reasonable assumptions, to lead to a weak price-setting mechanism. Elementary economic theory would hold that the part of the government with the greatest interest in relative prices is the department whose responsibility it is to pay for medical care services. Thus, the problem with state regulation of medical care inflation is ineffectiveness, not the difficulty of enacting regulation in the first place. Indeed, we already have evidence that this strategy is being widely attempted (Lewin, 1974).

The third strategy—restraining inflation by centralizing expenditures via national health insurance—presents a mixed picture. On the one hand, concentration of governmental responsibility for health expenditures is, on the basis of our theory, likely to promote serious interest by the government in anti-inflationary policy. On the other hand, the concentrated provider interests will be (and are) mobilized to resist precisely this feature of proposed national health insurance legislation. Again there is evidence to support our theory: most current providers resist the notion that health should be financed out of a single budget, whatever their views on the particular form of national health insurance. They point to Great Britain as a "starved" medical care system, where something in excess of 5 percent of GNP is expended on health care despite the fact that it is all publicly funded (Friedman, 1975). In contrast, health care expenditures in Sweden, Canada, and the United States are closer to 8 percent of GNP, despite the fact that the sources of financing for such expenditures range in the three countries from totally public (although not all at one level of government) to substantially private (Anderson, 1972; Fraser, 1974; Marmor et al., 1975). Concentrated or diffuse budgeting for health appears to be a significant issue raised by the Kennedy-Corman strategy.

To summarize, the greater the likely effectiveness of an anti-inflation policy, the less likely is its enactment. The market improvement strategy has some promise of effectiveness, but little likelihood. Public regulation at the state level has political appeal, but much lower probability of effectiveness. Controlling inflation through a single national health insurance program has some chance of effective constraint, but for that reason is likely to mobilize effective opposition.

The greatest chance of controlling relative medical inflation would appear to be through the back door of a national health insurance plan that is not necessarily passed for the purpose of controlling medical inflation and does not have a strong inflation control mechanism built into it; but which increases the effective pressure for controlling medical inflation in the future by increasing the portion of medical expenditures that flows through the federal budget.

In the specific area of controlling relative expenditure growth (as opposed to price inflation) in the hospital sector, supply control has considerable appeal as being both effective and politically viable specifically because its costs fall primarily on the prospective newcomers to the industry whose opposition to supply control is outweighed by the support of established hospitals that want to curtail competition.

Let us consider now how one might regard the suggestions for controlling inflation brought forward at the September 1974 DHEW Pre-Summit Conference on the problem.

The Conference on Inflation: Illustrations

Clearly, it is in the interest of most provider groups for there to be an ever-increasing demand for health and thereby ever-present inflationary pressures. This can be starkly illustrated by the recommendations of the 1974 Conference on Inflation in Health (U.S. DHEW, 1974). The recommendations to curb inflation were almost without exception inflationary and to the benefit of the provider groups. Following is a partial listing of the recommendations for curbing inflation, with our comments in parentheses.

1. Increase the federal budget for health service programs. (This action will increase the relative expenditures for health and will increase the inflationary pressures in the health care industry. While there may be, depending on the program, some substitution from the private sector to the public, thereby hurting some health care firms, increased federal activity will for the most part benefit health care providers.)

2. Contain operating costs to as close to parity with increases in the Consumer Price Index as possible. (This is the goal of anti-inflationary policy, but no method of implementing it is contained in this section.)

3. Restructure reimbursement. For example, reimbursement should be on a total budget rather than a line-item basis. This policy has been tried in some Canadian provinces with limited success (Andreopoulos, 1974).

4. Shift emphasis to ambulatory and preventive care. (While there may be some shift from the more expensive hospital care, the main effect is to bring more health care onto the "insurance gravy train." A good example—dental care—is given by Lave, 1976. The relative expenditure growth in health care is likely to be exacerbated and will put even greater upward pressures on medical prices. This policy may be desirable, but it will not reduce inflation.)

5. Initiate consumer education activities directed toward increasing consumer knowledge regarding what are realistic patient exceptions from the health care system. (Inflationary and expenditure impact is insignificant one way or another, but it does create some jobs for health care researchers.)

6. Provide consumers with information on fees and prices. (This recommendation will probably result in a one-time reduction in prices of small magnitude. It should be noted that the providers

showed considerable skepticism regarding this approach and suggested that it was, in fact, inflationary.)

7. Change the statutory definition of health maintenance organizations in order to allow for more flexibility in assembling benefit packages tailored to the needs and financial resources of particular population groups. (While this move may be desirable, it is not clear what effect it will have on health care inflation. Essentially this law allows HMOs to use optimal discrimination in pricing—a monopoly ploy to increase revenues and profits.)

8. The quality of health care cannot be allowed to become a casualty of zealous efforts to contain costs in the health sector. (Unfortunately, this is the crux of the matter, that increases in quality—more comfortable beds, better trained nurses, equipment which only brings very marginal increases in success rates—have been responsible for a substantial part of the increases in hospital care costs. *Not* to put a lid on quality improvement is *not* to put a lid on relative expenditure growth. On the assumption that hospital costs have risen because of increases in both quality and quantity demanded, then the desire to reduce relative expenditure increases without having any effects on quality improvement is a desire not to stop relative expenditure growth.)

9. Monitor the impact of and contribution to inflation in the health care sector. (This is a chance for the self-interested researcher to get in on the "anti-inflation gravy train." The main effect will be to increase trivially the relative amount of expenditures devoted to health care.)

10. Encourage comprehensive health planning coupled with regulatory power to reduce duplication of facilities via the innovative use of certificate-of-need and rate-setting mechanisms. (This is essentially the hospital supply proposal we have already discussed.)

11. Increase supply of primary care providers and, in particular, third-party reimbursement for the services of nonphysician providers should be encouraged. (The first part of the suggestion will probably work in the intended direction.)

12. Reconsider wage and price controls. (It was noted that a wide array of provider groups dissented from this view. For a discussion of how the controls worked, see Ginsburg, 1976.)

Conclusion

Economic theory suggests that the economic market will systematically underproduce public goods. This conclusion is often
used as a justification for governmental intervention. But the implication of this paper is that moving from the economic marketplace
to the political marketplace does not necessarily solve problems. In
the absence of some concentrated interest, the political market is
unlikely to adopt a policy simply because it constitutes a public
good (Alford, 1974). The political market (like the economic one)
will systematically underproduce public goods (and overproduce
public bads). The political process is unlikely to right the distributive wrongs of the economic marketplace when a similar set of
actors dominates both. The history of medical inflation and governmental response (or lack of response) to it is an illustration of this
fundamental problem.

The application of this theory to national health insurance
suggests sober estimates about the government's capacity to restrain
the nation's health care expenditures, which are increasing at the rate
of more than $10 billion a year. The experience of Canada and
Sweden suggests that government financing on a large scale alone
does not reverse the upward spiral in prices and expenditures.
Certainly this has been the case when the government uses an
insurance mechanism in which financing is diffusely shared among
patients and different units of government. There is evidence that
where financing is concentrated and service providers are directly
budgeted (rather than reimbursed retrospectively by insurance),
expenditures and the rate of medical inflation are lower. This has
been the case in Great Britain, with its National Health Service. In
the last fifteen years England has spent a third less of its resources on
medical care and experienced roughly a third the rate of inflation of
the other countries (Canada, Sweden, the United States). While no
one expects the United States to legislate a national health service,
the experience of Great Britain has important implications for the
degree of financing concentration desirable in a future national
health insurance program.

The Federal Government as Venture Capitalist: How Does It Fare?

JOHN K. IGLEHART

Kaiser Foundation Health Plan, Inc.,
Washington, D.C.

I N THE ANNALS OF FEDERAL PROGRAM DEVELOP-
ment, the Office of Health Maintenance Organizations (OHMO)
is a unique enterprise. The office is charged with the specific
assignment of creating new private businesses that ultimately must
succeed or fail by their own capitalistic devices. The very notion
that government should so boldly challenge private medicine says a
great deal about its dissatisfaction with the status quo, but perhaps of
more importance now is a report on how this federal experiment in
venture capitalism is faring.

First of all, one must recognize the formidable obstacles that loom
before a government agency that strives to crack a private market.
These obstacles stem from the complex nature of government itself,
its role as a redistribution agent, and its political inclination to be all
things to all people (or at least as many as can be accommodated at any
one time). Congress posed additional obstacles by its complicated
design of the Health Maintenance Organization Act of 1973.

The HMO concept emerged as a government initiative during the
Republican administration of Richard M. Nixon. The concept proved
politically and ideologically attractive to Nixon's conservative administration because of its reliance upon financial incentives rather than
regulation to contain spiraling health-care costs, thus reducing gov-

Milbank Memorial Fund Quarterly/*Health and Society*, Vol. 58, No. 4, 1980
© 1980 Milbank Memorial Fund and Massachusetts Institute of Technology
0160/1997/5804/0656-12 $01.00/0

ernment's role. But the HMO act, as Birnbaum (1980) points out, became ensnared in inflexible language, delayed rule-making, and bureaucratic wrangling, thus complicating OHMO's role as administrator. Organizationally, OHMO is part of the Public Health Service and currently falls under the Office of the Assistant Secretary for Health, Department of Health and Human Services (HHS).

The challenge of creating new businesses is a tall order for any organization. For an agency like HHS, it was a totally foreign undertaking. Three broad social purposes dominate the works of the department: administering income transfer payments to eligible individuals (aid to families with dependent children and Social Security, for example), financing medical care for eligible elderly and poor people (Medicare and Medicaid), and awarding grants to nonprofit organizations that are engaged in activities deemed worthy of public support (medical schools, for example) but cannot conceivably generate enough revenue on their own to become self-sustaining. Thus the orientation and skills of most HHS employees do not lend themselves readily to venture capitalism.

Karen Davis, deputy assistant secretary for health planning and evaluation, and Howard R. Veit, director of OHMO, characterized OHMO's mandate in a June 11, 1980, memorandum to Dr. Julius B. Richmond, assistant HHS secretary for health and U.S. surgeon general:

> As we considered HMO legislative issues and general program direction, we continually encountered the conflict between the social goals the HMO program was endowed with at its inception and the difficult and complicated task of creating viable, self-sufficient businesses. This conflict is difficult, but not always impossible, to reconcile. In general, OHMO and OHPE [Office of Health Planning and Evaluation] have recommended protecting the social responsibility features of the HMO statutes. You should be aware, however, that the "pro-competition" proponents in OMB [Office of Management and Budget] and the Congress will attempt to weaken these aspects.

Venture capitalism is a form of private investment in which government usually plays no central role except, in select instances, one of oversight through the Securities and Exchange Commission. Venture capitalism involves individuals or organizations that invest their money in high-risk development opportunities, hoping for a high return on equity. OHMO's development activities characterize some, but not all, features of venture capitalism. OHMO invests public dollars in high-risk situations with a hope that the return for society will be the creation of private organizations that are capable of delivering quality health care at a reasonable price.

A fundamental difference between the federal funding of HMO development and of other HHS health service projects is the matter of self-sufficiency. From the outset, HMOs are expected to work toward the day when they do not depend on federal dollars to operate, except for those that pay for services rendered through Medicare and Medicaid. Virtually all other health service projects funded by HHS are expected to depend entirely on the federal dollar for survival. When federal support is removed, the projects are abandoned, except in those instances when state or local governments are willing to assume the costs.

The task of creating new HMOs has taxed the capabilities of OHMO's small staff. Initially, OHMO felt most comfortable awarding grants to HMO project applicants, but staff lacked the expertise to offer the kind of financial planning and marketing advice so critical to the success of a new prepaid group practice. But there has been progress on this front. OHMO staff is in a better position today to offer technical assistance and also it is using industry experts in financial matters to help new plans. Veit recognizes that the future of the HMO industry hinges in good part on its ability to attract capable managers to the field. Also, the General Accounting Office (GAO), the monitoring arm of Congress, has worked closely with OHMO to increase the management skills of the program and its grantees.

OHMO has evolved in its six years of operation—and countless reorganizations—from essentially a grant-making office to an office that has come to recognize, if not yet totally implement, its complex mandate. In talking with me on March 23, 1980, Veit said:

> OHMO is much more analytical now than before, much tougher in its review of grant applications. But it's difficult in our program to separate the bad risks. It's a painful process to get staff to look with discernment at potential grantees. But we strive to be unrelenting on that score because funding bad grantees today only leads to failures tomorrow.

The difficulties of creating a private business usually are a revelation to HMO grantees as well. Many of the grantees represent consumer-based organizations that do not have staffs with the necessary business background to successfully launch a new enterprise. One HMO official described this dilemma in a personal interview April 14, 1980, but did not want to be identified; Veit himself, however, also subscribes to these views:

> We've found that the health-care field is not a field that has attracted a lot of people with corporate skills. HMOs are businesses that generate millions in income and expenses. You can't have a nice guy who is a social worker running that kind of an organization. Most of our grant applications derive from community groups that are striving to change the delivery system a little. OHMO has tried to adjust to this problem by becoming more aggressive itself in seeking out organizations that have some of the necessary skills to create HMOs.

OHMO's mandate is further complicated by the conflicting nature of its several roles. Besides serving as a venture capitalist, OHMO also is charged by law with promoting the HMO concept in the hope of stimulating development through private capital and with regulating federally qualified HMOs. Thus, the OHMO must serve as the prime HMO booster and the major overseer of HMO performance—conflicting assignments that cause no end to strife within the program. A federally qualified plan is an HMO that abides by operational requirements set out in the HMO act, including the offering of a comprehensive package of benefits. In return, the act provides access to the market through a requirement that all employers of 25 or more individuals must offer their employees an opportunity to enroll in a qualified HMO if one is available in the area. HMOs that accept federal funds and become operational must seek federal qualification.

Veit's directorship also is hindered by other realities of the bureaucratic life. Almost one-third of OHMO's full-time employees—62 of 177—work in the ten regional offices of HHS. These staff members, however, report to the respective regional health directors, who, in turn, are responsible to the assistant secretary for health, not to Veit. OHMO, like most government programs, also operates under the vagaries of a political system that is constantly reordering its priorities

—not the kind of environment needed to bolster health maintenance organizations in an uncertain market. Veit (1980) referred to this problem in a speech:

> The impact of the federal program could have been greater if the government's commitment to HMO growth had remained consistently higher during the 1970s. In 1975, there were ample funds appropriated by Congress to start new HMOs. In 1976 and 1977, scarce dollars for new programs together with poor administration by HEW [now HHS] impeded growth. In late 1977, the department began to reorganize the federal program. This, plus increased congressional appropriations in 1978, 1979, and now in 1980, has allowed us to bring many more new HMOs into development.

The foregoing list of obstacles that stand before OHMO is by no means an apology for its performance. Any individual who spends time observing or participating in the life of a government program soon recognizes that things never run as smoothly as one would prefer, the staff is never as capable as it could be, and funds never seem to go far enough. OHMO is certainly no exception to this rule. The marvel, perhaps, is that OHMO has accomplished anything as a tiny outpost favoring marketplace solutions in a department that tilts to regulation.

Performance

One measure of OHMO's performance is the growth of new prepaid health plans in the 1970s, though a cautionary note seems appropriate. Most plans started with federal funds are small. And though they serve as symbols of one direction of reform favored by government—prepaid group and individual practices—their impact on the system thus far has not been dramatic. Zealous rhetorical overkill in the early days of the program, even while Congress was still debating the legislation that led to the 1973 HMO act, far surpassed what could realistically be expected to occur in the relatively short time that has passed since then. The overwhelming number of members enrolled in HMOs today belong to plans started long before the federal government began its romance with prepaid group practice.

Since 1970, the number of HMOs has increased from fewer than 30 to 230. This includes federally qualified plans and plans that have not sought qualification. Enrollment nationally in prepaid health plans, or HMOs as they have been called since the federal government got in the act, has increased from 2.9 million to almost 9 million, according to OHMO. Since 1974, the federal government has awarded grants of $130 million and committed $175 million in loans. Of the 230 HMOs that now are providing care, 113 are federally qualified, a regulatory stamp of approval affixed by OHMO that was defined earlier. Of the 113 qualified HMOs, 80 have received federal grant and/or loan assistance. Veit (1980) notes that federally assisted HMOs are "for the most part, still small and still striving toward self-sufficiency. Although the federal program has already had a considerable impact on the growth of the field, 85 per cent of all members are in HMOs that have developed privately. The federal government has, however, put in place a number of new programs that represent substantial capacity for future growth."

OHMO, not surprisingly, has encountered failure, too. Any time government intervenes in a private market, it assumes risks that private investors are generally thought to be unwilling to take. OHMO has revoked the qualification of 7 plans,[1] leaving 113 so designated.[2] Thus, the current failure rate is 6.0 percent. The overwhelming cause of failure was inadequate plan management, according to OHMO, but lack of capital and poor location also were factors.

Another relevant measure of OHMO's performance is the failure rate on loans advanced to qualified HMOs to subsidize their operations until they become self-sustaining (Department of Health, Education, and Welfare, 1979). As of January 1, 1980, the Department of Health, Education, and Welfare (HEW) had extended $157 million in

---

[1] Sound Health Association, Takoma, Washington; Central Essex HMO, Orange County, New Jersey; Health Alliance of Northern California, Los Gatos, California; ChoiceCare Health Services Inc., Fort Collins, Colorado; Gem Health Association, Boise, Idaho; Group Health Plan of New Jersey, Hudson County, New Jersey; and HMO Concepts, Anaheim, California. After they failed as separate entities, Sound Health Association was taken over by Group Health of Puget Sound and Group Health Plan of New Jersey by Health Insurance Plan of Greater New York.

[2] Regarding nonqualified plans, an informal list prepared by OHMO's division of development estimates that 60 plans have failed since records were first kept in 1970. Judith M. Mears, a lawyer for the Kaiser Foundation Health Plan who conducted a survey on failures, concluded, on the basis of a 1979 census, that a total of 174 nonqualified plans existed between 1970 and 1979. Thus, she estimated a failure rate of 34 percent for nonqualified HMOs in the 1970s.

loans and loan guarantees to qualified plans. Of that total, $6.9 million remains outstanding from the qualified HMOs that ceased operations in 1979. That amounts to a 4.4 percent loan default rate for qualified HMOs in 1979.[3]

While Mears found it possible to calculate a fairly accurate rate of both federally qualified and nonqualified HMOs, she concluded that the data necessary to compute a failure rate for small businesses or service businesses are not being collected by any private or governmental entity. The rate that business people and personnel in federal agencies attribute to the Small Business Administration (SBA) is that one of every two small businesses goes out of business within the first two years of operation, but the SBA does not use this statistic in any of its official material.

One question Congress undoubtedly will ponder in early 1981 when it considers extension of the Health Maintenance Organization Act is how to judge a failure. Can the termination of an operational HMO be judged a total failure, given the knowledge that it is a risky venture? Were there valuable lessons learned that justify the public investment? Should the federal government reduce its potential for loss by investing only in HMOs that look like sure winners?[4]

One thing OHMO has learned through the failures is that the demise of an HMO is accorded far more publicity than is the bankruptcy of most small businesses. In a story from Fort Collins, Col-

---

[3] Mears, in her survey, found that a loan default rate of 4.4 percent falls about in the middle of a list of default rates for selected federal loan programs: farm ownership, 0.1 percent; rural housing, 0.2 percent; farm operating loans, 1.0 percent; farm emergency loans, 1.0 percent; Hill-Burton loans, 1.7 percent; FHA hospital loans, 1.7 percent; health professions student loans, 2.0 percent; FHA Title II (group practice facilities and physicians' offices), 3.5 percent; Small Business Administration loans, 3.8 percent; all HUD loans, 5.4 percent; nursing student loans, 5.4 percent; economic development loans, 7.1 percent; Federal Housing Administration nursing home loans, 9.6 percent; guaranteed student loans, 11.5 percent; direct student loans, 17.4 percent; Federal Housing Administration Section 235 program loans, 19.5 percent.

[4] OHMO's current development strategy calls for placing first priority on cities where health care costs are considered above the national average. OHMO places in this category the following areas: Boston-Lawrence-Haverhill-Lowell, Massachusetts; New York City and environs; Buffalo, New York; Newark, New Jersey; Philadelphia and Pittsburgh, Pennsylvania; Washington, D.C.; Baltimore, Maryland; Atlanta, Georgia; Miami, Tampa, St. Petersburg, Florida; Chicago, Illinois; Detroit, Michigan; Cleveland, Ohio; Milwaukee, Wisconsin; Houston and Dallas, Texas; St. Louis, Missouri; and Denver, Colorado.

orado, headlined "Health Maintenance Organization Collapses as Its Doctors Drop Out," the *New York Times* reported on January 2, 1980:

> Insured medical care for 30,000 people in northeastern Colorado is ending today because almost all the area doctors abandoned the local health maintenance organization. The doctors' decision to withdraw from ChoiceCare Health Services, Inc., left subscribers scrambling for coverage, federal officials fuming and creditors holding a debt of more than $1 million.

In Veit's view, the program has not been operating long enough to accurately calculate what its failure rate ultimately will be:

> The ultimate success of the program depends on the number of [HMO] programs that are both financially viable and deliver high-quality care. Determining success rates requires many years given the long development period for an HMO. Our experience shows that it takes three or four years to become operational, and an additional four to five years to reach the break-even point. Thus, it takes seven to nine years of development before we can talk definitively about success. (Veit, 1980)

On a more pessimistic note, Veit told a newspaper interviewer, "It's a miracle that more haven't failed. Like any business, an HMO that isn't run effectively will fail. In the coming years, we anticipate 5–10 failures a year" (*American Medical News,* 1980).

One of the more interesting results of federal HMO development is the evolution of a particular model—the individual practice association, or IPA as it is known in industry parlance. When Congress designed the HMO act, it lumped under the HMO definition a form of practice in which member doctors remain in their individual offices but are compensated on a prepaid basis. IPAs are formed by solo fee-for-service practitioners as a defensive measure, in fear of the economic consequences of the creation of a prepaid group practice in their area. IPAs generally are closely affiliated with the local medical society. Private physicians have taken advantage of the availability of federal funds to create IPAs. Strumpf (1980) found that the growth of IPAs from fewer than 5 before enactment of the HMO law to 89 today stemmed largely from federal funds, in the case of 42 plans, and from support by the Blue Cross and Blue Shield Association, in 15 other instances. He said:

When development is viewed from this competitive perspective, we find that 55 currently operational IPAs developed after a PGP [prepaid group practice] was established [in the same service community].[5]

Fee-for-service physician response to the federal HMO initiative has led to the development of more new plans than has the response from the business community, despite the increasing expressions of concern by businessmen about the rising cost of medical care (Demkovich, 1980). Those corporations that have become involved in the HMO movement have done so not by sponsoring their own HMOs but rather by encouraging their employees to enroll in already operating plans.

InterStudy (1979) made this point in reporting to the Health Care Financing Administration its progress under a grant for "Stimulation of Alternative Health Care Delivery System Development": "One of the original intents of the project, actual corporate development of an ADS [alternative delivery system], was found to be an impractical alternative for most firms."

The National Association of Employers on Health Maintenance Organizations (Employee Benefit Plan Review, 1979) reported a similar conclusion in its Survey of National Corporations:

There appears to be little interest among respondents to develop their own HMOs—even though this group would have access to the necessary capital—and of the survey respondents only 4.6 percent have developed a company HMO, and 93.4 percent indicated no interest in developing one.

The Future

Congress enacted legislation in 1973 that sought to promote HMOs, but the act was so laden with costly requirements that new organizations developed under it found competing against traditional insurers

---

[5] IPAs require physicians conditioned to fee-for-service patterns to change their practice modes in order to live within the fixed budget that prepayment dictates. The Physicians Health Plan of Minnesota, an IPA organized by the Hennepin County Medical Society, published a fascinating account entitled, "A Case Study of Utilization Controls in an IPA," which details how one organization coped with the challenge. The study was prepared for OHMO under Contract No. 342804.

almost an impossible task. In two subsequent sets of amendments approved in 1976 and 1978, Congress removed some of these requirements and relaxed others in the hope of stimulating more HMO development. New provisions also were added, reflecting the critical need to train HMO managers and bolster OHMO's capacity to provide technical assistance to developing plans.

These amendments included minor changes in the mandated benefit package, relaxation of the open-enrollment requirement, higher ceilings for grant awards, extension of the loan eligibility period, establishment of an HMO management training program and a technical assistance authority. Other amendments included a new requirement for employers to arrange for HMO payroll deductions and authority for HMOs to seek payment from workmen's compensation and other insurance for enrolled members who had double coverage.

The HMO act expires September 30, 1981, and the administration now is preparing its recommendations for extension of the law. The Carter administration has been resolute in its commitment to HMO development and there is no reason to believe that the president will change course on this question, despite a view held by his Office of Management and Budget that the HMO concept has demonstrated its effectiveness and now it is time for the private sector to assume responsibility for further plan development.

The major legislative issues involved in the extension are similar to the kinds of questions debated in 1976 and 1978. Should more flexibility be included in the mandated benefit package so that HMOs can compete more effectively? Should the development authorities be streamlined so that financial assistance flows without major disruption to HMO projects? A new thrust also will impact on the 1981 debate. A small but growing number of members of Congress believe a medical marketplace virtually free of federal sanctions would be the most favorable environment in which competition could thrive. These members may strive to remove requirements such as community rating in the hope of making HMOs more competitive. Most of the HMO industry would resist such a move because of the importance of community rating as a major distinguishing characteristic of prepaid group practice, because of its value in helping to achieve financial stability, and because it provides high-risk groups better access to HMOs.

In sum, government must recognize that it has created a unique program. OHMO is charged with using tax dollars to develop new private businesses, a mandate that places the office in a role uncharacteristic of a government agency. But in carrying out this assignment, OHMO cannot in all instances be a hard-nosed entrepreneur looking for the best risk because another dimension of its mandate is to increase access to care to the most vulnerable segments of American society. Balancing these mandates in a responsible manner will be a demanding assignment even under the best of circumstances.

References

American Medical News. 1980. Lack of Good Managers Called Biggest Problem Facing HMO Industry. June 13.

Birnbaum, R. 1980. Health Care Regulation and Competition: Are They Compatible? Health Maintenance Organizations. Paper delivered at Project Hope Symposium, Millwood, Va., May 22–25.

Cassidy, R. 1980. The HMO Flop That Gave Fee-for-Service a Black Eye. *Medical Economics* 57:73–77.

Demkovich, L. 1980. Business, as a Health Consumer, Is Paying Heed to the Bottom Line. *National Journal* 11:851–854.

Department of Health, Education, and Welfare. 1979. *National HMO Development Strategy through 1988.* DHEW Publication No. (PHS) 79-50111. Washington, D.C.: Government Printing Office.

Employee Benefit Plan Review. 1980. NAEHMO Survey of Health Care Coverage and Industry Involvement in Cost Containment. April.

InterStudy. 1979. Grant Application 18-p-97019 prepared for the Health Care Financing Administration. Excelsior, Minn.

New York Times. 1980. Health Maintenance Organization Collapses as Its Doctors Drop Out. January 2.

Strumpf, G. 1980. The Present Status of HMOs. Paper delivered at a seminar on Challenge of the Next Ten Years for HMOs Sponsored by the Esselstyn Foundation, Claverack, N.Y., June 19–21.

Veit, H. 1980. Future Roles for the Federal Government in the Development of HMOs. Speech before the Group Health Institute. Boston, May 4.

Address correspondence to: John K. Iglehart, Kaiser Foundation Health Plan, Inc., 900 17th Street, N.W., Washington, DC 20006.

HMOs, Competition, and Government

RICHARD McNEIL, Jr.

ROBERT E. SCHLENKER

This article considers the role of three sets of forces affecting the development of health maintenance organizations (HMOs) during the early 1970s: legal restrictions, market conditions, and the federal government's policy stance. Our review of the evidence suggests that the rapid increase in the number of HMOs during this period was primarily due to favorable market conditions in certain areas of the country combined with a highly encouraging federal policy toward HMOs. Legal restrictions do not appear to have been as serious a barrier to HMO development as was earlier believed.

In 1973–74, major new legislation was enacted at both the federal and state levels, ostensibly to encourage HMO development. Our review of this legislation suggests that, while it removes many of the old legal requirements which apparently were not serious barriers to HMO development, the new legislation imposes a host of new conditions and requirements on HMO participation in the health care marketplace. Ironically, some of these new features may impede the operation of the very market forces which encouraged the earlier HMO growth.

In 1970 the term Health Maintenance Organization (HMO) was coined, and HMOs were loudly and widely proclaimed as a major component of a new federal initiative to "restructure" the medical care delivery system.[1] Much of the HMO concept's appeal was based on evidence that HMOs could offer their members comprehensive care at lower costs than conventional fee-for-service

[1] The sine qua non of an HMO is prepayment for medical care in contrast to the fee-for-service mode's use of postpayment. More specifically, we define an HMO as an organization which accepts contractual responsibility to assure the delivery of a stated range of health services, including at least ambulatory and in-hospital care, to a voluntarily enrolled population in exchange for an advance capitation payment, where the organization assumes at least part of the financial risk or shares in the surplus associated with the delivery of medical services. This definition includes many of the so-called "foundation-type HMOs." The federal HMO strategy was officially unveiled in a March 1970 statement by Robert H. Finch, then Secretary of HEW (Lavin, 1970). President Nixon's February 1971 Health Message to Congress strongly reinforced the HMO strategy as a major federal initiative. Later that year, an HEW White Paper called for a national goal of 1,700 HMOs in operation by 1980 (HEW, 1971:37).

providers.[2] But just as important, HMOs were also seen as offering benefits extending beyond their membership in the form of a strong competitive stimulus for improved performance by the traditional fee-for-service sector. Competition from HMOs would, it was asserted, improve the efficiency of health care delivery and help contain rapidly rising medical costs for everyone. By the same token, most HMO advocates recognized (Havighurst, 1970; Ellwood et al., 1971) that effective competition from fee-for-service providers would be an important incentive for HMOs to maintain high-quality standards.

From the vantage point of the early 1970s the outlook for HMO development was mixed. On the one hand the cost and price record of the "prototype HMOs" relative to the fee-for-service delivery method indicated HMOs could compete effectively in the health care market. Yet on the other hand, the establishment of HMOs appeared to be blocked in many areas by consumer ignorance of the HMO concept, provider hostility, and what were thought to be serious legal barriers to HMO development created by various state and federal laws and practices.

In this article we examine two aspects of HMO development. First, we note the rapid recent growth in the number of HMOs and attempt to determine the relative importance of *market, legal,* and *policy* conditions in influencing this rapid HMO growth during the 1970–73 period.[3] We find that the available evidence is consistent with the hypothesis that the number of HMOs has grown primarily in response to favorable market conditions and high-level-policy encouragement from the federal government. Legal conditions, with two exceptions, do not appear to have greatly retarded HMO formation.

Second, in light of these results, we evaluate the major changes in legal conditions which occurred during 1973 and 1974.

[2]These contentions were supported by data on "prototype" HMO-like organizations such as the Kaiser Foundation Health Plan, the Health Insurance Plan of Greater New York (HIP), Group Health Cooperative of Puget Sound, and the Foundation for Medical Care of San Joaquin County. See, for example, Donabedian (1969) and Greenberg and Rodburg (1971); the most recent comprehensive review of HMO performance is by Roemer and Shonick (1973).

[3]Our definitions of "*market, legal,* and *policy* conditions" are given in the text which follows.

We conclude that while most of these new laws—ostensibly aimed at encouraging HMOs—do remove some legal barriers, they replace them with new ones. Paradoxically, the new laws intended to encourage HMOs may ultimately be more detrimental than those they replace.

HMO Growth in the Early Seventies[4]

As a starting point in examining HMO development, Table 1 summarizes our estimates of the increasing number of operational HMOs in recent years. In this table, in most of the data which follow, California is distinguished to highlight special trends in that state.[5] Table 1 shows that the number of operational HMOs has increased dramatically since the end of 1969. For the country as a whole, the number of HMOs increased fivefold in just five years. This precociousness is even more impressive in light of the length of time involved in starting an HMO. InterStudy's survey data indicate that for HMOs becoming operational during 1970–73, this process took about two and a half years.

Total HMO enrollment in the country was around five million in mid-1974, of which nearly 70 percent was in the two largest organizations, the Kaiser Foundation Health Plan and the Health Insurance Plan of Greater New York (HIP). Almost half the HMOs had fewer than 5,000 enrollees. Thus, while enrollment trends will become a major indicator of HMO success or failure over the long run, at this stage we feel it most appropriate to focus on the growth in the *number* of HMOs.

[4]Much of the information for this article (InterStudy, 1973–74; Schlenker, Quale, and McNeil, 1973; Schlenker, Quale, Wetherille, and McNeil, 1974; and Schlenker, 1974) is taken from InterStudy's ongoing program of HMO research.

[5]California's uniqueness stems, among other things, from a long history of HMO presence in the state (notably Kaiser) and from its Medicaid (Medi-Cal) policy which, in contrast to other states, encourages recipients to obtain their medical care from HMOs (or, as they are called under Medi-Cal, Prepaid Health Plans, PHPs). Considerable controversy surrounds this aspect of Medi-Cal, and many contend the program lacks appropriate safeguards for both the Medi-Cal recipients and the state. Supporters maintain (Medical Care Review, 1973) the program has been very successful in restraining the previously uncontrolled costs of the program.

TABLE 1

Estimated Number of Operational HMOs
(at End of Each Year)

	1969	1970	1971	1972	1973	1974
Total						
Number of HMOs	37	41	52	79	133	183
Percentage increase over previous period	—	11	27	52	68	38
Total excluding California						
Number of HMOs	21	25	34	51	75	102
Percentage increase over previous period	—	19	36	50	47	36
California						
Number of HMOs	16	16	18	28	58	81
Percentage increase over previous period	—	—	13	56	107	40

Conditions Influencing Recent HMO Growth

Although the number of HMOs has grown rapidly, Table 1 masks considerable variation across geographical areas. We have attempted to analyze these variations to assess the relative importance to HMO development of various legal, market, and policy forces. Because of the time lag involved in HMO start-up, we concentrated on conditions in existence around 1970–71.

Legal Conditions

As of August 1973, 25 states had one or more HMOs in operation. We compared this group of states to the 25 states without HMOs for those laws usually cited as barriers to HMO development. Since very few states changed these laws prior to 1973 (and many states still have not changed), a comparison of the two groups of states should give some indication of the influence of these state laws on HMO development. Table 2 shows that while there are some differences in legal conditions between the HMO and non-HMO state groups, there are no clear differences in the frequency

TABLE 2

State Laws Affecting HMOs[a]

	Strict insurance regulation	Some insurance regulation	Physician control	Open physician panel	Nonprofit only	Advertising prohibited	Professional corporate restriction	Certificate of need: outpatient	Certificate of need: inpatient
Total number of states with provision	3	33	14	9	40	15	3	11	20
By subgroup:									
25 states with HMOs	0	18	6	2	22	8	2	8	14
25 states without HMOs	3	15	9	7	19	7	1	3	6

[a]These laws are those usually cited as legal barriers to HMO development. "Insurance regulation" requires HMOs to meet various financial reserve requirements, although, in contrast to insurance companies, HMOs provide services and not dollar payments. "Physician control" refers to laws which require that physicians constitute all or a part of an HMO's controlling body. "Open physician panel" provisions are a part of some states' Blue Cross enabling act and require an HMO to allow the participation of any physician in the HMO. "Nonprofit only" indicates a requirement that a key component of the HMO (usually the plan entity) be organized on a nonprofit basis. "Advertising prohibited" indicates that the HMO cannot advertise its benefit package and rates. "Professional corporate restriction" indicates a restrictive application to HMOs of laws controlling the incorporation of physician groups. "Certificate of need" laws are discussed later in the text; basically, they require governmental approval prior to certain changes in services or expansion in facilities. For more details, see Schlenker et al. (1973: Chapter III).

with which the laws thought to severely restrict HMOs appear in the two groups.

This table shows that HMOs succeeded in becoming operational in states with every legal barrier except "strict insurance regulation." (We found only three states which we considered as having such regulation, Alaska, Nebraska, and North Carolina. As we shall see, other conditions could well be responsible for the absence of HMOs in these states at the time of the study.) State laws requiring "physician control" and "open physician panel" are the only legal conditions which seem to associate with complete HMO absence.[6]

InterStudy's mid-1973 survey of operational HMOs also indicates that these legal conditions are less important in limiting

[6]State legal conditions could, of course, slow the growth in the number of HMOs and affect their organizational form; and this would not be revealed by our comparison. For example, InterStudy's mid-1973 survey suggests that HMOs adopt special organizational forms to avoid laws against for-profit operation. Nearly half the HMOs indicated they were "nonprofit" but had for-profit subsidiaries.

HMO formation and development than originally believed. We asked HMO administrators to cite the factors they perceived as significant barriers to their HMO's formation and growth. Three-fourths saw gaining access to employer and other potential member groups as their most serious formation and growth problem. The second most serious formation barrier was opposition from other providers, followed by problems of obtaining financial support. For growth barriers, obtaining financial support was second, and provider opposition third. The fourth most serious barrier for both formation and growth was expanding physician staff. A legal barrier was, in general, felt by HMOs to be only the fifth most serious formation or growth barrier they faced.

Market Conditions

In contrast to legal conditions, market conditions seem strongly related to the presence or absence of HMOs in a state. The HMO and non-HMO state groups reveal striking differences in a number of variables indicating demand, supply, and price conditions in the medical care marketplace. Table 3 presents the averages of a group of these variables for the two groups of states. The data indicate that states with HMOs, as compared to the states without HMOs, tend to have higher incomes, larger and more urbanized populations, more physicians per capita, higher hospital costs per day and per capita, and greater public and private insurance expenditures. While such differences are, of course, far from conclusive, they are consistent with the hypothesis that HMOs will locate where they can best compete with the conventional medical care delivery system, and that they can best compete where consumers spend considerable amounts on medical care (and especially on hospital care) through insurance, out-of-pocket expenses, and taxes for government medical assistance programs.

Legal and Market Conditions in Urban Areas

State data provide only gross measures of conditions affecting HMO development. Local area conditions may be much more important. To explore this issue we have made a preliminary examination (Schlenker, 1974) of both legal and market conditions during the 1971–73 period in Standard Metropolitan Statistical

TABLE 3

HMO and Non-HMO State Group Comparison
for Selected Market-Related Variables

Variables	Average for HMO States	Average for Non-HMO States
Demographic-Economic[a]		
1. Total population, 1970	5.3 million	2.8 million
2. Population density per square mile, 1970	225	64
3. Percent of population in urbanized areas, 1970	59	30
4. Mean family income, 1969	$11,341	$9,570
Health Resources and Expenditures[b]		
5. Patient-care physicians per 100,000 persons, 1970	126	93
6. Short-term hospital beds per 1,000 persons, 1971	4.1	4.5
7. Hospital costs per day, 1971	$84	$67
8. Hospital costs per person, 1971	$94	$77
9. Insurance premium per person under 65, 1970	$105	$90
10. Medicare payments per enrollee, 1970	$328	$277
11. Medicaid payments per inhabitant, fiscal 1971	$27	$16

[a]These data are all from the 1970 U.S. population census.

[b]The physician data are from *Distribution of Physicians in the U.S., 1970* (American Medical Association, 1971); the hospital data are from *Hospital Statistics, 1971* (American Hospital Association, 1972) and the *U.S. Statistical Abstract 1972;* insurance data are from the *1972-73 Source Book of Health Insurance Data* (Health Insurance Institute); Medicare data are from *Medicare: Reimbursement by State and County, 1970* (HEW, SSA, Office of Research and Statistics, 1973); and Medicaid data are from *Medicaid and Other Medical Care Financed from Public Assistance Funds: Fiscal Year 1971* (HEW, SRS, National Center for Social Statistics, 1972).

Areas, SMSAs. A comparison of averages for SMSAs with HMOs versus those without revealed the same general pattern for legal and market variables as just presented for the state comparisons.[7] Further, regression analysis indicated that SMSA population size and hospital expenses per patient day were highly significant and positively related to the probability of both HMO presence and new HMO formations in an SMSA. At the same time the legal

[7]Legal conditions, of course, continued to be measured at the state level; each SMSA therefore took on the values of the legal variables of its state.

variables indicating open-physician-panel and control requirements were significant and negatively related to these probabilities. These results are consistent with our earlier findings; in particular, the strong relationship between hospital costs and HMO presence and formation supports the hypothesis that HMOs thrive where they can best compete with other providers by reducing the use of high-cost hospital care.

The regression analysis also indicated the importance of HMO presence in an SMSA prior to 1972 as a predictor of new HMO formation during 1972–73. In other words, once one or two hardy HMOs broke the ice, others tended to follow. Three quarters of the HMOs formed in 1972–73 located in SMSAs which already had one or more HMOs at the end of 1971. This phenomenon of innovation followed by imitation is quite common in a competitive market economy and was noted long ago by Schumpeter (1934). The new HMOs might have followed older ones because conditions favorable to the early HMOs also appealed to later entrants (perhaps more so because of the earlier HMOs' success in overcoming initial obstacles). Or, new HMOs might have followed because the early HMOs posed a competitive threat to other providers, causing them to retaliate by forming their own HMOs. In either case, the phenomenon of innovation followed by imitation lends support to the hypothesis that the pattern of HMO development represents a response to salient conditions in the marketplace.

Other data also support the "market response" explanation of HMO growth. InterStudy's 1973 survey of HMOs revealed, for example, a significant increase in the frequency of Blue Cross/Blue Shield sponsorship of HMOs over the 1970–73 period. This suggests that during this period the Blues may have been "testing the water" with HMOs and responding to a perceived competitive threat from HMOs to their traditional market position. Also, the sponsorship of HMOs by private corporations increased during the same period and this too could be interpreted as a response to market incentives by a group which was in the past usually outside the health care delivery field but tends to respond to market incentives. Finally, physician groups became increasingly involved in HMO sponsorship, especially during 1972–73, perhaps partly in response to the competitive threat posed by new HMOs sponsored by others.

Policy Conditions

Of the conditions which we examined as potential influences on HMO development, "policy conditions" are the most difficult to specify. By that term we mean the posture, other than as expressed in law, which government adopts toward HMOs within its jurisdiction. We distinguish "policy conditions" from "legal conditions" because "policy" is not always embodied in law, especially in the case of a new phenomenon such as HMOs. As we use the term, "policy conditions" indicates a general "governmental acceptance factor" which in turn is indicated by, for example, funding, promotional efforts, and speeches and writings by governmental authorities.[8]

An examination of the status of state and federal policy toward HMOs during the period of rapid HMO development in the early seventies suggests that federal policy probably had a very encouraging effect on HMO development, and that state policy, except in California, probably had very little influence on HMO development.

Federal policy. A federal policy of HMO encouragement manifested itself in two ways during 1970–73. The first was strong public statements endorsing the HMO concept. As noted above, the administration first officially outlined its HMO strategy in March 1970 and reinforced this in 1971 with presidential message and an HEW White Paper. These actions prompted wide discussion of the HMO strategy in the professional literature, (see Lavin, 1970; Ellwood et al., 1971; Saward and Greenlick, 1972). This rhetorical initiative undoubtedly raised the legitimacy of HMOs and suggested that more substantive federal assistance would soon be forthcoming.

The second manifestation of the positive federal policy toward

[8]It is also convenient to distinguish between "legal" and "policy" conditions because we are considering both state and federal government. State government has until recently had very little "policy" toward HMOs in the sense of a considered stance toward encouraging or discouraging HMO development. Yet as we have seen above, a number of states had laws which affected HMOs, even though those laws were typically enacted for other purposes. In contrast to the states' "law without policy," the federal government initially had a considered, coherent policy of encouraging HMOs but only limited federal law affecting HMOs.

HMOs during 1970–73 was modest funding. From fiscal year 1971 to 1973 the federal government expended $28 million in grants and contracts related to HMO development (HEW, 1974b). Of this amount, $12 million was used to finance resource development and technical assistance for organizations not directly involved in the provision of prepaid health services. The remaining $16 million went to direct planning and development grants to 79 organizations, of which 17 were operational by March 1974. Also during fiscal years 1971–73, ten additional operational HMOs received some form of technical assistance from HEW. The direct impact of these funds was modest. Federally funded HMOs account for only a small part of the HMO growth over those years, and the funded HMOs' existence cannot be attributed in most cases solely to federal funding. However, the funding and highly visible oratorical activity together were taken by many to presage greater federal encouragement of and assistance to HMOs in the future, and many organizations were thereby prompted to go ahead with HMO development.

State policy. In contrast to the clearly favorable federal policy, it is difficult to identify a state policy toward HMOs, much less to evaluate its influence. With the exception of California noted above, most states do not seem to have had a "policy" toward HMOs until at least 1973. As we have seen, most states have applied certain laws to HMOs which were thought to hamper HMO development. But the piecemeal application of these laws— which had been typically enacted much earlier with far different organizations in mind—hardly indicated anything as organized and coherent as the term "policy" implies. If anything, these laws suggest that until very recently most states have not had a "policy" of encouraging or discouraging HMO development.

HMO Development in 1970–73, in Summary

The main conclusion we derive from the legal, market, and policy data is that HMO formation and growth during 1970–73 was primarily a response to favorable market and federal policy conditions. In short, federal policy provided an encouraging backdrop, and HMO development then proceeded in those areas where HMOs could best compete with other providers.

This is not to say that legal conditions were unimportant, but they do not appear to have been as detrimental to HMO formation as was initailly assumed. However, in late 1973 and early 1974 major legal changes occurred at both the federal and state levels, heralding a new phase in HMO development. We turn now to consider these new legal conditions in light of the 1970–73 experience.

New Laws Affecting HMOs

Nineteen seventy-three and early 1974 brought much new HMO legislation at both the federal and state levels. Given the importance of market conditions which seems indicated by the evidence just presented, the standards for evaluating this new legislation must, in our view, also be market-related. Our concern is not simply whether these new laws will encourage or discourage HMO development, but whether these new laws will encourage or discourage *fair market competition* in the medical care delivery system by allowing HMOs and the fee-for-service mode to compete on equal footing and without compromising medical care quality. The basic principle underlying a fair-market-competition standard is that obstacles which unfairly bar HMO entry into the medical care market should be removed, but that HMOs should not receive any special advantages (such as undue subsidization) relative to the rest of the medical care delivery system. This standard has been well articulated in the recent policy statement on HMOs by the Institute of Medicine of the National Academy of Sciences (1974).

Certainly, "fair market competition" is not a completely objective standard. Reasonable people can differ as to whether specific laws are preferential to one group or not. In our estimation, most new HMO legislation reflects the view that competitive market forces cannot be relied on to ensure adequate medical care quality from HMOs. To varying degrees, the new laws constrain the HMO's cost-containment incentives in an attempt to protect the consumer against quality reductions. The evidence on this point to date is mixed, but suggests the danger is minimal. Studies of prototype HMOs have not found inferior medical care, and have often found the opposite (Roemer and Shonick, 1973). On the other hand, allegations of poor quality do surround some of the new

California PHPs. As the discussion below suggests, in our view most of the new legislation sacrifices too much in potential cost containment to gain quality safeguards, many of which may be either unnecessary of ineffective. The primary effects of many of these so-called safeguards may be, unfortunately, to slow the process of HMO formation and to raise the cost of HMO care (perhaps above competitive levels for a large segment of the market) without significantly increasing the consumer's protection against inferior medical care.

A further drawback of many of the new laws is that the beneficial requirements they do impose on HMOs are not also imposed on their competitors (insurers and providers). We hope, however, this imbalance will only be temporary, and future programs such as national health insurance will require all health care insurers and providers to adhere to minimal-quality and consumer-safeguard standards.

The discussion below considers first, at the state level, HMO enabling acts, certificate-of-need laws, and Medicaid. We will then turn to federal laws, specifically to Medicare and the HMO Act of 1973.

State HMO Enabling Acts

As pointed out earlier, in most states the piecemeal application to HMOs of various laws which were enacted with far different organizations in mind hardly constitutes anything as organized and unambiguous as a "policy." It was partly to correct this problem that state HMO enabling acts were advocated and passed. As reported by Holley and Walker (1974a; 1974b), by mid-1974, 17 states had such laws; seven states enacted their legislation in 1974, seven in 1973, two in 1972, and one in 1971.[9] In addition, similar legislation was pending in several other states.

While it is too early to determine the effect of these new laws on HMO development, our analysis suggests that their contribution to HMO development will be mixed. On the positive side,

[9]The states included in this list, with the year of enactment in parentheses, are: Arizona (1973), Colorado (1973), Florida (1972), Idaho (1974), Illinois (1974), Iowa (1973), Kansas (1974), Kentucky (1974), Michigan (1974), Minnesota (1973), Nevada (1973), New Jersey (1973) Pennsylvania (1972), South Carolina (1974), South Dakota (1974), Tennessee (1971), and Utah (1973).

most enabling acts require the state to monitor the quality of care the HMO delivers, require HMOs to have an established mechanism for processing enrollee grievances, and require some form of enrollee participation in the HMOs' policy-making body. All these seem to be positive provisions for protecting consumer interests. In addition, nearly all of the enabling acts also release HMOs from restrictions on advertising and the corporate practice of medicine, though these restrictions do not seem to have greatly burdened many HMOs.

However, the new enabling laws also impose new and more burdensome requirements on HMOs which probably will not advance consumer interests. For example, several states' enabling laws impose financial-reserve requirements on HMOs similar to those applied to insurance companies. While appropriate for insurers, these requirements are not appropriate for an HMO, which contracts to provide medical services and not dollar benefits. Some enabling laws also require state approval of an HMO's rates; most fail to exempt HMOs from certificate-of-need laws, which were designed for traditional hospitals (and are further discussed below). Several laws also require HMOs to have various open-enrollment provisions, which can be expected to significantly increase an HMO's costs and decrease its ability to compete, since few states impose analogous requirements on insurance companies or traditional providers. Few state enabling laws have "dual choice" [10] provisions, which would increase HMOs' access to the market, and in only one state to date (Michigan) does the dual-choice provision apply to more than state employees.

In our view, many of these regulatory requirements will do little to protect consumers and will unnecessarily limit opportunities for HMO development. For instance, in Arizona the HMO enabling act imposes new requirements of $50,000 deposits and $100,000 reserves per HMO and a 1 percent tax on net charges. These requirements hindered at least one organization in its efforts to form an HMO. Yet while imposing these financial requirements, the Arizona enabling act is silent in the areas of quality monitoring, grievance procedures, and enrollee participation in policy making.

[10]"Dual choice" is a provision requiring employers to offer employees an option to apply their health benefits to either an HMO or a conventional health insurance plan. As discussed later, this is a key provision of the federal HMO Act.

Nevada is another example. In the regulations evolving from the enabling act, fledgling HMOs are required to have a minimum net worth of $100,000; purchase a surety bond of not less than $250,000; maintain a blanket fidelity bond of at least $1,000,000; and establish a monthly reserve equal to 3 percent of collected enrollee payment. These new requirements appear to have driven two formational plans from the market and threaten the continued operation of a third. Thus, paradoxically, in many states an HMO "enabling act" may not increase the consumer's protection from shoddy HMOs or encourage fair competition between HMOs and other modes of health care delivery, but may instead decrease the likelihood of effective competition from HMOs.

State Certificate of Need Laws

Certificate-of-need laws require hospitals and certain health facilities to obtain approval, a certificate of need, from a regulatory authority prior to undertaking new construction or certain modifications in services.[11] These laws originated as a legislative response to the continuing increases in the cost of hospitalization. Advocates of certificate-of-need legislation saw these cost increases as a result of several factors: oversupply of hospital beds, the overutilization incentives of third-party cost reimbursement, and the excessive zeal of nonprofit hospitals in undertaking new capital expenditures for elaborate but economically inefficient facilities. Twenty-three states had certificate-of-need laws as of January 1974, and most of these were applied to HMOs. Judging by the number of certificate-of-need bills now pending, it seems very likely that more states will be adopting certificate-of-need legislation in the future. In addition, as of April 1974, 32 states had reached agreements with the federal government for implementation of Section 1122 of the 1972 Social Security Amendments (P.L. 92-603), which in effect establishes a certificate-of-need requirement under federal law for Medicare and Medicaid reimbursement of capital costs.

Although the rationale for and probable effectiveness of certificate-of-need laws in curbing hospital costs is not the subject

---

[11]An analysis of these laws, with particular attention to their potential impacts on HMOs, can be found in Havighurst (1973; 1974).

of this article, they have been questioned (Havighurst, 1973) by others. The applicability of such laws to HMOs rests on even weaker logical footing, since the central characteristic of the HMO is its incentive to minimize the cost of needed medical care. An HMO's viability depends on its ability to *compete* with other providers. However, it seems likely that the very forces within the traditional system whose stubborn resistance to efficient utilization and cost considerations brought on the passage of certificate-of-need laws in the first place will eventually control the control mechanism. When those controls are then applied to HMOs as well, the outcome is likely to be a reduction of effective competition from HMOs and other innovative health delivery approaches.[12] Anecdotal evidence suggests that this has already occurred in some states.

While most of the HMOs InterStudy surveyed in mid-1973 had formed before many certificate-of-need laws were in operation, many had felt the inhibitory force of these laws on their growth. In states with certificate-of-need laws in effect or pending, 48 percent of the responding HMOs cited such laws as moderate or severe barriers to their growth. Although the overall impact of certificate-of-need laws remains to be seen, it appears unlikely at this point that they will contribute to fair market competition.

Medicaid

Although Medicaid is a joint federal-state program, most of the responsibility for program operations is lodged at the state level. The 1969 Social Security Act Amendments made approving mention of prepayment plans for providing Medicaid services, but participation by HMOs in Medicaid was complicated by requirements that all Medicaid eligibles in a state were to receive the same scope of services, that those services were to be available throughout the state, and that Medicaid eligibles be allowed to choose where they would receive their medical attention. The 1972 Social Security Act Amendments (P.L. 92-603) allowed the states to waive these requirements. Unfortunately, specific regulations

[12]Professional Standards Review Organizations (PSROs) are another control mechanism subject to this danger, since providers from the traditional system will be able to rule on the "quality" of care provided by their competitors in HMOs and elsewhere.

for implementing the Medicaid-HMO provisions of the Amendments were not proposed until 1974 (Federal Register, 1974b), suggesting a less than maximal effort to encourage HMOs to participate in Medicaid.

In view of these facts it is not surprising that HMO participation in Medicaid is not great outside of California. According to the responses of 112 organizations to InterStudy's July 1974 enrollment survey, about 6 percent of the about 5 million HMO enrollees are Medicaid recipients. Although nearly half the HMOs in that survey had some Medicaid recipients enrolled, over half of these HMOs were in California. However, as discussed below, the attractiveness to HMOs of participation in Medicaid may increase as the result of the preference given by the federal HMO Act of 1973 to HMOs with Medicaid members.

If Medicaid participation does increase, this will not necessarily mean an improvement in fair market competition among delivery systems. The states vary considerably in the requirements they impose on both HMOs and fee-for-service providers. Oregon and Maryland illustrate (HEW, 1973) the different financial incentives states provide for HMO participation in Medicaid.

In Oregon an HMO must absorb all financial losses and can keep none of any savings it achieves, while in Maryland an HMO bears no losses and can receive half the savings. Measured against our view of fair market competition, both methods err, although in opposite directions. Oregon may be too harsh on HMOs; Maryland too lenient. To be consistent with our fair market standard, an HMO should absorb any loss it incurs in meeting its contractual obligations. By the same token, when an HMO can meet its obligations at an agreed-upon capitation rate, the HMO should be allowed to retain any savings. Unfortunately, this ideal is not yet a part of the Medicaid program.

Medicare

As noted above, historically most of the important laws affecting HMOs were at the state level; the emphasis has now shifted to the federal level. The remainder of this article focuses on the two most important recent federal actions affecting HMOs: recent Medicare modifications and the 1973 HMO Act. Our subsequent discussion draws heavily on the work of McClure (1973; 1974) and the Institute of Medicine (1974).

Medicare is presently the federal government's largest health program. As with Medicaid, HMO involvement in Medicare has not been extensive. While close to half (46 percent) of the 112 HMOs responding to InterStudy's mid-1974 survey enrolled Medicare beneficiaries, these beneficiaries accounted for less than 5 percent of all HMO members. In our view, the Medicare program fails to meet fair-market-competition criteria, but for different reasons than the laws previously discussed. This is best shown by an examination of Medicare's policies for HMO reimbursement. Although only one reimbursement method is in use now (under section 1833 of the Social Security Act), two additional alternative reimbursement methods were authorized by Section 1876 of the 1972 Social Security Amendments; but regulations for these methods were still being developed in early 1975.

The "old" cost-reimbursement method. HMOs now enrolling Medicare beneficiaries are reimbursed on a cost basis. Reimbursement must be related to the allowable costs of providing covered services. The HMO neither absorbs any losses nor obtains any surpluses and thus has no financial incentive to provide care efficiently to Medicare enrollees.

The "new" cost-reimbursement method. Under the new cost-reimbursement method provided for by the 1972 Social Security Amendments, an HMO can be paid an advance capitation payment for both parts A and B of Medicare. However, this mechanism is still essentially cost reimbursement, because the capitation payment will be *retrospectively* adjusted to reflect the HMO's Medicare-allowable expenses for providing care to beneficiaries. Again the HMO can neither keep any savings nor sustain any losses.

The risk-sharing reimbursement method. The other new reimbursement alternative is a risk-sharing plan which theoretically would bring an HMO's efficiency incentives partially into operation. Unfortunately, however, few HMOs will be able to qualify for participation under this arrangement in the near future. The proposed regulations (Federal Register, 1974c) provide that to be eligible for a risk-sharing contract an urban HMO must have a current enrollment of 25,000 members and have had an enrollment of at least 8,000 for each of the two preceding years. For rural HMOs the current enrollment must be 5,000 and for each of the preceding three years have exceeded 1,500. HMOs meeting these requirements are called "mature" HMOs. Other HMOs, denoted as "developing," are expected to use a cost-reimbursement method. Most of the 112 HMOs responding to InterStudy's mid-1974 enrollment survey were located in urban areas, only 18 reported an enrollment of over 25,000, and even some of these could not meet the requirement of at least 8,000 enrollees for each of the two preceding years.

Even if many HMOs could qualify for the risk-sharing method, they would have little financial incentive to do so. Under this reimbursement mechanism, any losses the HMO sustains must be borne by the HMO. However, any savings are split between the HMO and the Medicare Trust Funds, with the added stipulation that any savings beyond 20 percent of costs go entirely to the Medicare Trust Funds.

Thus, given the eligibility problems of the risk-sharing mechanism, and the small potential for financial reward it offers, we expect few HMOs to undertake that relationship with Medicare. This leaves cost reimbursement as the alternative. From our point of view, the problem with cost reimbursement is not that it is burdensome for an HMO, but that it is irrational, given the HMO's incentives.[13] Cost reimbursement treats an HMO like a fee-for-service provider, bypassing and possibly disabling the HMO's prepayment incentive for efficiency. In our estimation, this denies to the Medicare program the efficiency advantages of HMOs and will tend to subvert HMO efficiency incentives or even encourage cost maximization. It might even be possible for an HMO to use its "reasonable cost" Medicare reimbursement to subsidize its other non-Medicare enrollees and thereby gain an unfair competitive advantage over fee-for-service providers.

[13]Other federal policies have shown a greater awareness of HMOs' uniqueness. See the Cost of Living Council's regulations for HMOs (Federal Register, 1974a) under what was to be Phase IV of the Economic Stabilization Program. These regulations were never implemented.

The unattractiveness of risk sharing under Medicare is evident in data from InterStudy's July 1974 survey. Fifty-two HMOs then enrolled some Medicare beneficiaries, and 36 more intended to do so by July 1975. In all, however, only *two* of these 88 HMOs indicated they expected to participate in a risk-sharing contract. Forty-four expected to use one of the cost-reimbursement arrangements, and the remaining 42 were undecided or did not answer. While it is certainly desirable to extend the benefits of HMO services to Medicare beneficiaries, cost reimbursement will not further fair market competition between HMOs and the fee-for-service sector. This is especially ironic since the federal HMO strategy began with the proposal (Finch, 1970) to use the Medicare program as a catalyst for HMO development.

The Health Maintenance Organization Act of 1973 (P.L. 93-222)

The most significant new federal policy affecting HMOs is the HMO Act of 1973 (P.L. 93-222). The act establishes a precedent for governmental attempts to encourage structural change in the health care delivery system. Because this legislation had bipartisan support, it could legitimize and encourage many kinds of health-delivery innovations in addition to HMOs, and could thereby prove to be landmark legislation.

Since the act has been law only since December 29, 1973, it is too early to gauge its impact on fair market conditions for HMOs. Regulations have been developed only for portions of the act. Despite its recency, however, some indications of the act's impact can be gained from the statutory provisions and regulations (Federal Register, 1974d) and from InterStudy surveys of operational and planned HMOs conducted in May and July of 1974 to determine HMOs' reactions to the new law.

In examining the act according to fair-market-competition standards, we divided its provisions into four general topic areas: (1) funding, (2) consumer protection, (3) enabling, and (4) regulation. The HMO Act is worded so that it applies only to those HMOs which choose to become "certified" under the act. However, we believe (as discussed below) most HMOs will feel compelled to certify. Certification requires that the HMO be in compliance with the regulation and consumer-protection aspects of the act, and certification is required before an HMO can benefit from the act's funding and enabling provisions.

Funding. In our view, the funding aspects of the act will probably be of only modest significance. As first introduced by Senator Kennedy in Senate Bill 14, the act provided $5.2 billion for HMO development. By the time the HMO Act became law it had been pared to an authorization for $375 million over a five-year period, of which $50 million is specified for research and evaluation studies of quality assurance. Experience from 1971 to 1973 discussed above suggests that funding at this level will probably not have a major impact. This is, however, desirable under our fair-market-competition standard. Except in cases where more drastic action is necessary to bring health care to underserved groups, fair market competition requires that government policy aim at encouraging conditions which allow HMOs to enter and compete their way into the market, rather than having their way paid for them.

Unfortunately, however, the funding provisions also introduce certain market distortions. For instance, the act distinguishes between nonprofit and for-profit HMOs. The former are eligible for grants, contracts, and loans, but not loan guarantees, while the latter are eligible only for loan guarantees and then only when serving medically underserved areas. The loan program will make available federal money to nonprofit HMOs at the Treasury rate plus an add-on for administrative costs. For-profit HMOs will be borrowing private money under federal guarantee but at significantly higher market rates. This is discriminatory against for-profit HMOs and creates an incentive for new HMOs to adopt the organizational contortions we noted earlier that are presently used by many nonprofit HMOs to claim that status.

Consumer protection. We feel that in the long run the most effective safeguard for HMO consumers is the existence of fair market conditions which give consumers the opportunity to make a free and informed choice among HMOs and between HMOs and other providers. This freedom of choice coupled with programs aimed at measuring the quality of care received in *both* fee-for-service and HMO settings should ultimately be the most effective protection for the HMO consumer. However, long-run safeguards are not

enough; short-run abuses should also be averted. Ideally, government intervention to protect consumers should insure against
market-safeguard failures but, at the same time, should enable the
market to deliver those safeguards ultimately. Achieving this ideal
is a difficult balancing act. If too many safeguards are applied (as
appears to be the case with many state HMO enabling acts), HMOs
will be unnecessarily hindered in entering the market. If too few
safeguards are used, allowing well-intentioned (or even ill-
intentioned) but slipshod organizations to operate, the quality of
care may suffer. We feel the consumer safeguards of the HMO Act
effectively balance these two opposing forces.

Under the act, a certified HMO is required to make its
services accessible and available to enrollees. When medically
necessary, services must be available and accessible 24 hours a
day, seven days a week. Certified HMOs are also required to have
a fiscally sound operation, and adequate provision against in-
solvency satisfactory to the Secretary of HEW. In addition,
certified HMOs must have grievance mechanisms for enrollees,
and are not allowed to expell an enrollee for reasons of health
status.

The act also specifies that certified HMOs must have a
quality-assurance system and report pertinent data to the
Secretary. While there has been little empirical evidence that the
quality of HMO care is worse than the traditional system, and
some evidence that it is better, there is the theoretical argument
that HMOs may underserve their members. To guard against both
the appearance and possibility of underservice, it is important to
have quality safeguards and to concentrate on *outcome* rather than
process measures of quality. However, since quality assurance and
reporting entail additional expense and are not at this time required
of other providers (PSROs may change this), and since the
measurement of quality is still more art than science, we feel it is
desirable to keep these requirements mimimal until all providers
are required to meet them.

Perhaps one of the most powerful and simple safeguards in the
act prohibits an HMO from enrolling more than 75 percent of its
enrollees from a medically underserved population (where the underserved are defined to include Medicare and Medicaid
enrollees). This provision will prevent HMOs from enrolling large

numbers of the underserved unless the HMO has also been successful in attracting other enrollees. This consumer safeguard should strengthen market competition as well as protect the underserved.

Enabling. Besides funding, the act offers HMOs other benefits from certification. The most important (a) preempt various restrictive state laws, (b) require employers who offer their employees health plans to allow employees to apply their benefits to HMO membership (referred to as "dual choice"), and (c) allow advertising of the nonprofessional aspects of an HMO's services. We refer to these provisions as the "enabling" aspects of the act.

The dual-choice provision is of most importance to the HMOs, as evidenced in the responses shown in Table 4 of 97 operational HMOs to InterStudy's May 1974 survey on their reactions to the HMO Act.[14] Nearly two thirds of the responding HMOs indicated dual choice was a significant advantage to be gained from certification under the act.[15] Far fewer HMOs viewed the funding or preemption benefits as significant advantages.

Even with the potential gains from certification, only half the HMOs responding to the survey indicated they intended to apply for certification. Most of the rest were undecided. A major reason for this uncertainty becomes clear when one examines the regulatory aspects of the act and their potential for reducing HMOs' ability to compete effectively.

Regulation. The major regulatory aspects of the act are:

(1) A very rich basic benefit package. The HMO Act not only requires the generally recognized minimum essential benefits of preventive and therapeutic physician services, emergency and inpatient hospital services, diagnostic X-ray and laboratory services, and out-of-area emergency coverage, but also re-

[14]Organizations planning HMOs provided similar responses to a survey conducted in July 1974. For the sake of brevity, we report here only the results for the operational HMOs.

[15]This is consistent with InterStudy's 1973 survey results reported earlier, which indicated that HMOs perceived gaining access to employee groups as their greatest problem in forming and growing.

TABLE 4

Enabling Provisions of the HMO Act
(Percentage of Respondents Indicating Relative
Attractiveness of Selected Provisions)

Provision	Significant Advantage	Moderate Advantage	No or Slight Advantage	No Response or Undecided
Funding: grants, contracts, loans, loan guarantees	36	18	41	5
Preemption of restrictive state laws and practices	12	21	61	6
Dual-choice requirement for employers	62	19	13	6

quires that HMOs offer many other services such as short-term mental-health serivces and alcoholism and drug-abuse services. Seventy-one percent of the HMOs responding to our survey said they could not meet these requirements without increasing their present benefit package and, hence, their premium.[16]

(2) Permanent regulation. Section 1312 of the act gives the Secretary permanent regulatory power over any HMO which becomes certified. No time limit or escape clause is provided whereby the HMO could remove itself from such regulation. For example, if a certified HMO (even one receiving no federal funds) found the minimum basic benefit package too highpriced and unmarketable in its service area, there is no way that it could seek relief. No such regulatory conditions have to date been imposed on health insurers or other providers.

(3) Open enrollment. The act requires that a certified HMO have an open-enrollment period of not less than 30 days a year during which it accepts individuals up to its capacity in the order in which they apply, without regard to health status. This provision could greatly increase HMO costs relative to other insurers with which they must compete, since open enrollment is

[16]The act does allow the use of co-payments for the provision of specific services, although only in very specific and limited ways.

not required of other insurers. One study (McClure, 1974) found that an HMO's costs for persons joining during open enrollment were 80 percent greater than for other enrollees.[17]

(4) Community-rate rating. Except for some administrative cost differences, HMOs are to charge the same premiums to all their members. Obviously, this means low users of services "subsidize" the high users. Such subsidization may be desirable from a societal viewpoint, but such requirements are usually not placed on insurers or other competitors of HMOs.

(5) Other miscellaneous requirements. The act also requires each certified HMO to have one third of its policy-making board be enrollees, requires that (after three years) group-practice-based HMOs obtain at least half their revenues from HMO activities, limits HMO purchases of reinsurance, and imposes other reporting, quality-assurance, and continuing-education requirements. Again, while many of these requirements are societally desirable they are usually not imposed on insurers and providers which compete with HMOs.

Obviously, meeting all the above requirements will not be costless for HMOs, and, in most cases, similar costs will not have to be borne by those who compete with HMOs. InterStudy's May 1974 survey shows that the HMOs recognize these potential problems, especially with the open-enrollment and community-rating requirements, as shown in Table 5.

In light of the cost increases likely to be caused by the richness of the basic benefit package, we were surprised that most HMOs did not see this as an important disadvantage, particularly since nearly three-fourths of the HMOs also said this would require changing their minimum-benefit package. Perhaps this optimism is based on a hope that potential enrollees will recognize and desire to pay for the increased services which the act will require.

[17]It is possible for an HMO to obtain a waiver of the open-enrollment requirement if it can show that open enrollment has or would result in the enrollment of a "disproportionate" number of high-risk persons which will "jeopardize its economic viability." This could mitigate the negative effect of the open-enrollment requirement, but is also gives more arbitrary power to government regulators and increases the complexity and uncertainty for HMOs in making cost projections and establishing premium rates.

TABLE 5

Regulatory Provisions of the HMO Act
(Percentage of Respondents Indicating Relative
Unattractiveness of Each Provision)

Provision	Significant Disadvantage	Moderate Disadvantage	No or Slight Disadvantage	No Response or Undecided
Permanent regulatory power given to HEW Secretary	23	26	33	18
Minimum basic benefits	12	28	58	2
Open-enrollment and community-rating requirement	40	21	33	6
Requirement that one-third of policy-making body be enrollees	18	16	61	5
Ongoing quality-assurance-program requirement	3	13	78	5
Requirement that medical group's principal activity be prepaid group practice	37	10	42	10

In sum, it seems likely that the ambivalence toward certification which many HMOs indicated in the survey is due to their reluctance to accept the burdens of the regulatory provisions of the act. This, however, raises a crucial dilemma. The dual-choice provision of the act may, in effect, compel HMOs to seek certification. The provision will require employers to offer their employees the option of joining an available certified HMO. Offering a non-certified HMO would not meet this requirement, and would probably create additional administrative costs for the employer. Thus, non-certified HMOs could have great difficulty gaining access to employer groups in areas with certified or potentially certified HMOs. HMOs may thus feel compelled to seek certification, even though certification is likely to increase their costs, possibly to the point that it will be extremely difficult to compete with traditional insurers and providers. Thus the HMO Act could well stifle fair market competition by forcing the majority of HMOs to become high-priced, "Cadillac" HMOs.

There are other aspects of the act which, while desirable on the surface, might have detrimental effects on competition. For example, the priority in funding given to HMOs which enroll the underserved may lead HMOs to seek increased Medicare and Medicaid enrollment. While this is laudable in many respects, we have indicated the pernicious incentives which Medicare's cost-reimbursement system for HMOs creates. Another potential danger is that the certification costs built into the act and the resulting increased competitive pressure could cause HMOs to underserve as a means of holding premium rates down to competitive levels. Ironically, this is precisely what those who advocated the costly regulatory requirements for certification.

While we have not discussed all the ramifications or details of the HMO Act, it is clear that the act escapes simple characterization. It has several very positive characteristics from a fair-market-competition viewpoint. It is a precedent for governmental encouragement of structural change in the delivery system to improve the market's operation. The funding provision of the act, while somewhat biased, should stimulate competition without overly subsidizing HMOs. The act also contains valuable protections for the consumer and an assist for certified HMOs by removing some of the more serious marketing and state legal barriers. However, in our view. the act has drawbacks which offset many of its positive features. While many of the regulatory provisions of the act would be desirable if applied to all health care providers and insurers, their unilateral imposition on HMOs could seriously weaken HMOs' ability to compete in a large segment of their potential market.[18]

Conclusions

No single delivery mode can incorporate incentives for achieving all the quality, cost, and distribution goals our society has set for health care delivery in the United States. Given this impossibility, we feel the best approach is a system which uses different delivery modes—based on different incentive structures—actively competing with one another.

[18]Rhode Island's recently enacted catastrophic health insurance plan law (HEW, 1974a) appears to adopt a more even-handed approach by requiring *all* insurers and providers to meet certain minimal conditions.

At this point, the future of HMOs and meaningful competition in the health sector is uncertain. Our evidence from the 1970-73 period suggests that HMOs can successfully compete with the fee-for-service delivery mode even when conditions are less than strictly fair. Now, however, the conditions for HMO development have changed. Ironically, many of the new federal and state laws which purportedly are designed to encourage HMOs may inhibit rather than promote competition and pluralism in health care delivery because those laws apply certain constraints only to HMOs.

Yet even this situation is subject to an even greater change in the conditions for competition in health care delivery. The most massive intervention in the health care marketplace yet attempted appears imminent in the form of national health insurance. This intervention presents tremendous potential for either improving or crippling effective competition in health care delivery. The uniform application to all health care insurers and providers of many of the provisions now applied solely th HMOs under the HMO Act would do much to promote effective and beneficial competition.

Richard McNeil, Jr.
InterStudy
123 East Grant Street
Minneapolis, Minnesota 55403

Robert E. Schlenker, PH. D.
InterStudy
123 East Grant Street
Minneapolis, Minnesota 55403

Research for this article was supported in part under a Health Services Research Center grant from the Bureau of Health Services Research, Department of Health, Education, and Welfare (Grant No. HS 00471-06). Paul M. Ellwood, Jr., M.D., made valuable comments on a previous draft, and the latter portion of this article draws heavily on the work of Walter J. McClure, Ph.D.

References

Donabedian, Avedis
  1969   "An evaluation of prepaid group practice." Inquiry VI. 3.

Ellwood, Paul M., Nancy N. Anderson, James E. Billings, Rick J. Carlson, Earl J. Hoagberg, and Walter McClure.
1971   ''Health maintenance strategy.'' Medical Care 9 (May–June): 291–298.

Federal Register
1974a   ''Phase IV Health Care Regulations.'' Federal Register 39 (March 27): 11378–11380, 11390–11393.

1974b   ''Medical Assistance Program Proposed Contracting Requirements.'' Federal Register 39 (June 5): 20042–20044.

1974   ''Federal Health Insurance for the Aged and Disabled: Health Maintenance Organizations.'' Federal Register 39 (August 27): 30935–30941.

1974d   ''Health Maintenance Organizations.'' Federal Register 39 (October 18): 37308–37323.

Finch, Robert H.
1970   ''Statement by Robert H. Finch, Secretary of Health, Education and Welfare, on Medicare and Medicaid Reforms.'' Washington, D.C.: Medicare and Medicaid Guide, Supplement No. 11, March 28, 1970, Commerce Clearing House, Inc.

Greenberg, Ira G., and Michael L. Rodburg
1971   ''The role of prepaid group practice in relieving the medical care crisis.'' Harvard Law Review 84 (February): 887–1001.

Havighurst, Clark C.
1970   ''Health Maintenance Organizations and the market for health services.'' Law and Contemporary Problems 35 (Autumn): 716–795.

1973   ''Regulation of health facilities and services by 'certificate of need'.'' Virginia Law Review 59 (October): 1143–1232.

1974   Regulating Health Facilities Construction (ed.). Washington, D.C.: American Enterprise Institute for Public Policy Research.

HEW
1971   Towards a Comprehensive Health Policy for the 1970's. A white paper (May). Washington, D.C.: U. S. Government Printing Office.

1973   ''Analysis of prepaid Medicaid contracts for comprehensive health benefits.'' HEW internal memo (August).

        ''Rhode Island Catastrophic Health Insurance Plan.'' Research and Statistics Note No. 33. Office of Research and Statistics, Social Security Administration (December 9).

1974b   Health Maintenance Organization Program Status Report. Washington, D.C.: Health Services Administration, (March, processed).

Holley, Robert T., and Robert W. Walker
1974a   Catalog of 1973 State Health Maintenance Organization Enabling Bills. Monograph. Minneapolis, Minnesota: InterStudy (February).

1974b   Catalog of State Health Maintenance Organization Enabling Bills: January through June, 1974. Monograph. Minneapolis, Minnesota; InterStudy (August).

Institute of Medicine
1974   HMOs: Toward a Fair Market Test. A policy statement. Washington, D.C.: National Academy of Sciences (May).

InterStudy
1973–74 A Census of HMOs. Published quarterly by InterStudy.

Lavin, John H.
1970   ''HEW's new drive to change health care delivery.'' Medical Economics, May 25.

McClure, Walter J.
1973   ''Detrimental effects of applying the present Medicare amendments to Medicaid.'' Memo. Minneapolis, Minnesota: InterStudy (November).

1974   ''A critique of the Health Maintenance Organization Act of 1973.'' Memo. Minneapolis, Minnesota: InterStudy (February).

Medical Care Review
1973   ''California Medicaid.'' Medical Care Review 30 (March): 282–287.

Roemer, Milton I., and William Shonick
1973   ''HMO performance: the recent evidence.'' Milbank Memorial Fund Quarterly, Health and Society 51 (Summer): 271–317.

Saward, Ernest W., and Merwyn R. Greenlick
1972   ''Health policy and the HMO.'' Milbank Memorial Fund Quarterly 50 (April): 147–176.

Schlenker, Robert E., Jean N. Quale, and Richard McNeil, Jr.
1973   Socioeconomic and Legal Factors Associated with HMO Presence: An Examination of State Data. Monograph. Minneapolis, Minnesota: InterStudy (October).

Schlenker, Robert E., Jean N. Quale, Rhona L. Wetherille, and Richard McNeil, Jr.
1974   HMOs in 1973: A National Survey. Monograph. Minneapolis, Minnesota: InterStudy (February).

Schlenker, Robert E.
1974   Why are HMOs in some urban areas and not in others? Minneapolis, Minnesota: InterStudy (November).

Schumpeter, Joseph A.
1934   The Theory of Economic Development. Cambridge, Massachusetts: Harvard University Press.

HMOs, Competition, and the Politics of Minimum Benefits

DONALD W. MORAN

Former Legislative Assistant to
Congressman David A. Stockman

OBSERVERS OF FEDERAL POLICY-MAKING HAVE long noted the tendency of policy fads to acquire a long train of fellow travelers and advocates of convenience as they march eastward across the Potomac. Over the last seven years, for example, the national goal of energy independence has been putatively pursued by a mysterious coalition of corn farmers with alcohol stills, supplicants to the Highway Trust Fund, and ailing automotive giants. National security has always been a favorite, justifying everything from welfare steamships to hothouse sugar mills. When added to the drive for "free trade, but fair trade," any Washington lawyer worth his salt can weave a patriotic bunting to clothe even the most humble special interest appeal.

Health care policy, of course, has never been immune from this sort of private interest masquerade. In the 1970s, the push for cost containment was used to whitewash all manner of otherwise antisocial behavior on the part of the government and the various provider groups scrambling for the federal health dollar. Although the Congress has apparently rejected expanded regulatory efforts designed to control hospital costs, it still smiles daily on a wide range of appeals from provider and consumer groups that are justified as cost-reducing measures.

Milbank Memorial Fund Quarterly/*Health and Society*, Vol. 59, No. 2, 1981
© 1981 Milbank Memorial Fund and Massachusetts Institute of Technology
0160/1997/81/5902/0190-19 $01.00/0

In the last two years, a new banner has been raised on the federal health policy scene in the form of proposals to inject *competition* into the market for health care financing. Predictably, a wide range of interests have now taken to automatically incorporating an appeal to competition into their justifications for more even-handed (i.e., favored) treatment within the heavily regulated health care delivery structure. Given the novelty of the notion, such efforts have met with mixed success. To date, in fact, the only real victories won under the competition banner have been the growing list of dispensations—such as certificate-of-need (CON) exemption and favorable treatment under Medicare—awarded to health maintenance organizations (HMOs) because of their perceived accordance with the competitive model.

To most observers such legislation is not considered to be of a special interest nature; on the contrary, HMOs, because of their assumption of normal investment risk in the health care marketplace, are viewed as fundamental elements of the brave new world envisioned by competition advocates. The Carter administration, for example, in a position paper on competition and its role in health care, cited its efforts to foster the growth of HMOs as the main evidence of its commitment to the competitive ideal. Moreover, all the empirical evidence available to date in support of the viability of the competitive model is based on experience in those markets, such as Minneapolis and the West Coast, where the establishment of HMOs has generated economic competition between prepaid plans and the traditional fee-for-service (FFS) system. All in all, far from being just a special interest entree for HMOs, the competitive model appears to be inextricably linked to the fate of the HMO movement.

A Market of Competing Prepaid Plans

According to Alan Enthoven, the *doyen* of the "competition" movement, and many other proponents of the market strategy, a market composed solely of competing prepaid health care plans is the best feasible formulation of the strategy. In his view, the market must in fact be biased toward the formation of prepaid plans lest unique characteristics of the market for health care financing render the market strategy unworkable.

First, according to Enthoven, the market for health care services

is fraught with consumer information deficiencies. In order to overcome the inability of consumers to choose between complex presen-
tations of widely differing health insurance offerings, the market
should be constrained so as to limit the number of choices to a set
of roughly similar plans competing on the basis of price and quality
for a standard set of benefits (1980a:81).

This, in turn, will cause the market to tend toward a structure of
competing, vertically integrated provider groups. Because competitors
will not be allowed to segment the market through product differentiation, only those who successfully control both investment and
service utilization will survive. Explicit utilization controls, such as
provider decisions to withhold or delay care, will in general be more
successful in restraining utilization than more indirect methods, such
as copayment requirements or deductibles that are small relative to
the total cost of service. Thus, it is anticipated that comprehensive,
prepaid plans will emerge the victor in any head-to-head battle with
more loosely organized FFS providers once the allowable product
offering has been suitably constrained (Enthoven, 1979:2, 1980a:5).

Nor, according to Enthoven (1979:4–6; 1980a:80), are information
defects the sole justification for imposing minimum benefit constraints
that ultimately lead to market dominance by prepaid plans. In the
absence of fairly high minimum benefit requirements, the market
would suffer from severe preferred risk selection. That is, low-risk
persons would gravitate toward lower-option plans providing only
bare-bones emergency coverage, while high-risk persons would gradually sift out into the high-coverage plans. The results would be that
the insurance character of the market would be broken, and the cost
of providing comprehensive benefits would soon be prohibitively high.

A related problem is that of "free riders," who could be expected
to "game" the system if choices were wide and annual changes between
plans were allowed. The notion is that those who are well would
select low-cost coverages until such time as high-cost elective surgery
or treatment were imminent. At that point, they would switch over
to a comprehensive plan, receive the needed services at little or no
additional cost, and then return to the low-option plan during the
subsequent enrollment period. Hence, high-option plans would find
themselves experiencing costs far in excess of collected premiums
(Enthoven, 1979:2; 1980a:79).

In summary, Enthoven would hold that *only* a market where benefit
choices were severely constrained—hence a market that would over

time perforce evolve into a sort of "duelling HMO" model—can introduce competition into health care financing without creating a whole new raft of problems.

Another argument for the competing prepaid plan model of competition has been advanced by McClure (1979, IV:50–59). Noting the traditional tendency of physicians' groups to act in concert on economic issues, he raises the specter of pervasive provider collusion and subsequent market failure, unless steps are taken to prevent the providers in the community from unanimously resisting the efforts of financing plans to effect cost controls. To prevent such collusion, McClure argues that strict limits should be placed on the percentage of physicians that can be involved with any one plan in each HMO area. In addition to the effect of forestalling collusion, of course, such a step would provide a direct stimulus toward a market of competing closed panel health care plans.

These criticisms may be valid, but the legislative future of *competition* is not necessarily bright. It may well prove, as these analyses suggest, that a market of competing prepaid plans offering standardized benefit packages is the optimal form of competition. There is still, however, the question of how to get from here to there. For, while the models with which the competition notion is being sold are, at the least, internally consistent, the same cannot be said of the *political process* through which any solution of this sort would be implemented.

If anything, the track record of the Congress to date suggests that the key design elements of the new market system—the rules by which providers compete—will be the brokered outcome of a process whereby existing market participants will attempt to give as little away as possible in exchange for the opportunities and problems of a more wide-open market for health care goods and services. In such an environment, I will argue, legislation contemplating a market solely composed of prepaid plans along the lines enunciated by Enthoven and McClure is the *least likely* outcome of congressional deliberation over injecting competition into the health care field.

The HMO Movement: Competition with Whom?

One major reason why a market composed solely of competing HMOs is unlikely to be generated by an act of Congress lies in the fact that

HMOs will not be judged in a vacuum, solely on arguments related to the desirability of internalizing investment risk or on the incentives for HMOs to promote preventive care strategies. Rather, they will be judged on the basis of whether their track record to date offers strong and compelling evidence that what HMOs sell is itself so inherently desirable that all other types of competitors should be barred from the race. On this point, the historical record is, at best, mixed.

The HMO movement—or more generically, the development of health care financing on a prepaid capitation basis by a closed panel of health care providers—did not begin as a competitive response to the presence of FFS practitioners; instead it began for the opposite reason: a dearth of other means of providing health care to impoverished or isolated communities.

The modern precursors were born in the slums of the eastern seaboard when mutual aid societies of ghetto immigrants pooled their resources to hire physicians who otherwise would not practice in the ghetto for financial reasons. Although such plans were common in the nineteenth century, they eventually faded away as traditional physicians, in response to the alleviation of poverty in the ethnic communities after the turn of the century, moved into these areas to establish more traditional FFS practices.

The next major growth area for prepaid plans was the physician-sparse West Coast, where the huge influx of workers to man the vital defense industries during the Second World War far outstripped the ability of local physicians to provide needed health care services. Kaiser Industries, for example, faced with a lack of adequate physician manpower to provide care for its imported workforce in its steel plants and shipyards along the coast, sponsored the establishment of Kaiser Plans in Oregon and California, with enrollment at first restricted to its own employees.

After the war, these plans went public and began to effectively compete against the traditional physician community for patients. Yet, the original motive for creation of all of these plans can hardly be described as competition for patients in the health care marketplace. Instead, the plans were at first effective natural monopolies, created because markets abhor a supply vacuum.

In fact, the only prepaid plan of any size created before 1947 in direct competition to traditional practice was the Ross-Loos Plan in Los Angeles, established in 1929. Yet, this plan neither sought nor achieved a major market share among the insured population; instead, it was content to accept those families willing to eschew the free choice of a traditional physician, offered by other insurers, in favor of the prepaid plan.

The real competitive drive for patients in these markets came, not from the prepaid plans, but rather from the traditional medical community, which viewed the prepaid plans, both from an economic and professional perspective, as threats to continuation of their prevalent mode of practice. The competitive response of traditional medicine proceeded on a number of fronts.

The most common was a long string of probable antitrust violations designed to starve the prepaid plans out of the marketplace. The Oregon State Medical Society, for example, made a habit, until admonished by the Justice Department, of expelling all members of the medical society who did business with the prepaid plans. In general, the professional response, as embodied in the American Medical Association's (AMA) Code of Ethics as early as 1932, was to declare contract practice and competition for patients unethical for a member physician and to discipline transgressions through formal and informal procedures.

It is thus ironic that organized medicine *as a body* entered into a strong economic competitive effort with the prepaid plans by promoting their own prepaid plan alternatives, generally known either as individual practice associations (IPAs) or foundations for medical care (FMC)s, to draw patients interested in prepaid plans away from the HMO heretics. A classic case in point, described by Goldberg and Greenberg (1977), is the competitive response of the local medical society to the entrance of the Kaiser Plan into the Pittsburg, California, area in 1953. Citing Gabarino (1960), they note that Kaiser's decision to appeal to the giant U.S. Steel plant in the area for enrollments produced a hurried decision to form a "Doctor's Plan" to be marketed to the employees before their deciding vote on health benefits selections. The physicians sponsored full-page newspaper ads and even went so far as to park participating doctors and their wives in the company parking lot to leaflet the membership, augmented by a sound truck exhorting the employees: "retain your family doctor"; "don't be a captive patient." In the end, the fact that the "Doctor's Plan" lost the deciding vote by a 4 to 1 margin does not diminish the obvious competitive zeal of the traditional medical community.

At about the same time, the desire of the Kaiser Plan to dilute criticism from the traditional medical community induced it to undertake a number of seemingly competitive ventures. First, it instituted a requirement of "dual choice," whereby the Kaiser Plan would only be offered to employees if the employer also agreed to offer a second plan giving employees the option of selecting FFS practitioners. This backfired to a certain extent because it allowed dominant FFS insurers to effectively freeze Kaiser out by refusing to have their plans offered as a choice alongside Kaiser. For example, in Portland, Oregon, the Oregon Physician's Service, the local Blue Shield plan, simply refused to participate in dual-choice arrangements; while the competing Blue Cross plan would participate only if it was guaranteed a 75 percent enrollment share.

A second effort, generated by the active refusal of many hospitals in HMO plan areas to provide admitting privileges to HMO physicians, was the decision by Kaiser to build its own hospitals instead of relying on local facilities used by FFS practitioners. While both these actions are consistent with the notion that Kaiser was attempting to solidify its competitive position in the marketplace, the alternative hypothesis cannot be rejected: that the decision by Kaiser and other large HMOs to draw back into their own facilities and, in the Kaiser case, to eschew head-to-head competition with FFS insurers for total employee group enrollment evidenced a desire to de-emphasize *economic* competition between prepaid plans and the traditional sector in favor of an enhanced promotion of the differences between prepaid plans and the traditional sector in terms of *medical practice style*. As Goldberg and Greenberg (1977:78) note in describing the California market:

> In some respects, for instance, Blue Cross competes more vigorously with Blue Shield than it competes with Kaiser since Blue Cross and Blue Shield must compete initially for the designation of the employer's health insurance offering. It is also interesting to note, however, that Kaiser generally does not react to any competitive response Blue Cross might make because Kaiser already offers comprehensive benefits and reviews carefully hospital admissions and length of stay. Furthermore, Kaiser has a policy against advertising and charges what it believes to be the lowest premium consistent with its standard of medical care.

This approach to competition on the part of Kaiser, and to a certain extent the other large, established HMO plans, provides the key to analyzing the likely fate of HMOs under a relatively unconstrained regime. For unlike the FMCs, IPAs, and other physician-sponsored HMOs that have sprung up in response to Kaiser, Group Health, and other major prepayment plans, the traditional HMOs refuse to meet head-to-head on price with traditional insurers; rather, they effectively compete against the entire fee-for-service system via product differentiation.

The rationale for the sort of competition preferred by the traditional HMOs is captured nicely by Christianson (1978:1):

> The notion that competition among health care providers can help control costs would seem to contradict the historical evidence. In the past, competition among providers for patients has contributed to the excessive performance of surgery, the proliferation of expensive and underused equipment, and the construction of excess hospital beds [citation omitted]. Since these and other outcomes of "provider competition" have contributed to rising health care costs, why should competition between traditional providers and alternative organizations for delivering care, such as HMOs, now be encouraged?

The answer, according to Christianson, is that this second sort of competition "can restructure the incentives and influence the decisions of traditional participants in the medical care marketplace to the benefit of business and other consumers." Thus, as HMO advocates Ellwood, Malcolm, and Tillotson (1979:1) conclude:

> The competitive health system strategy requires three main elements:
> —creating forms of health delivery systems that are more efficient than the present system, and that are hence able to compete on price, benefits, access, and style of medical care;
> —such units must be installed across the country; and
> —once the majority of health care providers in any given community are involved in competing alternative delivery systems, the workability of the approach can be evaluated.

Thus, they came down squarely on the side of a finding of inherent desirability in the HMO style of practice. Moreover, they effectively concede that a wide-open market for health care financing, unless operated under the sort of constraints proposed by Enthoven and McClure, would fail to generate the desired competition model in the natural evolution of things. That is, the proposed constraints, whether or not they are sufficient conditions for the establishment of a market of competing prepaid plans, are at least necessary conditions.

In order for the Congress to accommodate this vision, then, it will be forced to rig the rules of any competitive game in order to ensure that prepaid plans win. Given the likely resistance of other groups (e.g., traditional insurers, hospitals, and physicians), it would take a strong conviction on the part of the Congress that prepaid health care delivery had intrinsic merits. To date, the history of federal involvement in the HMO movement offers little evidence that such a conviction will soon materialize.

HMOs, Competition, and the Congress

The congressional fascination with HMOs began during the Nixon administration, as the result of that administration's frantic search for a method of appearing to deal with exploding costs under Medicare and Medicaid without atypically resorting to heavy-handed, sector-specific cost control regulation.

HMOs, at least in theory, filled the bill nicely. They were private enterprises, at risk in the free marketplace, and held out the promise of keeping the politically powerful traditional medical practitioners in line with a decentralized barrage of good, clean Republican competition. Yet, because of their reformist aura, they could be sold to a Congress drifting increasingly leftward due to the political polarization attendant on the administration's other preoccupation, Vietnam. In fact, in Nixon's special health message to the Congress in February of 1971, touting HMOs as the solution to the problem of rising medical care costs, the word *competition* is conspicuously absent. Instead, Nixon extolled their potential as a "new method for delivering health services," characterized as having a "strong financial interest in preventing illness." The proposed demonstration projects designed to test their effectiveness under a dual choice model would generate a "health care supermarket" in which the notion that there were economies of scale in the group practice of medicine could be tested. By 1973, when legislation effecting Nixon's proposed demonstration program was imminent, the rhetoric grew bolder: HMOs were now a "promising innovation of group medical centers" that would ultimately "reform the health care delivery system."

Even while debating the HMO demonstration program, the Congress had already enacted legislation allowing HMOs into mainstream federal health policy by establishing a favorable arrangement for prospective payment of HMOs enrolling Medicare and Medicaid beneficiaries. The *quid pro quo* at that time, of course, was that HMOs were subjected to facilities review and approval under Section 1122 of the 1972 Social Security Act Amendments. In the same year, the Senate passed and sent to the House a bill that went far beyond the administration's original proposal, calling for $1.3 billion to launch a full-scale commercialization project for HMOs and other prepaid plans.

The House, accepting for the moment the administration's conviction that such an effort was far too costly, failed to consider the measure; and it died when the Ninety-Second Congress adjourned.

By 1973, however, the House was ready to go to work and produced a bill modeled more closely along the lines of the original administration proposal. Yet, several new wrinkles crept in, setting the stage for a debate that continues to this date. In its efforts to make the bill more flexible, the administration was pushing for the broadest possible definition of an organization eligible for assistance in order to promote diversity in plan structure (and, not incidentally, to open the door for assistance to physician-sponsored plans, lest the AMA and its legislative muscle derail the entire effort).

The Congress, however, urged on by such groups as the American Public Health Association, approached the bill like a committee bent on designing a horse and produced a far narrower definition of a "qualified HMO" than the administration had hoped for. The bill produced by the House-Senate conference committee established a definition of an eligible plan that was so restrictive only some 20 of the 133 extant HMOs would qualify. The balance were relegated to the lesser status of "health service organizations" and "supplementary HMOs," whose access to the federal funds—and to the highly important overrides of troublesome state laws—was sharply restricted compared with the benefits attendant on federally qualified HMOs.

This outcome was probably the result of the high degree of confusion then prevalent over what HMOs were, what the bill was likely to do, and what the future direction of federal efforts affecting the overall delivery system would be. For example, the Senate committee report on the bill states the objective of the legislation as an effort to "increase options available from the point of view of the consumer" but "not . . . to remake the delivery system." Yet, paradoxically, the committee believed that HMOs would in the future "largely eliminate many of the problems presented by the prevalent fragmented solo practice model."

A second seeming paradox is found in the bill's treatment of the copayments question. The HMO Act allows federally-qualified HMOs to require only nominal copayments for covered services. Copayments, of course, are instituted for the sole purpose of introducing price sensitivity—i.e., price rationing—to services that might otherwise be overutilized. Yet, the report explicitly states the intent of Congress that such copayments should be "no barrier to care"; instead, they were "solely a device to enable an HMO to market its benefit package at a competitive price." The net effect of this provision was to proscribe copayments as a means of controlling utilization but to condone them as a sort of under-the-table premium increase for qualified plans.

The Congress did, however, seem to have an inkling of the likely natural market outcome of its experimental delivery system, as demonstrated by a reference to the distinction between qualified and "supplemental" HMOs. The committee argued for its decision not to provide the latter with start-up funds on the grounds that they would occur naturally in the marketplace without help; qualified plans meeting the committee's specifications, on the other hand, were not expected to survive without significant direct federal support.

Thus, far from being interested in the potential of HMOs for generating competition, the Congress was instead attempting to outwit the normal functioning of a competitive marketplace and install in the field its own horse, which, while more reminiscent of a camel, was nevertheless expected to win the race with liberal applications of financial dope. Subsequent federal efforts in the HMO arena lend credence to the view that despite the rhetoric, federal efforts to promote HMOs have precious little effect in promoting competition in the marketplace.

In 1979, for example, the Health and Environment Subcommittee of the House Interstate and Foreign Commerce Committee produced and pushed through the House a bill reauthorizing the Health Planning Act. The most controversial feature of the bill was a section providing a sweeping exemption from certificate-of-need laws for all "providers of ambulatory and inpatient care on a prepaid basis." This broad exemption was justified by its sponsor, Congressman W. Philip Gramm (D-Texas), in the name of competition; i.e., that the degree of investment risk assumed by HMOs and other such plans was, due to the normal operation of market forces, an effective discipline against overinvestment in facilities and equipment, obviating the need for a surrogate regulatory discipline.

The broadness of the definition of an entity eligible for the Gramm Amendment exemption was not unintentional. It held out the promise that any health care financing entity which assumed risk for its own investments could effectively exit the regulatory maze of facilities franchising and compete in the open market. By further exempting from CON (certificate-of-need) requirements the activities of non-HMO hospitals that provided services primarily to such providers, the Gramm Amendment language was, in effect, a procompetitive loophole through which a truck could be driven.

While the broad language of the Gramm Amendment survived the House, it proved too much for the House-Senate Conference Committee, which severely restricted the exemption's scope by allowing the exemption only for HMOs with enrollment in excess of 50,000 persons. Only a handful of HMOs—notably such giants as Kaiser, Group Health Association of Puget Sound, the Health Insurance Plan of New York, and the other long-established traditional HMOs—were thus released from the market entry barriers of the certificate-of-need laws. The balance, including new plans that might start up to compete against the established HMOs, remained subject to the CON entry restraints.

In fact, it could be argued that, given the persistence of CON requirements for new prepaid plan entrants, the 1979 Health Planning Act exemption, far from being procompetitive, granted the traditional HMOs a major new tool to preempt the field in those areas in which they were already established, obviating the need for whatever new HMO-style entities might otherwise materialize in competition.

The Minimum Benefits Route

The contention that the Congress would willingly bequeath the entire market for health care services to competing prepaid plans is very difficult to support based on this history. While halting steps have been made in the direction of promoting HMOs that might not otherwise arise, these efforts have been justified more in terms of remedying prior discrimination against prepaid plans than because they are preferred competitors per se (see, for example, Goldberg and Greenberg, 1977).

It is possible, however, that during the course of consideration of legislation to promote competition in medical care markets, the Congress might unconsciously predispose the market toward the competing prepaid plan model by imposing either high minimum benefit requirements or outright benefit package standardization. As noted earlier, the inability of financing entities representing loosely organized FFS providers to constrain service utilization to the level achieved by prepaid plans could place them at a decided disadvantage over time.

Enthoven would argue that this would be a desirable outcome. Enthoven (1980a:45–50) distinguishes the practice styles of FFS practitioners and prepaid plans as the tendency of FFS providers to perform services that increase costs in excess of marginal benefits. Thus, unless FFS practitioners could adjust their practice styles to the utilization levels experienced by prepaid plans, he would argue that FFS plans should *not* survive in a cost-conscious competitive market.

Here, I believe, lies the crux of the problem. In essence, Enthoven argues that many of the amenities that accompany the FFS practice system today—such as short waiting times for services; free choice of physician and hospital; and the exercise of individual preferences respecting, for example, decisions of whether or not to hospitalize—bear costs far in excess of their true utility to consumers. As such, they are quirks of the current incentive structure rather than the outcome of conscious consumer choice.

An apposite view would be that this thesis should be put to the test in the marketplace. Stockman (1980) has argued that failing to allow individuals to choose among a wide range of different delivery modalities and practice styles would forestall the tremendous potential for innovative approaches to health care financing that might otherwise arise. Moreover, he argues that these amenities have, in certain instances, positive value for consumers.

The trade-off then—if there is one—is between different sorts of costs associated with different market formulations. On the one hand, a wide-open market with only minimal benefit package constraints would promote provider innovation. The standard benefits market, by contrast, would forestall many of these innovations, which would largely result from product differentiation. On the other hand, the wide-open market would induce individuals to sort themselves out to some extent on the basis of perceived risk and degree of risk aversion. In such a market, Enthoven argues, comprehensive benefit plans could not survive (1980a:79).

The question, then, is whether the costs associated with obviating product innovation are greater or less than the costs associated with creating a bias against plans that offer relatively comprehensive benefits. Interestingly, the Congress has, at least to date, tended toward the view that comprehensive benefits per se are a more desirable feature than freedom for innovation. As the record shows, however, this congressional tendency generates additional costs that must be factored into the equation.

Minimum Benefits and the Congress: Medicare and Medicaid

Posturing about comprehensive national health insurance aside, the Congress has shown a bias toward expansive definitions of allowable benefits under those programs where the federal government has control over benefit specifications.

Since at least 1950, the Congress has been hard at work adding ever wider benefits to government-financed health programs. The original Aid to Families with Dependent Children (AFDC) program, enacted in 1935 under the Social Security Act, contained a simple income disregard for the amount of bona fide health care expenditures, i.e., expenditures for health care were deducted from the income of families in determining eligibility. In close cases, this practice effectively passed through, dollar-for-dollar, the health care spending of the poor. The Social Security Act Amendments of 1950 converted spending for medical care for the poor to a vendor payment system. Thus, rather than merely passing through medical care expenditures, the Social Security system made direct payments to health care providers for needed health care services for the AFDC-eligible poor. In 1960, the Kerr-Mills Act expanded both benefits and eligibility under the vendor payments program, including, for the first time, low-income aged persons without children in the home. Six years later, this program was dramatically expanded by the enactment of Medicare and Medicaid.

As originally conceived, Medicare was to be simply a program of hospital insurance for the aged. By the time it emerged from the House of Representatives, however, physicians' services were also covered. The Medicaid component, calling for a sweeping program of medical care services to low-income Americans, was also added by the House version. Since enactment Medicare has been amended seven times, and Medicaid nine times. In each instance, either eligibility has been expanded or required benefits have been substantially upgraded.

In 1968, Medicare benefits, originally covering ninety days of hospitalization annually, were upgraded by adding a *second* ninety days of coverage, called the "lifetime reserve," upon which the aged could call in any given year if the original ninety-day coverage was exhausted. At the same time, Medicaid was amended to include the "early and periodic screening, diagnosis, and treatment" (EPSDT) program, a major effort to provide a full range of comprehensive care to eligible children.

Shortly thereafter, in 1972, two large new blocks of eligibles were added to Medicare—those receiving disability insurance and those with end-stage renal disease. In addition, those receiving Supplemental Security Income, except in certain instances, were made eligible for Medicaid.

During the balance of the 1970s, virtually every Congress has added on to this growing laundry list of coverages and benefits. Chiropractors' services and the services of podiatrists are allowed in many instances. Psychiatric services have been expanded widely, particularly in Medicaid, and optometrists, skilled nursing facilities, and dentists have been able to have their services added on to the list.

Even in the budget-conscious 96th Congress, efforts were made to add to the federal programs laundry list. Legislation passed the House calling for, among other things, the expansion of both eligibility and mandatory services for children under Medicaid, the addition of the treatment of planter's warts, the provision of pneumococcal vaccine, new home health benefits, expanded dental services, ad infinitum. When budgetary considerations threatened enactment, the ingenious ploy of loading in benefit additions to the Omnibus Budget Reconciliation Act—the bill designed to reconcile spending with budget totals by *reducing* federal outlays—nearly succeeded. In the end, a number of the proposed additions survived the House-Senate conference on the budget.

The Implications for Legislation to Promote Competition

The most direct indication of the unfortunate congressional tendency to load up the cart with new goodies is the Health Maintenance Organization Act itself. In order to qualify for federal subsidies and the boon of "dual choice" requirements for employers, "qualified HMOs" must offer an incredible array of services, including extensive mental health coverage, treatment for alcohol and drug dependency, home health services, family planning, infertility services, and optometry services for children. To the extent that few, if any, other insurers offer anywhere near this package, federally qualified HMOs often find themselves, despite cost-reducing utilization patterns, at a severe competitive disadvantage. In fact, many have held out the benefit requirements of the HMO Act as one of the major impediments to the nationwide development of health maintenance organizations. Even advocates of a market of competing prepaid plans, notably McClure (1979, IV:120–121), have commented on the disadvantages of too narrow a definition of elegible entities and benefit offerings.

Given this tendency on the part of the federal government to promise all things to all people, those who promote high minimum benefits or standardized packages must be given pause. For over and above the questions of the potential for market innovations and of whether wider choices would offer consumers greater utility (for an excellent discussion of this point, see Meyer, 1980:7–10), there is the plain political question of whether Congress, faced with the task of determining what the minimum package would be, would so load up the requirements as to make the task of financing health care fabulously expensive.

To be sure, Enthoven (1980a:143–144), among others, is not unaware of this potential problem. He notes that a means must be found to minimize the "gatekeeper" role of government in this and other respects. Yet, this problem is not merely a technical design point that can be forever resolved during consideration of enabling legislation. For, if the government is given a determining role in deciding what the market shall offer, it will retain that right in perpetuity. Moreover, as the evidence to date shows, it will not fail to exercise that right frequently in the name of equity, i.e., constituency-group appeasement.

The Stakes Are Far Too High

If anything, legislating minimum benefits in a program that covers all Americans will have a far more pervasive effect than the experience to date in Medicare, Medicaid, and the HMO Act. The great majority of competition schemes envision that whatever qualifying requirements are enacted for plans will, by virtue of leveraging the Internal Revenue Code and the Social Security Act, become a blueprint for virtually all saleable health insurance in the United States.

Faced with such a prospect, the various provider constituencies— and the victims of peculiar diagnoses known affectionately on Capitol Hill as the "Disease-of-the-Month Club"—will be motivated by more than sheer convenience or desire. They will be motivated by the impulse for survival. For to be left off the minimum benefits list will be, perforce, to shift for themselves in a world where whatever federal preferences they now have will be dissolved. To chiropractors, podiatrists, psychologists, naturopaths, faith healers, and other practitioners outside the "physician" umbrella, getting into the game via congressional mandate will make the difference between prosperity and perpetual fringe status.

It is possible that the heavy political pressure of the traditional organized groups and institutions—including, of course, the HMOs, who have not been notorious for welcoming mandates to include nontraditional providers—will keep these groups off the list for a time. Yet, sheer economic necessity will force these groups to return again and again until they are finally successful. Arm in arm with those desperately needing kidney dialysis, interferon treatments, and every other imaginable group of "outs," they will form a coalition to force reopening of the minimum benefits question. Eventually— and inevitably—the wheel will be greased.

The "Third Best" Options

Given this political reality, it may well be time to set aside the pursuit, among health care theorists, of the optimal "second best" market structure—of either the constrained market form preferred by Enthoven or the regulatory "second best" promoted by such commentators as Altman and Weiner (1978). Instead, it may be necessary to turn to a "third best," from which can be distilled a solution that provides for some constraints on adverse selection and free riders; some constraints on plan innovation and product differentiation; some bias against FFS solo practitioners; and some risk that, left to themselves in an open system, the American people may spend more, rather than less, on health care.

Unless such an accommodation is reached, the result of pushing procompetition legislation through the Congress may well be far different from what the proponents anticipate. Either the legislation will melt under the heat generated by warring factions, or else whatever market-based incentives the approach might generate will be buried under the special interest trophies won in the competition for inclusion on the minimum benefits list. It is hard to see how either outcome would be an improvement over the present morass.

References

Altman, S.H., and Weiner, S.L. 1978. Regulation as Second Best. In Greenberg, W., ed., *Competition in the Health Care Sector: Past, Present, and Future.* Washington, D.C.: Federal Trade Commission.

Christianson, J.B. 1978. *Do HMOs Stimulate Beneficial Competition?* Excelsior, Minn.: InterStudy.

Ellwood, P.M., Malcolm, J., and Tillotson, J.K. 1979. The Status of Competition in the Health Industry. Unpublished manuscript.

Enthoven, A.C. 1979. Why We Cannot Have a "Free Market" in Health Insurance. Why Some Rules Are Needed to Produce Good Results. Unpublished manuscript.

——— 1980a. *Health Plan.* Reading, Mass.: Addison-Wesley Publishing Co.

——— 1980b. Supply Side Economics of Health Care and Consumer Choice Health Plan. Unpublished manuscript: American Enterprise Institute Conference on Health Care, September 26.

Gabarino, J.W. 1960. *Health Plans and Collective Bargaining.* Berkeley: University of California Press.

Goldberg, L.G., and Greenberg, W. 1977. *The Health Maintenance Organization and Its Effects on Competition.* Washington, D.C.: The Bureau of Economics, Federal Trade Commission.

McClure, W. 1979. *Comprehensive Market and Regulatory Strategies for Medical Care.* Excelsior, Minn.: InterStudy.

Meyer, J.A. 1980. Health Care Competition: Are Tax Incentives Enough? Supply Side Economics of Health Care and Consumer Choice Health Plan. Unpublished manuscript: American Enterprise Institute Conference on Health Care, September 26.

Stockman, D.A. 1980. Can Fee-for-Service Medicine Survive Competition? *Forum on Medicine* (January), 21–25.

Address correspondence to: Donald W. Moran, 212 E. Alexandria Avenue, Alexandria, VA 22301.

Deciphering Deinstitutionalization: Complexities in Policy and Program Analysis

STEPHEN M. ROSE

School of Social Welfare,
State University of New York
at Stony Brook

S OCIAL POLICY and reform-oriented social programs of the last fifteen years seem to require continuous decoding and re-examination. Not only has there been a substantial gap between promise and general outcome (Warren, Rose, and Bergunder, 1974), but also the rhetoric of progressive reform has frequently created expectations of social change that have not been met; often the results amount to betrayals of the intended beneficiaries, if not of the policy makers themselves (Rose, 1972). Indeed, the most common pattern in the American experience of social reform since the Kennedy years has been one of liberal optimism, political mobilization behind loosely conceived programs, demonstration projects, more generalized funding, and then a quiet slide into criticism and cynicism. The Juvenile Delinquency, Community Action, and Model Cities programs, among others, were begun in an atmosphere of conflict; the programs then declined, while endless battles occurred within localities as agencies fought to maintain their control over previously negotiated domains, and eventually became absorbed into the federal bureaucracy.

The fate of deinstitutionalization policies, however, has differed somewhat from that of other contemporary programs. Some cor-

0160-1997-79-5704-0429-32 $01.00/0 ©1979 Milbank Memorial Fund

respondence has existed between promise and performance. These programs began with all the rhetorical force of initiatives in other policy areas, and at about the same time, but not all of them have been dismantled. Deinstitutionalization policies, although they have met increasing criticism that ranges from skeptical to hostile in tone, have held their own in varying degrees. Two clear-cut questions remain: What relation exists among deinstitutionalization theory, policy, and practice? And why has this policy survived and grown while other broad-scale social reforms are declining or dead?

Deinstitutionalization on a large scale has been attempted in four areas of public social policy: in juvenile delinquency, adult criminal justice (where efforts to prevent institutionalization through "diversion" programs have received more attention than early release efforts),[1] mental retardation, and mental health. The last areas, mental illness and mental health, have become the broadest, with policies and programs at the federal, state, and local levels. They are also the most controversial and may be the most complex to decipher, since data are available to prove almost every contention about the programs.

Deinstitutionalization is a major departure from previous psychiatric practice. In fact, institutions such as state hospitals, state schools for the retarded, reformatories for juvenile offenders, and prisons have been the mainstay of policy and treatment practice since Dorothea Dix's campaigns in the first third of the nineteenth century (Rothman, 1971). Before 1955, various forms of segregative institutions were the preferred mode of treatment for people suffering from the very serious forms of mental disability, as well as for delinquents and adult offenders. Achieving their construction was as significant a reform as closing them down now appears to be.

Defining a New Policy

Most simply, deinstitutionalization is a formal policy of the federal government, first articulated as a direction for public policy in 1960 and 1961 and then proclaimed as a political goal by President John

---

[1]Scull (1977), however, cites a study called *The Quiet Revolution,* by Robert Smith, which indicates large-scale discharge of delinquents.

F. Kennedy in 1963. The Joint Commission on Mental Illness and Health's *Action for Mental Health* (1961) asserted that psychiatric patients were not being helped by their incarceration; in fact, it argued that long-term stays in hospitals were debilitating, producing institutionalized behavior and a tendency toward chronic illness; hospitals were extremely costly and therapeutically little more than large-scale custodial warehouses. The commission recommended that all efforts be directed toward preventing hospitalization, curtailing its length when it was unavoidable, and returning patients to community life, where ideally they would be rehabilitated through community-based services. Services funded through the community mental health centers (CMHC) program were to be delivered through locally based, comprehensive, mental health service centers; these facilities would be designed to prevent mental illness, to catch problems early before they became serious, and to prevent existing problems from becoming chronic by providing aftercare. At the same time, the states would save at least part of the cost of operating large custodial institutions, which would be phased out and replaced by smaller local facilities; the federal government would also help finance local programs planned through state and local agencies.

The program received rapid bipartisan political support since it represented both a progressive social reform and a tremendous saving.

The numerical results of deinstitutionalization to date are evident in a rapid decline in the inpatient populations of state and county hospitals, amounting to a reduction of over 62 percent nationally from 1955 to 1974 (Comptroller General, 1977). Projected savings to the states from this practice are discussed below, but evidence of benefits to psychiatric patients, especially those hospitalized over long periods, is not to be found anywhere in the professional literature. Conversely, those who have reported on the programs, from the office of the comptroller general of the United States to numerous special commissions and investigators (in New York, for instance, the Moreland Commission and the special prosecutor's office), have exposed fraud and abuse and exploitation of former patients (see Hynes, 1977; Comptroller General, 1977; New York State Assembly, Joint Committee, 1975).

This article will attempt an analysis of deinstitutionalization policy and will focus on the sector of community mental health care, its approach to reform, its programs and practice, its accomplishments and difficulties, and criticisms of its operations or results. My aim will be to raise questions about the actual function and efficacy of deinstitutionalization as a strategy of social reform.

Problems in Evaluation

Among the more difficult tasks in evaluating deinstitutionalization is determining who benefits from its status as a reform policy. Both the ideology of the community mental health movement and the stated intentions of the programs define the mentally disabled as the primary beneficiaries, although policy statements do mention the need to reduce costs to state governments. Some data indicate, however, that large groups of former patients have not benefited at all and may even have been harmed by the policy. The rising recidivism rates, along with rising rates of new admissions, indicate that deinstitutionalization has failed substantially in preventing mental breakdown or hospitalization, while at the same time tremendous progress has been made in reducing the overall number of inpatient beds in state hospitals. How can we account for the remarkable success in achieving the latter goal and the devastating defeat in moving toward the former? Moreover, what criteria can be used to assess these matters, or from what perspective can we select the proper data or the proper approach to evaluation?

These problems, difficult in their own right, become even more so when we examine the issue of "legitimation" (or traditional social approval). For a century, mental disability or dysfunction has been considered a medical problem; recently the influence of the psychiatric viewpoint has precluded almost any other form of thought about mental dysfunction. People in severe mental or emotional distress are called "sick," are placed in hospitals, and are "treated" by health care teams, usually headed by a physician, which rely on medication as a primary form of therapy. Other typical therapeutic modalities within the state hospital system also focus on defects in the individual as an explanation for mental disability, yielding what are intrapsychic or intrapersonal responses. This point of view prevails beyond treatment rooms and hospitals to the apparatus for program planning and defining policy as well. The shift from custodial care to community-based care amounts more to a substantial relocation of existing treatment practices than to a redefinition of the nature of the problems and a subsequent redetermination of needs and programmatic responses. Factors critical to daily social existence—such as supportive and healthful housing environments, sufficient income to sustain life and promote rehabilitation, and support services from within the community—were at first ignored as deinstitutionalization was put into practice. This form of neglect cannot be imputed to either simple ignorance or intent; instead, it must be understood as flowing from a psychiatric predisposition to focus on the medical and psychiatric needs of hospitalized and former patients, as if subjective existence were social life itself.

Historical Background

Surprisingly, major disagreement has arisen over the question of when policies resulting in the discharge of large numbers of patients began, and what role was played by the advent of psychotropic drugs in bringing about the general policy that began to be articulated on a national scale in 1961. Mental health care in state hospitals had changed little from the turn of the century until the period immediately following the Second World War, when the impetus for change came from outside the mental health professions:

> Military leaders were astonished to find almost two million draftees rejected from the services for mental disorders or deficiency; the admirals and generals had had no idea that there were so many mentally unreliable persons. Even though rejection rates before training significantly restricted the supply of able-bodied servicemen, the military accepted the psychiatrists' judgments in these cases and thus enabled psychiatry to expand its role and authority in the medical services. (Musto, 1975: 58–59)

A series of steps that included the creation of special hospitals for veterans and the development of a new mental health unit, later the National Institute of Mental Health (NIMH), marked the beginning of the first major federal-level involvement in mental health policy, an area previously a part of the domain of the states.

National involvement increased rapidly after the Joint Commission on Mental Illness and Health published a research report that was the culmination of five years of work, begun in 1955. *Action for Mental Health* set forth the basic goals of what were later to become national theory, policy, and practice standards for community mental health care:

> The objective of modern treatment of persons with major mental illness is to enable the patient to maintain himself in the community in a normal manner. To do so, it is necessary (1) to save the patient from the debilitating effects of institutionalization as much as possible, (2) if the patient requires hospitalization, to return him to home and community life as soon as possible, and (3) thereafter to maintain him in the community as long as possible. Therefore, aftercare and rehabilitation are essential parts of all service to mental patients. (Joint Commission, 1961: xvii)

The major focus of public reform in mental health officially became the state psychiatric hospital, which was proclaimed the source of the problem and was slated for immediate cutbacks and eventual elimination. In fact, the state hospital system had already begun to decline by 1961; Scull (1977) has shown that inpatient populations of state and county hospitals reached their peak of 558,000 in 1955. By 1963, when the CMHC program was articulated in President Kennedy's now famous "bold new approach" speech, the population had reached 504,600 (Scull, 1977: 67; Comptroller General, 1977: 8); it has been declining ever since.

Reasons for the Policy of Deinstitutionalization

Just as important as when deinstitutionalization began is why it commenced when it did. Those who strongly supported community mental health care saw it as a humanitarian reform designed to improve mental health services and help prevent both mental illness and institutionalization. They decried traditional psychiatry and its custodial practices, or "warehousing," and considered the new approach to be a "revolution" in the field. Bellak (1964) is only one example of those who supported this view. Bassuk and Gerson believe that the role of the new drugs complemented external political pressures toward deinstitutionalization: "The pressure was further augmented by the desire of state legislatures to reduce the financial burden of state mental hospitals" (Bassuk and Gerson, 1978: 47).

Others think that the motivation for altering institutional psychiatry was entirely economic, that the asylums had indeed become warehouses with little noticeable effectiveness and monumental cost. The proponents of this view also comment on the growing admission rates at state hospitals, which increased 52 percent between 1955 and 1972, while some point out the looming inevitability of large-scale capital construction costs for new institutions to house the growing numbers of inpatients (Musto, 1975; Scull, 1976, 1977). Reduction of the inpatient population became an economic necessity. Reich and Siegal (1973: 38–39) describe the situation in this way:

> Due to years of starvation financing, the state hospitals by and large were unable to provide their patients with currently acceptable or adequate standards of psychiatric care . . . .
>
> The states, under court pressure to upgrade facilities, faced a dilemma. The cost of overhauling buildings and providing programs for institutions which had been underfinanced for 50 years would be immense. At a time when state budgets were tightly squeezed and increased taxation was politically unpalatable, the millions of dollars necessary for improved psychiatric services to the chronically mentally ill and retarded were simply unavailable. Another means of caring for chronically mentally dysfunctional patients would have to be found.

Whether the change resulted from a humane new concept of mental health care or from more crude fiscal motives, the problem of understanding why deinstitutionalization was undertaken is further complicated by the equally polarized views expressed in the literature about the role of psychotropic drugs. The Joint Commission, dominated by the medical profession, cites the positive position: "Drugs have revolutionized the management of psychotic patients in American mental hospitals, and probably deserve primary credit for reversal of the upward spiral of the State hospital inpatient load" (Joint Commission, 1961: 39). Bellak (1964) takes a middle-of-the-road position, arguing that such drugs made community mental health care a practical policy. Scull (1976) and Mechanic (1969) take the more critical view; both say that the medication argument is simplistic, reinforces the medical view of insanity as illness, and "is empirically inaccurate and inadequate in other ways as well" (Scull, 1976: 178) as a rationale for deinstitutionalization.

Historical irony adds to the confusion. The first major change in mental health practice, which some refer to as the first psychiatric revolution, was the establishment of the mental hospital or asylum. After many years of legal and legislative battles, twenty-eight of the thirty-three states established state mental hospitals during the first half of the nineteenth century. The Jacksonian period brought with it an air of uncritical optimism that took over the field of mental health as well as most other areas of society. In the newly emerging asylums, the medical superintendents were projecting 100 percent cure rates (Arnhoff, 1975: 1278). According to Bassuk and Gerson (1978: 47), "by 1900 more than 100 new state institutions were built." Rothman (1971: 110) describes their orientation to mental illness as complex, if not contradictory. On the one hand, "every general practitioner in the pre-Civil War era agreed that insanity was a disease of the brain," while, on the other,

> medical superintendents' explorations of the origins of insanity took them into practically every aspect of antebellum society, from economic organization to political and religious practices, from family habits to patterns of thought and education. And little of what they saw pleased them . . . . Everywhere they looked, they found chaos and disorder, a lack of fixity and stability. The community's inherited traditions and procedures were dissolving, leaving incredible stresses and strains. (Rothman, 1971: 114)

After more than a hundred years we have come full circle, and the new revolution in psychiatry is necessary to deal with the problems posed by the old one. Physicians still believe that insanity is a disease either of the brain or in it, but the focus of problem analysis in the new era is also on the environment, if only on the environment of the asylum (Goffman, 1961). Essentially, the medical view of mental illness has gone unchanged, and the transformation that did take place was one of type rather than kind—one in which the same basic types of service would be delivered through a new community-based delivery system. Put another way, the nature of the change was to move predominantly old, medically defined, inpatient services to new outpatient facilities. The hospital came under attack as if it somehow existed independently of the profession that managed it, proclaimed its virtues, and supervised its decline, while always rationalizing its existence—a process that allowed for continued medical control. A further irony, which Bassuk and Gerson (1978: 47) note, is that the initial development of the new state hospitals was economically motivated; they were seen as a cost-effective treatment setting that was preferable to smaller but more numerous county institutions.

Community Mental Health Centers: Policy and the Program

At the center of the new federal master plan for preventing mental illness, preventing chronicity, and restoring long-term patients to community life was the comprehensive community mental health center (CMHC). Mobilization of political support for this service delivery system was tremendous, since the program had received some earlier stimulus from innovators within the mental health system (Milbank Memorial Fund, 1959).

The CMHCs were charged in the first legislation with providing five essential services (inpatient, outpatient, partial hospitalization, emergency services, and consultation and education). They were to provide aftercare services for those released from institutions, provide alternative short-term inpatient service for those who had to be hospitalized, and reduce the need for hospitalization by providing emergency services to people in crisis. The CMHCs were the heart of a federal program of grants to support the construction of facilities and, later, for staffing.

Each CMHC was designed to serve a gerrymandered geographic area or catchment with a population of 75,000 to 200,000 people. (For a critical discussion of the neglect to define the key term "catchment" adequately, see Panzetta, 1971.) The National Institute of Mental Health estimated in 1963 that it would take approximately 1500 such centers to serve the entire population of the United States. The rate at which they were established has been slowed somewhat over the years, but "as of July, 1975, NIMH had awarded construction and/or staffing grants of $1.2 billion to 603 CMHC's. When all 603 CMHC's become operational, they will serve areas covering about 41 percent of the U.S. population. As of July, 1975, 507 CMHC's were in operation" (Comptroller General, 1977: 68).

Problems with the CMHC Program

Although the fact received little attention from the media or from policymakers during the first ten years of the community mental health center movement, most activity inspired by community mental health care and brought about by federal policy was at the level of the state, where deinstitutionalization proceeded rapidly after 1963. The data from the comptroller general's five-state study (Table 1) show that the inpatient population declined by 38 to 84 percent. Data from the state of New York, where the number of patients decreased from over 90,000 in 1955 to 39,223 in 1974, confirm this picture (Lander, 1975: 19). Bassuk and Gerson's (1978: 49) data from 1955 to 1975 are also consistent with these estimates: "There was a 65 percent decrease in the census of resident patients in state mental hospitals, from 559,000 to 193,000."

TABLE 1

Decline in Mentally Ill Inpatient Population, 1963–1974

State	Population		Reduction	
	1963	1974	Number	Percent
Maryland	8,100	5,000	3,100	38
Massachusetts	17,500	6,000	11,500	66
Michigan	20,100	6,000	14,100	70
Nebraska	3,700	600	3,100	84
Oregon	4,060	1,260	2,800	69
Total	53,460	18,860	34,600	65

Source: Comptroller General, 1977: 9.

The same pattern appears to have continued from 1963 to the present. As CMHCs were expanding in size and number, state hospitals were housing fewer and fewer inpatients and, in some cases, even being phased out of existence (Chase, 1973). According to public testimony by NIMH officials, a decrease in state hospital populations and the phasing out of these institutions were a main goal of the CMHC program and its primary justification (Chu, 1974: 777). From the beginning, the CMHC movement was portrayed as a means of reducing state hospital populations by 50 percent within ten years. Sources as widely disparate as, on the one hand, NIMH and the comptroller general's office, and, on the other, the Nader group and Scull, present similar evidence. Its implication is clear: thus far, in relation to its primary goal and its essential rationale, the CMHC program has failed.

A team of NIMH researchers reported in 1973 that they could not establish a clear and consistent relation between CMHC development and change in the inpatient population at state psychiatric hospitals (Musto, 1975: 69). The comptroller general's report states:

> NIMH data on sources of referrals to CMHCs also indicate that the CMHC program was having only a limited impact on reducing public mental hospital populations. For example, for 1974 NIMH reported that about 29,300, or about 3.8 percent of the 780,400 additions to CMHC's were referred by public mental hospitals. Public mental hospitals accounted for fewer referrals to CMHCs than any other referral source reported, except for the clergy. (Comptroller General, 1977: 69)

This same report (1977: 72) contains a further indictment of the CMHC program:

> In general, the CMHC program has developed apart from the public hospital system. Many CMHCs did not view reducing the use of State mental hospitals as a primary goal and therefore did not direct much effort toward this goal. The lack of a formal link between the CMHCs and the public mental hospitals helped fragment responsibility for the mentally ill released from mental hospitals. It also appears to have hindered the accomplishment of two CMHC program goals—reducing the use of mental hospitals and providing a coordinated system of care for the mentally ill.

The Nader group report (Chu and Trotter, 1974) makes the same charges. Chu, its co-author, concluded (1974: 775)

> that community mental health centers have largely failed to fulfill any of their major stated goals. They have not supplanted state hospitals; they are not usually accessible. . . . They have continued the two class (rich and poor) system of care by frequent exclusion of indigent patients as well as those with the most severe problems . . . and centers are not held accountable to NIMH, which means they continue to receive NIMH funds whether or not they are fulfilling NIMH goals.

Providing Aftercare

On March 1, 1976, the New York State Assembly's Joint Committee to Study the Department of Mental Hygiene submitted *Mental Health in New York,* a comprehensive study of public mental health services; it did not even mention CMHCs as pertinent to public mental health care in the state or in programs it surveyed in four other states. The direction of the 1975 amendments to the federal CMHC legislation, providing for the development of aftercare in supportive living environments and a series of related services coordinated by the CMHCs, also failed to influence CMHC practice substantially, as the comptroller general's report indicates. How can we account for this phenomenon? How can a major mental health policy, articulated by the federal government and supported by the state governments, have no direct bearing on the bulk of publicly funded mental health care in the public sector?

This last question is a difficult, but necessary, one to pursue. What makes it difficult is the apparent failure of deinstitutionalization policies to provide even minimally adequate aftercare and community support services anywhere in the nation. Instead, the rhetoric of deinstitutionalization seems to mask a brutal political and economic reality—the general abandonment of mentally disabled people who have been further debilitated, mentally and physically, by institutionalization. Evidence indicates that the new policy has brought with it a new set of mental health problems, including massive numbers of people needing rehospitalization; gross inadequacies in community resources for aftercare and rehabilitation; large-scale scandal, exploitation, and abuse in the new industry of operating community facilities; increased drug and alcohol dependency among released patients; and an apparent social and psychological decay among patients released into nursing homes, adult homes, or "welfare hotels." The extent to which this last provocative claim is accurate was made clear by a special prosecutor appointed by the state of New York to investigate abuse in the nursing home and adult home industries. His report severely criticized the concept of community mental health care and cited the failure of federal, state, or local officials to develop adequate community-based services for former patients: "The discharge of mental patients from psychiatric hospitals without insuring the delivery of aftercare services makes deinstitutionalization a procedure for patient aban-

donment, rather than a progressive program of patient care"
(Hynes, 1977: 41).

Organizational Coordination

Abandonment of organizational responsibility, as well as of patients,
characterizes deinstitutionalization:

> Deinstitutionalization has not received the full and well-coordinated
> support of many State and local agencies administering programs that
> serve or can serve the mentally disabled. Moreover, agencies serving
> population groups that do or could include the mentally disabled have
> not included deinstitutionalization of the mentally disabled in their
> program plans nor have they made it a specific operating objective or
> priority. Furthermore, they have not provided financial or other sup-
> port needed to help mentally disabled persons (1) avoid unnecessary
> admission or readmission to public institutions, (2) leave such facilities,
> or (3) receive appropriate help in communities. (Comptroller General,
> 1977: 24)

Mental health departments have refused responsibility for
housing, welfare, or medical or other social needs, while other agencies were frequently not involved in discharge planning or in the
development of joint programs. In a study of nine cities that focused
on interagency cooperation and coordination, made when CMHCs
were growing most rapidly, Warren, Rose, and Bergunder (1974)
found that community mental health agencies were the least competent or interested in initiating or responding to invitations to collab-
orate, while other agencies demonstrated interest only in protecting
or enhancing their own domains.

The effect of the agencies' attitudes has been disastrous for
former patients and for the communities into which they have been
placed in large numbers, yet no practical mechanism for assuring
that agencies will carry out their responsibilities has emerged.
Thompson (1975: 60) notes, "Anyone who has spent any time
evaluating residential care is aware of the inadequacy of many of
these facilities. Often this inadequacy is not openly discussed by
mental health policy makers for fear that somehow it will be blamed
on them." Reich and Siegal (1973: 54) argue pointedly that "no
adequately prepared organizations or facilities exist to handle all of
the new dischargees." They conclude (1973: 55) that the policy

originally perceived as radically innovative and humane has turned into its opposite: "To discharge helpless, sick people into the street is inhumane and contributes to the decline of the quality of life in the urban environment." The overall effect of the policy prompted the *New York Times* to say that deinstitutionalization has served to transfer the back wards to the back alleys (Musto, 1975: 70).

The Role of Drugs

As if this problem were not complex enough, the debate intensifies when we turn to the role of psychoactive and/or neuroleptic drugs. As already mentioned, substantial data indicate that the process of discharge began in 1955, after such drugs were introduced into some hospitals, but well before they came to be seen as the panacea for mental illness. Bellak (1964: 3), an ardent proponent of community mental health programs, is hesitant to call the drugs a cure-all but says that "nevertheless, they have made community psychiatry a reality." Musto (1975: 70) supports this contention, but from a more critical stance: "The hospital census has been reduced by means ranging from hospitals' abundant use of drugs to the massive discharge of patients, many of them elderly, to proprietary nursing and foster homes." Perhaps the most powerful indictment comes from within the ranks of psychiatry, in a paper by Crane (1973: 124):

> In the last decade, hospital beds have been increasingly phased out; and, to take their place, new community mental health centers have been opened or existing facilities have been expanded throughout the nation. According to the medical profession, this new program for the treatment of the mentally ill would not have been possible without neuroleptics. . . . Inadequate programs for the management of these mentally handicapped persons have created new and unexpected problems, and, in an effort to solve them, the psychiatric community has become more and more dependent on the use of neuroleptic agents. One of the consequences of this reliance on psychopharmacology has been the tendency to minimize the potential danger of long-term exposure to powerful chemical agents. Thus, permanent neurological disorders have become very common among patients treated with neuroleptics, but little effort has been made to come to grips with this problem.

231

Bockoven and Solomon designed a study to compare two groups of patients discharged from psychiatric hospitals, one before the current levels of drug use and one after. The study was based on two five-year follow-up evaluations, the first between 1947 and 1952, and the second between 1967 and 1972. They found no substantial difference between the two groups, an unexpected result "in view of the absence of psychotropic drugs during the entire five years [of the first study], compared with extensive use of psychotropic drugs . . . for both initial treatment on admission and the entire period of aftercare" (Bockoven and Solomon, 1975: 800). The failure of community mental health agencies to develop adequate or appropriate aftercare programs is linked by these authors (1975: 801) to overfixation on drugs: "The presence of adequate rehabilitation and social maintenance programs would decrease the tendency to rely on psychotropic drugs as the mainstay of aftercare."

In the eyes of these and other critics, drug dependence is more a problem of the profession prescribing them than of the population seduced or coerced into taking them. According to Crane (1973: 125), "drugs are prescribed to solve all types of management problems, and failure to achieve the desired results causes an escalation of dosage, changes of drugs and polypharmacy." Neuroleptics are used to control behavior or to facilitate management, and to solve psychological, social, administrative, and other difficulties that are nonmedical in nature. Scull (1976: 86) calls this drug dependence "the technological fix" and argues that the research methodology used to justify the use of such drugs was shabby and unscientific. Research conducted by Tobias and MacDonald in 1974 confirms this assertion; on the basis of forty studies, they concluded "that because of methodological flaws, no inferences can be drawn" (see Scheff, 1976: 303).

The situation would be bad enough if the only problem were overzealous use of drugs by a profession that depends on them to produce manageable behavior in patients so that state hospital beds can be emptied in response to political policy. Unfortunately, the problem is deeper: long-term use of such drugs as the phenothiazines may prolong social dependency and create harmful and irreversible neurological damage. Crane (1973: 127) notes that the predominant form of this damage, usually called tardive dyskinesia, has been attributed to psychotropic drugs for at least ten years and that more than a hundred papers had been published about it by 1973, but with little impact on the profession of psychiatry. Gardos and Cole support this view. From their review of the literature, they conclude that as many as 50 per cent of the chronic patients discharged to aftercare "may not need to be on antipsychotics, either because they would do well without medication or because they would not do well on drugs for reasons including failure to find optimum drug or dose level, noncompliance, or toxicity" (Gardos and Cole, 1976: 34). They also discuss tardive dyskinesia, and speculate that the number of people neurologically damaged by this by-product of psychotropic medicines may be larger than has previously been estimated, because the ailment can exist in a suppressed form while the drug is still being taken.

Among the other failures of drug-dependent aftercare is the refusal to acknowledge the relation among barren, empty lives created by massive discharges into hostile communities, grossly underdeveloped community support services, and increasingly high levels of rehospitalization. Recidivism rates rose nationally from 47 percent in 1969 to 54 percent by 1972 (Comptroller General, 1977: 22). In New York, the figures are even higher, reaching almost 65 percent in 1974 (Lander, 1975: 2–3), compared with 27 percent in 1955. Since admissions have doubled in the same period, the actual number of people released from hospitals is awesome. According to Bassuk and Gerson (1978: 49), "admissions to state hospitals increased from 178,000 in 1955 to a peak of 390,000 in 1972 and had declined only to 375,000 by 1974. . . . Moreover, a growing proportion of the admissions were readmissions (in 1972, 64 percent of them): about half of the released patients are readmitted within a year of discharge."

In spite of the severe problems produced by deinstitutionalization, and in spite of criticism of the quality of life available to former patients discharged without either support systems or adequate social and financial resources, the policy and practice continue. Someone must benefit from them; since evidently it is not the former patients, it seems logical to examine the costs and benefits to the states that are closing the back wards of their psychiatric hospitals.

Economic Reality

As indicated in the early sections of this paper, a different perception of deinstitutionalization can be based on political and economic analysis. Its proponents' essential argument is that the policy of deinstitutionalization is best understood as a political and economic measure designed primarily to sustain near-bankrupt state governments and to establish the basis for transferring funds from public services to the private sector. Before the passage of community mental health legislation and the funding of the CMHC program, mental health services were paid for almost exclusively by state tax dollars. The adherents of the political-economic view note that the rising level of admissions to state hospitals, estimated to be a 100 percent increase between 1955 and 1972 (Musto, 1975: 70), would have added to the states' already substantial fiscal burden the necessity for undertaking new capital construction. As early as 1955, they point out, state governments were able "to maneuver to obtain the cost savings it offered. Some of the largest savings immediately realizable came from the cancellation of planned new construction, and decisions to do this were widespread" (Scull, 1977: 139).

Further savings would be realized through increasing federal involvement, which stimulated discharges and attempted to encourage the shifting of funds from inpatient care to outpatient or aftercare. The 1965 Social Security amendments, for example, enacted Medicare and Medicaid programs that included coverage for skilled nursing-home care to facilitate the discharge of older people to private facilities; they supported inpatient treatment of elderly mentally ill patients in general medical hospitals and funds for outpatient psychiatric care. In addition,

> the act authorized inpatient mental hospital benefits for the mentally ill. This was to encourage States to discharge the elderly who, with financial assistance and supportive services, were able to live in the community. It was intended that the Federal assistance for the institutionalized mentally ill would enable the States to shift their funds to developing alternatives to care in mental hospitals and to improve the care provided in such facilities to help persons return to communities. (Comptroller General, 1977: 207–208)

Many states did not do this. In New York, in 1974, the average part of mental health budgets allocated to aftercare was 6.5 percent; at Pilgrim State, the largest hospital, the amount was only 1.1 percent (Legislative Commission on Expenditure Review, 1975).

In 1966, the amendments to the Comprehensive Health Planning and Public Health Services Act mandated that at least 15 percent of state formula grant allotments for public health services be directed toward community-based mental health services. This legislation was the forerunner to the 1967 Partnership for Health amendments, which required that at least 70 percent of public health services funds for mental health be set aside for providing services in communities (Comptroller General, 1977: 210).

Financial Incentives to Deinstitutionalization

In 1972, through the Social Security amendments, the federal government further stimulated state governments to make discharge and early release their mental health policies, and intensified the growing tendency to replace state hospital wards with private skilled nursing facilities (SNF) or intermediate care facilities (ICF). This legislation "provided for financial penalties on States not implementing effective programs for controlling unnecessary use of mental hospitals, skilled nursing facilities, and ICFs, including institutions for the retarded" (Comptroller General, 1977: 213). The Supplemental Security Income (SSI) program was also authorized under the 1972 amendments but did not begin as a standard program of federal assistance until 1974. It provided the funding for cost-of-living payments to discharged patients at a level beyond what the Aid to Disabled program was able to do. Other legislation in 1975 (Social Security, Special Health Revenue Sharing, CMHC amendments) continued to stimulate community-based services, empty state hospitals, and transfer funds from public to private sector facilities and programs.

The states were in a position to act on humane policy promises, while reducing the overall proportion of state expenses devoted to mental health and shifting the cost of care from state to federal funds. A major saving resulted from discharging large numbers of mental patients from the state hospitals. One estimate (Comptroller General, 1977: 5) of the annual average cost of caring for a person in a public mental hospital in 1974 was $11,250. In New York, during the same period, the cost per person was $13,835. The cost of outpatient care in New York, or aftercare combined with outpatient care, during 1974 was $531 per person per year of state mental health department funds. This fantastic saving was offset somewhat by the fact that a person discharged from the hospital was necessarily referred to SSI; this meant that residents of New York who were placed in adult homes received a monthly check of $386.70 (before October 1, 1977, when an additional $18.00 of personal allowance money was added). The monthly cost to the state for each SSI recipient living in an adult home was $219.00, while the federal share was $167.70. On an annual basis, the cost to the state of New York for such a person consisted of $2,628 of SSI funds (or less if the person was placed in a boarding home or hotel), plus $531 of mental health funds. If an overestimate of $1,500 is added for various services, the total still comes to just over $4,600, some $9,000 less than the annual per person cost of hospitalization. In New York alone there are 50,000 fewer inpatients in 1979 than there were in 1968, and more than 65,000 fewer than in 1955; the amount of state money saved thus becomes all too apparent as a motivation for complying with federal incentives to deinstitutionalize. In 1968 dollars, the amount saved would be somewhere in the vicinity of $585 million per year, without projections of the additional costs from rising admissions figures and possible capital construction.

A number of studies of savings as a result of community-based care have been made in the past five years. Ironically, most of them do not specify that total costs, including those incurred by the federal government, have gone up, and that one major reason for overall increases involves paying for profit margins assumed by private-sector domination of the residential market for housing dischargees from state hospitals, a point discussed below. The comptroller general's office reviewed a number of cost-benefit studies and discussed the findings in its report. Three factors were selected as central to reducing the cost to the public: housing, employability, and primary source of funds; for instance, the cost of community care could be greater than the cost of state hospital care when the person involved was in an intensive-care setting or a private facility, unemployable, and dependent on public funds for support. Overall, however, savings were substantial—an average net saving of $20,800 per person, with one state showing a saving of $39,400, both calculated over a ten-year period (Comptroller General, 1977: 5). These figures include the costs of skilled nursing and intermediate-care facilities, which lower the savings substantially when compared with the costs of adult homes or boarding home situations. In New York in 1976, a relatively small percentage of people were placed in such high-cost facilities rather than in nonmedical group residences or boarding homes. Using the national average, however, multiplied by the number of inpatients discharged since 1965, we can see that an estimated cost savings to the *states* in the ten-year period from 1965 to 1974 would be approximately $5.4 billion, again without regard to accelerated admissions rates and added capital construction costs.

The cost-benefit analysis cited by the comptroller general's office, which estimated that $20,800 per person would be saved over a ten-year period, was prepared by Murphy and Datel (1976). They based their calculations on criteria for deinstitutionalization that included comprehensive and continuing care in a community setting, progress toward independent living, and improved integration of community services. They also pointed out that the client population was made up of "successful" cases of discharge: "Recidivists were dropped from the analysis, as were clients likely to be reinstitutionalized, since they represented a failure in the community services system" (Murphy and Datel, 1976: 166). They reached two conclusions: first, that "federal sources are shown to carry much of the load on maintaining deinstitutionalized clients," and, second, that "benefits accruing to state funding sources through deinstitutionalization far exceed those accruing to federal funding sources" (Murphy and Datel, 1976: 166). A third conclusion is warranted: given the stipulations, the savings are grossly understated. This finding is supported by a comparative study by Sheehan and Atkinson of the costs of services in Texas. The authors concluded: "The real beneficiaries of the present system are the state legislatures, as the cost of supporting community inpatient services and state hospital backup care for those who need it is less than the cost of providing inpatient care through the state hospital alone" (Sheehan and Atkinson, 1974: 244).

In the apparent trade-off made in federal intervention into state budgets and mental health policies, budget aid is exchanged for more centralized decision making and for control over private sector involvement. Each time the federal government became more involved in the deinstitutionalization process, states saved money in exchange for discharging patients, contracting with the private sector to use public funds, and indenturing themselves to federal control through participation in shared funding programs such as SSI, Medicare and Medicaid, and Health Revenue Sharing. In order to save dollars for other state purposes, the state budgetary process has become dependent on federal funds. What would happen to state fiscal capability if the federal government were to withdraw from or be unable to maintain contributions to SSI, Medicaid, and other programs? Given the federal government's fiscal power over the determination of policy and programs, if required, the social control apparatus of the states has become absorbed into the larger control needs of the federal government.

The Private Sector Interests

The issue of the private sector has yet to be discussed. Its interest has been to invest in mental health service provision and/or other activities, which until deinstitutionalization were publicly funded. The success of private sector interests, both large- and small-scale, can be comprehended by remembering that hundreds of thousands of people have come into and been discharged from state hospitals since 1955, and many of them have had no family or other resources to rely on for housing or other services. Nursing homes, intermediate care facilities, adult homes, old hotels, and boarding home operations became a booming economic investment. The results in hard money terms are substantial: "Data from a survey completed in April, 1974, by the National Center for Health Statistics, HEW, showed a 48 percent increase in the number of nursing home residents with mental disabilities since 1969—from 607,400 to 899,500" (Comptroller General, 1977: 11).

The extent of fraud and other forms of criminal exploitation of nursing home residents in the state of New York prompted the governor to appoint a special commission to investigate the situation, and then a special prosecutor to follow up that investigation. Whether or not the individual owners were honest in reporting charges, the growth and income of this industry are phenomenal: "According to NIMH estimates, nursing homes are the largest single place of care for the mentally ill. They represent 29.3 percent, or $4.2 billion, of the estimated total direct care costs for the mentally ill of $14.5 billion in 1974" (Comptroller General, 1977: 11). To claim any value for deinstitutionalization, in light of the proportion of people placed in nursing homes, is even more ludicrous when we realize that far more than 50 percent of the nursing homes are larger in size than the back wards of the state hospitals from which the patients came; according to data collected in 1974 on nursing home residents, more than half were placed in homes with 100 or more beds, while an additional 15 percent were placed in homes with more than 200 beds (Comptroller General, 1977: 16). Critics refer to this practice as reinstitutionalization (as opposed to recidivism or rehospitalization). My argument is not against nursing homes or intermediate care facilities as such; certainly some people do need extensive medical supervision. Rather, my point is that such care is not related to the rhetoric of community living and need not be part of the profit market.

After nursing homes had been established as a successful enterprise and as a corollary of deinstitutionalization, the numbers of patients being discharged did not diminish: different types of facilities emerged to house them, with lowered levels of care provided and smaller SSI payments allocated. Given lower profit margins, the market factor required that larger numbers of people be placed. The results, particularly for former patients and "oversaturated" communities, have become commonplace. Reich and Siegal (1973: 46) describe the situation in New York:

> Several private entrepreneurs saw in the policies of the State Department of Mental Hygiene an opportunity for financial gain. Under the facade of community service they refurbished unsuccessful old hotels and motels and arranged with the state hospitals to accept any patients the hospitals wished to discharge. The result is that many of these proprietary homes have become unsupervised state hospitals. Many of the patients were on high doses of tranquilizers, causing them to be apathetic, disinterested, and unable to function at any level. Young mental hospital dischargees became isolated in the homes because they were unable to relate to the average age of the other residents (over 65). Patients gathered in the lobby, gazing blankly into space, rocking back and forth, staring at a television set which had been turned off. If the clients deteriorated in proprietary homes, they were often turned out on the street when the state hospitals did not re-admit them.

In the four years after that was written, the situation continued to deteriorate, prompting the *Village Voice* on October 31, 1977, to run the headline, "State Abandons Mentally Ill to City Street."

The Nader group reported similar findings: "Mounting evidence from around the country indicates that large numbers of patients are being transferred en masse to nursing or so-called foster homes or welfare hotels, where conditions are frequently worse than those in state hospitals" (Chu, 1974: 777). Rather than rely on discharge numbers as an indication of progressive development, Lamb and Goertzel (1971: 29) asked in a follow-up study, "To what extent have [former patients] shed their mental patient role and identity?" Investigating the typical placement in California boarding homes, they concluded:

> These facilities are in most respects like long-term state hospital wards isolated from the community. One is overcome by the depressing atmosphere, not because of the physical appearance of the boarding home, but because of the passivity, isolation and inactivity of the residents. . . . Thus, boarding homes are for the most part structured so that they maximize the state-hospital-like atmosphere. The boarding home operator usually needs or wants a group of quiet, docile, "good" patients. The monetary reward system of the boarding home encourages this, for the operator is being paid by the head, rather than being rewarded for rehabilitation efforts. (Lamb and Goertzel, 1971: 31)

Chase (1973) discovered one chain of board and care homes that had thirty-eight facilities in California alone, twenty-five elsewhere, twelve general hospitals, and other holdings yielding a net revenue in 1972 of $79.5 million. In the context of profit, and of the mental health or public welfare agencies' refusal to take responsibility for following up, inspecting, and raising charges against exploitative landlords, or for providing services, most former patients have been left to survive on their own, whether in a single room in a former resort hotel, in a nursing home or intermediate care facility, or in a boarding home. The bleak nature of their everyday lives constitutes what Klerman (1974: 786) has called a trend toward community chronicity, or marginal social existence and psychological disability maintained in a community residence, but apart from other people.

The abuse, leading to state investigations and federal congressional hearings, has become so widespread that it has paralleled the general medical abuse of Medicaid and Medicare programs, but without many of the useful services they delivered. In surveying the extent of transfers from state hospitals to private nursing and adult homes, Scull (1977: 150) concluded:

> One indirect consequence of decarceration has been a much greater involvement of the private sector in spheres of social control which were formerly the exclusive province of the state. The pattern of socialization of loss and the privitization of profit, already well established in the military-industrial complex, is now imprinting itself on new areas of social existence. Particularly in America, an effort is under way to

transform "social junk" into a commodity from which various "professionals" and entrepreneurs can extract a profit. Medicare and the nursing home racket are merely the largest and most blatant examples of this practice.

Conclusions

The Medical Paradigm

In *The Structure of Scientific Revolutions,* Thomas Kuhn (1970) discusses the notion of a "paradigm," which he defines as a set of theoretical assumptions that arise to explain enigmatic phenomena and, if they fit the needs and interests in a field, gradually become accepted as reality itself. Put another way, once room is made within the social structure and ideological framework in a given area, the new paradigm emerges to redefine that field. Once it is accepted, the underlying structure of assumptions begins to recede from conscious concern into the background, where it retains its explanatory potency but is increasingly submerged as what has now become "normal" thought and practice. Changes that develop over time turn out, in fact, to be marginal, methodological, or incremental, and uniformly within the paradigm-receded-from-consciousness. Even evaluations of theory and methodology remain bound by the paradigm, capable of assessing only the efficiency rather than the nature of a given practice.

In the social development of a field, the paradigm expands in this way until it confronts an irreconcilable internal or external problem; either scientific "anomalies" or unanswerable questions arise, or the social utility of the paradigm is called into question. In either case, but particularly in the latter, either a significant qualitative change will occur (what Kuhn considers a "scientific revolution"), or the reigning paradigm will successfully, yet temporarily, co-opt or incorporate the threat. According to Berger and Luckmann's (1967: 24) description of this effort, "Even the unproblematic sector of everyday reality is so only until further notice, that is, until its continuity is interrupted by the appearance of a problem. When this happens, the reality of everyday life seeks to integrate the problematic sector into what is already unproblematic." Perhaps it will be useful to briefly examine deinstitutionalization in this context.

At the level of overarching paradigms or large-scale assumption structures related to the person in our society, the theme of individualism is important; it is an accounting of an individual's well-being—or lack of it—based on the interrelated conception of the person's motivation, behavior, and psychological make-up. *In Mental Illness and the Economy,* Brenner (1973: 245) puts it this way:

> The general cultural theme of individualism has had a pervasive impact on our understanding of both mental hospitalization and economic success and failure. Traditionally, it has been taken for granted that, since the mentally hospitalized patient is psychiatrically ill, mental hospitalization could be explained in accordance with prevailing theories of mental illness. These theories assumed that mental illness could be described within two broad categories, functional and organic. . . . In both of these models, the broad social environment was largely ignored.

Brenner points out the parallels in "common-sense" knowledge about individual behavior (health versus sickness) and economic position (success versus failure), identifying as a common thread disregard of the historical development of the social and economic order.

What is implied in this assumption is that, since individuals are internally accountable or responsible for their behavior, within the prevailing paradigm, responses to social or economic behavior are typically also based on premises about the individual, or about aggregates of individuals presumed to be similar by virtue of their social behavior or economic position. Furthermore, economic stability (or lack of it) or economic policy is unrelated to individual emotional or psychological condition. In the case of mental illness, the causal relations assumed to exist are only between observed behaviors classified as symptoms and the disease categories that have been created as aggregates of or receptacles for those same symptoms.

In the field of mental health, the reigning paradigm has incorporated the individualist theme from the broader ideology and historically redesignated it in medical and/or psychological terms, having appropriated the territory from an earlier individualistic definition of demonic possession. Whether the individual defect in the person has been considered organic or psychological, the dominant medical perspective has continuously claimed it as within the province of medical control, and designed for it various organic or psychotherapeutic methods of treatment aimed primarily at the person or, at best, his or her family environment. As mentioned earlier, medical determination of the best methods of treatment has consistently been regulated by the economic needs of the state; this relationship began with the founding of the state asylums and continued through their expansion into unwieldy and costly custodial warehouses to their present dismantling. At the same time, both the medical establishment and the state government have claimed that the economic basis for change was in fact a response to a therapeutic innovation that gave rise to the organizational rearrangements that followed.

The historical development of community mental health care follows this pattern almost exactly. The state hospitals, claimed by some to be the results of the first psychiatric revolution, were established at a time of rising medical influence, which was superseded by the emergence of the states as entities economically more viable than localities. The nineteenth century saw the asylum movement and its initial premise of "moral treatment" give way to custodial care and the preliminary notions of maintenance therapy. Around the turn of the century, when moral treatment was believed medically bankrupt but the asylums and hospitals were considered socially useful, organic and functional descriptions of psychoses emerged as paramount. This change in approach is tantamount to incorporating a problem posed within a paradigm into an acceptable degree of advancement of practice. The development of the psychoanalytic tradition, still grounded in the paradigm of individual defectiveness, created a brief period of internecine or intramural struggle, still bounded by medical domination. Throughout the twentieth century, we have seen the demise of all hope for mental hospitals as curative or restorative institutions, but we are far from universally understanding why they have been substantially diminished.

From within the prevailing medical paradigm of mental health, not surprisingly, the rationale for reducing inpatient populations and creating a community mental health policy is treated as a therapeutic innovation. According to this outlook, the internal problems posed by the acceptance of institutionalization as the preferred therapeutic tool for severe mental illness led to the development of a new model. The organizational rearrangements that ensued, in other words, came about because of a humanitarian thrust from within. Community mental health care was a "natural development," so to speak, of the continuous search for better methods of treatment, another example of internal readjustment, this time to an externally imposed challenge to the utility of the paradigm. Aiding this process of internal adaptation was the factor of general social legitimation; that is, medical control over mental health problems had gained social acceptance, or acquiescence, even if its current practices were being scrutinized and threatened from political and economic standpoints.

Those bound by this confined orientation toward social and economic reality eagerly point to the more than 50 percent reduction in inpatient populations of state hospitals within one decade as a victory. What they cannot account for so successfully is the utter failure to accomplish the other goals: primary prevention (that is, the prevention of mental illness), the prevention of hospitalization, or the prevention of rehospitalization. What they cannot comprehend is their own social-historical nature and that of their location within the same social context as their patients. They therefore cannot perceive that economic necessity, which Brenner and others have shown to be correlated with mental hospitalization rates, has been as directly correlated to the demise of the state hospital system as it has been to the incidence of mental disablement or dysfunctioning. They also find it difficult to see that the present organizational rearrangements—the decline of the hospital system and the related rise of the CMHCs—were precipitated by economic and political factors, rather than the reverse: in this view, the mental health professions see themselves as the tail wagging the dog.

The policy of deinstitutionalization demonstrates the power of reigning and socially stabilizing paradigms; organizational rearrangements are made in the name of humane social change, while, simultaneously, traditional orientations and practices are maintained in new settings. The lives of the intended beneficiaries of the change continue to be interpreted in medical terms, but only until problems can no longer be avoided. The contemporary problem, which creates all the criticism of community mental health care, is the twofold failure of the CMHCs: to prevent new hospital admissions and to sustain discharged patients in the community. These two factors, like the problems posed by institutionalization, have relevance both internal and external to the mental health professions. Internal problems are posed by recidivism and the failure of the CMHCs to deal adequately with state hospital dischargees, while the failure of the new methods to control costs brought about by new admissions and recidivism, coupled with inflation, is external. The situation of economic necessity giving rise to political intervention remains as unseen now as it was in 1961, the last time a presidential commission reported its findings.

We will soon enter another new era in the field of mental health, one that will be presented with some of the same enthusiasm and rhetoric as the last. The "new" new era, already on the horizon with offices in NIMH and small-scale projects in a limited number of states, is that of Community Support Systems (CSS) programs. This new development is obviously an effort to recognize the failures of the old new era to anticipate and plan for concrete problems of daily life among those pushed out of hospitals into deprived and exploitative living environments. Utilizing the comptroller general's criticism of community mental health care, the new program has moved forward with tremendous energy to induce the federal government and the states to consolidate and increase efforts among various agencies, which have passed the buck from one to another in excusing failures to meet either therapeutic or economic expectations. The outcome of CSS programs, of course, cannot be predicted with great accuracy. We can speculate, however, that these programs, too, will fail to fulfill their stated objectives, to the extent that they are delegated to agencies restricted by the prevailing paradigm. Since that is at least the most likely outcome, the problems will remain. Much, if not most, of the energy of CSS program implementation will be devoted to what Kuhn called "mopping up operations," such as "demonstrating" extensive pathologies within individuals that prevent them from taking advantage of newly available service opportunities.

Deinstitutionalization as a Broader Issue

The analytic tasks required to comprehend deinstitutionalization become even more complex when we include the areas of mental retardation, delinquency, and adult corrections. Substantial diversity exists; in some cases, much more nonprofit housing and consumer involvement is present (as in the area of retardation), or diversion programs have become formalized as parts of the policy and program structure. How can we account for the varied patterns of utility and effectiveness of the same general policy with different groups of target populations? What has the experience been with juvenile delinquency and adult criminals? Perhaps most important, after analyzing deinstitutionalization as a social reform, how can we organize a system of reparations for those already considered its beneficiaries?

The questions raised here require a multidisciplinary, multifield investigation, one that compares the historical development of deinstitutionalization across the four policy and program fields, and focuses on the role of federal, state, and local governments, on rhetoric, policy development, and interorganizational relations, and on fiscal incentives. At the same time, it will also have to assess the role of the private sector and the voluntary agencies.

Finally, the role played by the courts must be examined. Although since 1972 they have systematically ruled in favor of deinstitutionalization for mentally ill and mentally retarded people, they have done so on the basis of material that asserted that community placement was, *by definition,* preferable to state hospital incarceration. Now that we know that such a conclusion is at best premature, and often incorrect, the role of the courts may change. Certainly that possibility was raised by the decision in a 1975 class action suit, *Dixon v. Weinberger,* in which a United States district court judge ordered a local government to finance the establishment of alternative facilities to the hospital and "accept responsibility for creating and paying for such community resources" (*Hospital and Community Psychiatry,* 1976: 205).

As Lottman (1976) points out, however, even progressive court victories stipulating efforts to design and provide adequate services have failed to yield the projected benefits because of their inability to define and implement adequate procedures to ensure compliance. Some of the recent court battles also indicate a hesitation or reluctance to challenge the psychiatric paradigm, whether traditional or contemporary. For example, court orders to place patients in the least restrictive alternative settings have been argued without adequate assessment of the quality of life in available community placements, while right-to-treatment cases serve to coerce states to put more money into conventional, psychiatrically defined, treatment modalities within state hospitals. The use of the courts, in other words, can either support or contest prevailing practices, depending on how aware plaintiffs and their lawyers are of the social context within which civil liberties cases are argued. As with existing policy and programs, even the evaluation of the role of the courts will ultimately depend on the conceptual paradigms used to construct the analysis.

References

Arnhoff, F. N. 1975. Social Consequences of Policy Toward Mental Illness. *Science* 188: 1277–1281.

Bassuk, E. L., and Gerson, S. 1978. Deinstitutionalization and Mental Health Services. *Scientific American* 238 (2): 46–53.

Bellak, L. 1964. *Handbook of Community Psychiatry and Community Mental Health.* New York: Grune and Stratton.

Berger, P., and Luckmann, T. 1966. *Social Construction of Reality: A Treatise in the Sociology of Knowledge.* Garden City, N.Y.: Doubleday.

Bockoven, J. S., and Solomon, H. C. 1975. Comparison of Two Five-Year Follow-Up Studies: 1947–1952 and 1967–1972. *American Journal of Psychiatry* 132: 796–801.

Brenner, M. H. 1973. *Mental Illness and the Economy.* Cambridge, Mass.: Harvard University Press.

Chase, J. 1973. Where Have All The Patients Gone? *Human Behavior* 2 (October): 14–21.

Chu, F. D. 1974. The Nader Report: One Author's Perspective. *American Journal of Psychiatry* 131: 775–779.

_____, and Trotter, S. 1974. *The Madness Establishment: Ralph Nader's Group Report on the National Institute of Mental Health.* New York: Grossman.

Comptroller General of the United States. 1977. *Returning The Mentally Disabled to the Community: Government Needs to Do More.* Washington, D.C.: Government Accounting Office.

Crane, G. E. 1973. Clinical Psychopharmacology in Its 20th Year. *Science* 181: 124–128.

Gardos, G., and Cole, J. O. 1976. Maintenance Antipsychotic Therapy: Is the Cure Worse than the Disease? *American Journal of Psychiatry* 133: 32–36.

Goffman, E. 1961. *Asylums: Essays on the Social Situation of Mental Patients and Other Inmates.* Garden City, N.Y.: Doubleday.

Hospital and Community Psychiatry. 1976. News and Notes, 27: 205–215.

Hynes, C. J. 1977. *Private Proprietary Homes for Adults: An Interim Report.* New York: New York Deputy Attorney General's Office.

Joint Commission on Mental Illness and Health. 1961. *Action for Mental Health.* New York: Basic Books.

Klerman, G. 1974. Current Evaluation Research on Mental Health Sciences. *American Journal of Psychiatry* 131: 783–788.

Kuhn, T. S. 1970. *The Structure of Scientific Revolutions.* Chicago: University of Chicago Press.

Lamb, H. R., and Goertzel, V. 1971. Discharged Mental Patients: Are They Really in the Community? *Archives of General Psychiatry* 24: 29–34.

Lander, L. 1975. The Mental Health Con Game. *Health/PAC Bulletin* 65 (July/August): 1–10, 16–24.

Legislative Commission on Expenditure Review. 1975. *Patients Released from State Psychiatric Centers.* Albany, N.Y.: State of New York.

Lottman, M. 1976. Paper Victories and Hard Realities. In Bradley, V., and Clarke, G., eds., *Paper Victories and Hard Realities: The Implementation of the Legal and Constitutional Rights of the Mentally Disabled.* Washington, D.C.: Georgetown University Health Policy Center.

Mechanic, D. 1969. *Mental Health and Social Policy.* Englewood Cliffs, N.J.: Prentice-Hall.

Milbank Memorial Fund. 1959. *Progress and Problems of Community Mental Health Services.* New York: Milbank Memorial Fund.

Murphy, J. G., and Datel, W. E. 1976. A Cost Benefit Analysis of Community versus Institutional Living. *Health and Community Psychiatry* 25 (March): 165–170.

Musto, D. 1975. Whatever Happened to Community Mental Health? *The Public Interest* 39 (Spring): 53–79.

New York State Assembly, Joint Committee to Study the Department of Mental Hygiene. 1975. *Mental Health in New York.* Albany: New York State Assembly.

Panzetta, A. F. 1971. *Community Mental Health: Myth and Reality.* Philadelphia: Lea and Febiger.

Reich, R., and Siegal, L. 1973. Psychiatry Under Siege: The Chronically Mentally Ill Shuffle to Oblivion. *Psychiatric Annals* 3 (November): 35–55.

Rose, S. M. 1972. *Betrayal of the Poor: The Transformation of Community Action.* Cambridge, Mass.: Schenkman.

Rothman, D. J. 1971. *Discovery of the Asylum: Social Order and Disorder in the New Republic.* Boston: Little, Brown.

Scheff, T. J. 1976. Medical Dominance: Psychoactive Drugs and Mental Health Policy. *American Behavioral Scientist* 19: 299–317.

Scull, A. T. 1976. Decarceration of the Mentally Ill: A Critical View. *Politics and Society* 6 (2): 173–212.

———. 1977. *Decarceration: Community and the Deviant: A Radical View.* Englewood Cliffs, N.J.: Prentice-Hall.

Sheehan, D. N., and Atkinson, J. 1974. Comparative Costs of State Hospitals and Community Based In-Patient Care in Texas. *Hospital and Community Psychiatry* 25: 242–244.

Thompson, S. 1975. Observations on After-Care from a Political Perspective. *Psychiatric Annals* 5: 187–189.

Warren, R. L., Rose, S. M., and Bergunder, A. F. 1974. *The Structure of Urban Reform.* Lexington, Mass.: D.C. Heath.

Address correspondence to: Stephen M. Rose, Ph.D., School of Social Welfare, State University of New York at Stony Brook, Stony Brook, New York 11794.

The Development of
Ambiguous Federal Policy:
Early and Periodic Screening,
Diagnosis and Treatment (EPSDT)

ANNE-MARIE FOLTZ

This paper examines why Congress's first major program for comprehensive health care to needy children took five years to begin even partial operation. An examination of the 1967 program's legislative history reveals that Congress paid little attention to EPSDT's implications: it was left ambiguous whether health (Title V) or welfare (Title XIX) would administer; costs were never clearly stated; eligibility and scope of services to be provided were left vague. Despite pressure from welfare rights interest groups, these ambiguities delayed the preparation of regulation and guidelines which never did succeed in resolving the question of overlapping jurisdiction and costs. In addition, many states' resistance to paying for the program further held up implementation.

The paper concludes that: (1) Congress's and HEW's unwillingness to face up to the real costs of health programs threatens long-term public and state support for such programs; (2) division of responsibility between health and welfare lessens the impact of a program; (3) grant-in-aid programs give states the power to distort the intent of federal health policies; and (4) where states fail to implement such policies, initiatives may pass to consumer advocacy groups.

In late 1967, the United States Congress passed the Early and Periodic Screening Diagnosis and Treatment (EPSDT) programs of the Social Security Act, potentially the most comprehensive child health care program the government had ever undertaken. However, this program was not implemented immediately; regulations emerged from the Department of Health, Education, and Welfare (HEW) only in November 1971; final guidelines were issued in 1972, and full implementation was deferred until July 1973. Even before that date, it was clear that most states would not comply with HEW's regulations and guidelines,[1] and as of December 1973, HEW (1974) reported that only half the states could be said to be implementing the program state-wide without problems.

[1] For example, in March 1973, the National Welfare Rights Organization in a letter to Caspar Weinberger, Secretary of HEW, cited "Massive non-compliance," based on HEW's own reports. See also Tolchin (1973) and Georgetown Law Journal (1971: 976).

M M F Q / Health and Society / *Winter 1975*

This paper will analyze what went on at the federal level to explain why these federal initiatives took so long to be carried out. Issues such as the cost of the program, the administering agency, and the extent of services and children to be served were not clarified in the legislation. The resulting ambiguities left the Department of Health, Education, and Welfare with the difficult, if not impossible, task of drawing up a set of regulations and guidelines which could satisfy administrators, state officials, interest groups, and Congress.

Background: Health Care for Children
Through Government Programs

Part of the ambiguity lay in the almost reluctant way in which the federal government had gotten into the business of providing health services to children. Programs had gradually been added to the federal responsibility and they varied greatly according to their emphasis. Some were concerned with preventive services, others with comprehensive care, still others with diagnosis and treatment of specific crippling diseases.

As Schlesinger (1967) has noted the first federal program to provide care for mothers and children through grants-in-aid to the states was the Sheppard-Towner Act of 1921. Its broad provisions for "promoting the welfare and hygiene of maternity and infancy" did not clarify what services were to be provided. Meanwhile the states and localities had developed on their own preventive care to limited groups of children through well-child conferences run by both voluntary and public agencies.

Screening as a federal policy goal appeared in the 1935 Social Security Act Title V legislation establishing a program for Crippled Children (CC). It sought to enable each state to extend and improve:

> such state services for locating crippled children, and for providing medical, surgical, corrective, and other services and care, and facilities for diagnosis, hospitalization, and aftercare, for children who are crippled or who are suffering from conditions which lead to crippling. . . . (Section 511)

To locate such children, some sort of screening procedure is implied. Locating crippled children or children with conditions which might lead to crippling could have taken one of two forms: either a broadly conceived interpretation to set up state-wide screening procedures, or a more narrowly defined one to set up registries of crippled children. The former, today known as "outreach," was not attempted by the states under this program. With the encouragement of the Children's Bureau, which administered the CC program, each state created registries of crippled children to demonstrate how many had been found. These registries proved to be more activity reports than reports on the health status of children and eventually most states dropped the registries.

Preventive care and screening were implicit in an equally important section of Title V, Maternal and Child Health Services, which was a successor to the Sheppard-Towner Act. In many states the legislation's goal of "promoting the health of mothers and children" was understood to mean not only the supervision of maternity clinics and hospitals, but also the promotion of well-child conferences. Thus, two types of screening developed from Title V: through MCH, the well-child conference; and through CC, registries of crippled children. Preventive care was provided by the MCH services through supervision of maternity clinics, through consultations with local health officials, and through the establishment of well-child conferences. Diagnosis and treatment were provided by the crippled children's program. However, by 1955 only 6.5 percent of the nation's children under 21 were reached by these programs (refer to Table 1).

During World War II, the Emergency Maternity and Infant Care program (EMIC) gave the states funds to carry out both curative and preventive services for wives and children of armed forces personnel in the lower pay grades. The well-child conferences of the Title V programs were expanded to care for the additional mothers and children. Despite the program's apparent success, it was nonetheless abandoned after the war with all the other emergency wartime programs (Sinai and Anderson, 1948).

The sixties saw the burgeoning of federally funded health programs for children as well as other age groups. The Title V programs were expanded to include federal grants for local projects: in 1963 the Maternity and Infant Care Projects provided funds for localities to carry out comprehensive maternity and infant care; in 1965 the Children and Youth Projects provided similarly to

TABLE 1

Children Served by Title V Maternal and Child Health
and Crippled Children's Programs and the Title XIX Program
as a Percentage of U.S. Population Under 21,
1940, 1955, and 1970
(based on data drawn from sources cited below)

| | Percentage of U.S. Population Under 21 | | |
	1940	1955	1970
Maternal and Child Health	3.0	5.8	6.9
Crippled Children	.5[a]	.4	.6
Total Title V Programs	3.5	6.2	7.5
Title XIX Program	—	—	9.4[b]

[a]Data are for 1939 since statistics were not collected for 1940.

[b]Children served by this program may also have received services through Title V programs.

Source: HEW (1957:7; 1971a:7; 1971b: Tables 7-9, 11; 1972c:1); U.S. Department of Commerce (1940: Table 2; 1956: Table 19; 1970: Table 50); U.S. Department of Labor (1941:40).

selected localities for comprehensive health services for children and youth; in 1968 dental care and intensive infant care projects were also authorized. Localities were also helped to establish health services through the OEO programs which funded neighborhood health centers and provide health services for head start programs.[2]

Medicaid, or Title XIX of the Social Security Act, although not a program aimed specifically at children, rapidly became their largest public medical program after its establishment in 1966. By 1970, expenditures for children under Title XIX were $968 million compared to $328 million spent by the Title V programs (Cooper and McGee, 1971: 9). Title XIX of the Social Security Act reimbursed the states for providing health care to welfare recipients and, if the states elected to have such a program, to those who were "medically needy." Each state set its own standards for medical need just as it set standards for eligibility for welfare, but it was intended to include those who were categorically eligible and who

[2]For a list of federal, state, and local government health programs for children in 1966, see HEW (1966: Table A-1). Health services administered by the federal government in 1972 are presented in Minnesota Systems (1972: 3-10).

faced high medical expenses although they were not poor enough to receive welfare payments. Children under 21 could also be included in any state's Medicaid program regardless of categorical eligibility, but only 17 states chose this option. Services provided under the 1965 Title XIX legislation included inpatient and outpatient hospital services, and physician's and other remedial services. Preventive care or screening services were not spelled out in the legislation (Social Security Act, Section 1905a). They could be provided, but in practice, most states did not reimburse for them.

Administration of the federal programs were assigned to different federal agencies. All the Title V programs had been assigned to the Children's Bureau and although this bureau moved from one federal agency to another over the years, it remained intact until 1969. In the states, Title V programs were usually administered by health officials. Title XIX, which became the major federal program for health services for children, was administered by a division within the Bureau of Family Services which grew into the Medical Services Administration (MSA) of the Social and Rehabilitation Service (SRS).[3] Most states placed the administration of the program in their welfare departments, although Mississippi set up an independent agency and five states placed it in the health department (HEW, 1970: 395-398).

All federal programs were to be directed toward children who did not have access to regular medical services. In the Title V legislation of 1935 this took the form of directing aid to areas suffering from "economic distress," or to rural areas where no medical care was available (Section 511). The provisions of health services through Title XIX (Medicaid) of the Social Security Act which were expanded by the 1967 amendments to include EPSDT, were directed only to those children eligible through the AFDC Program (Title IV), or classified as "medically needy" by the states (Sections 401-410 and 1905). At no time was the federal law interpreted as having legislated health services for all children. When Congress discussed the Emergency Maternity and Infant Care (EMIC) Act of 1943, it rejected the Children's Bureau's first request for funds

---

[3]Strictly speaking, MSA does not administer Title XIX. It is considered to be a federally assisted state-administered program. However, MSA's duties of monitoring the states' programs and sending policy directives make it look as if it is administering the program, even though states have in the past ignored some of the directives without losing federal funding.

because "there was no requirement of lack of financial ability as prerequisite to the benefits" U.S. Congress, House of Representatives, Report of Committee on Appropriations, February 24, 1943:6, as cited in Sinai and Anderson (1948: 113).[4] Only when Congress was reassured that the program was restricted to needy children did it appropriate the funds. This federal decision to focus programs on poor children rather than on all children was to complicate the administration and implementation of health programs, because it established a two-class system of health care: private for the haves and public for the have-nots, even though well-child conferences had traditionally been open to anyone who wanted to use them without a means test.[5]

The Beginnings of EPSDT

By 1967 health services for needy children were being carried out by many different federal, state, and local agencies, as well as by voluntary groups and parent-teacher associations. Standards were set by those agencies as well as by the American Academy of Pediatrics, committees of state medical societies, and the American Public Health Association. The time was ripe for a comprehensive plan for preventive health services which would include screening and treatment for children, most particularly those who did not receive care through the private sector. Evidence had been accumulating for years that preventive services would decrease infant and child mortality and lessen the likelihood of crippling diseases, but no government program had yet attempted to provide these services in a comprehensive fashion.

The establishment of a program of preventive services for children confronted the federal government with four major ques-

[4]Various other proposals have been heard from time to time. For example, in 1972, Senator Ribicoff of Connecticut was considering a "kiddycare" bill which would have provided national health insurance for all children the way that Medicare provided a national health insurance for those over 65 regardless of need. Several other members of Congress during its 93rd and 94th sessions were known to have child health insurance bills "in the wings."

[5]The "Bureau of Child Hygiene has been opening child heath centers in various parts of the state where *children of all classes* may be brought for free monthly examination and inspection" (Ingraham, 1926: 115). Emphasis added.

tions which had to be resolved in the course of legislation, administration, and implementation of the program. These questions were: (1) Which children were to be reached? (2) What would be the extent and quality of health services offered? (3) How much could or should be spent on the program? and (4) Through what administering agency was the program to be implemented? The cost would, of course, affect both the extent and quality of care and the numbers of children to be reached. These four questions do not seem to have been addressed in an orderly or exhaustive fashion by those planning the program. As a result, the program that has became known as EPSDT created considerably more controversy during the five years after it was signed into law by President Johnson in 1968 than it did during its eight-month legislative gestation.

The idea for federally sponsored periodic screening for low-income children first appeared in 1966 in a program analysis prepared in the Secretary's Office of HEW. The case finding was to lift a burden from the population by saving children from handicapping conditions. Three possible programs for the screening and treatment of low-income children were suggested: one program would serve an estimated one million newborn children in health-depressed areas at a cost of nearly $30 million; another would serve five million children including newborns and those aged one, five, and nine who live in health-depressed areas at a cost of $150 million; and finally the third would serve all the nation's 104,000 premature infants at a cost of a mere $5.3 million (HEW, 1966: III, 22). This was the first and last time a federal document put a specific price tag on a specific nationwide screening or preventive care program for specified child populations. As for the administration of this program, it was suggested that "it could be organized as an extension of the present Crippled Children's Program. Funds for such a program could come through the Title XIX 'Medicaid' program. . . ." (HEW, 1966: III, 18), with the suggestion that Title XIX be amended to include diagnostic examinations. The seeds of administrative ambiguity were thus planted in this first report.[6] The

[6]Title XIX was barely under way at the time the Program Analysis was written, and its authors may have wanted to hedge their bets since its scope, administration, and direction were unclear. At least one author has said that it was their intention that the program should be administered by Title V with Title XIX acting as a pass-through mechanism (personal communication, George A. Silver, M.D., June 3, 1974).

scope of services was not discussed in any detail.

President Johnson, in his address to Congress on the Welfare of Children on February 8, 1967 (U. S. Congress, 1967a) recommended that increased funds for the care of needy children be doubled to a total of $221 million. He also asked that the number of needy children being seen and treated under the Crippled Children's program be doubled to one million. Whether these increased appropriations and expanded legislation were aimed at the same populations was not clear from the President's message.

EPSDT Legislation—H.R. 5710

Some clarification appeared eight days later when the President's ideas were incorporated in legislation introduced by Representative Wilbur Mills. The Social Security Amendments of 1967, or H.R. 5710, provided broad-ranging changes in the Social Security Act programs, of which the child health provisions formed only a small part. When the House Ways and Means Committee invited comment from interested parties, the bill was described as including "revisions in the Old-Age, Survivors and Disability Insurance; provisions relating to health care for the aged and others (Title XVIII and Title XIX); provisions relating to public assistance; tax provisions relating to senior citizens, etc." (U. S. Congress, 1967b). Only those who already knew that nearly half of those eligible for care under Title XIX were under 21 would have noticed that the hearing could have anything to do with children.

The provisions for Early and Periodic Screening, Diagnosis and Treatment (EPSDT) of needy children consisted of three amendments: two to Title XIX and one to Title V, of the Social Security Act. The major amendment to Title XIX (now frequently referred to as the EPSDT amendment) was worded as follows:

> . . . effective July 1, 1969, such early and periodic screening an diagnosis of individuals who ar eligible under the plan and are under the age of 21—to ascertain their physical or mental defects, and such health care, treatment, and other measures to correct or ameliorate defects and chronic conditions discovered thereby, as may be provided in regulations of the Secretary. [Sec. 301 (b)(1)]

The intent of this legislation was to encourage staes to extend their coverage of care for children to preventive ervices. At the time, only seven states specifically provided for this care in their state plans (HEW, 1967: 44).

The other amendment to Title XIX called for cooperation between the Title XIX and the CC and MCH programs of Title V. This amendment provided for the state Title XIX agency to enter into agreements with any agency receiving payment for part or all of its costs under Title V; that it use such an agency in furnishing care and services; and that it make provision for reimbursing such an agency for the care and services furnished. This agreement of cooperation was not new to Title XIX. When Medicaid was passed in 1965, it had included a provision for the state Title XIX agencies to enter into agreements with the state agencies responsible for administering or supervising health services and vocational rehabilitation. The novelty was that the Title V agencies were specifically mentioned, the agreement was to include reimbursement and the Secretary of HEW would write regulations clarifying the scope of the relationship [Section 1902 (a) (11) (A) and (B); (A) was the original statement; (B) was the 1967 addition].

The third amendment, an amendment to Title V, said that state health plans with regard to the Crippled Children's program must:

> ... effective July 1, 1967, provide for early identification of children in need of health care and services, and for health care and treatment needed to correct or ameliorate defects or chronic conditions discovered thereby, through provision of such periodic screening and diagnostic services, and such treatment, care, and other measures to correct or ameliorate defects or chronic conditions as may be provided in regulations of the Secretary. [Section 301 (a) (2)]

This mandate to carry out preventive care replaced the weaker langage in the earlier Crippled Children's provisions for locating crippled children. Authorizations for the program were to be increased from $55 to $65 million (U. S. Congress, 1967b: 93). In its explanations of the act's provisions, HEW said that the amendment to Title XIX plus the "proposed increase of $15 million [sic] in the authorization for 'Crippled Children's Services' and the requirement . . . that such services include periodic screening and diagnosis would greatly strengthen the nation's programs for children" (U. S. Congress, 1967b: 26). HEW had not mentioned how the program was to be administered or how many children were to be served.

These three amendments constituted what has become known

as EPSDT, the Early and Periodic Screening, Diagnosis and Treatment Program. EPSDT went through three phases in its legislative history: as H.R. 5710 when it was discussed in hearings before the House Ways and Means Committee in March and April 1967; as H.R. 12080 when in August it emerged from the Ways and Means Committee Report; and still as H.R. 12080 in hearings before the Senate Finance Committee during August and September of the same year. During each phase, the issues of program cost and administration were taken up while the questions of scope of services and eligible population were more frequently ignored.

The First Public Discussion—H.R. 5710 Hearings

Hearings on H.R. 5710, held before the Ways and Means Committee during March and early April 1967, extended for nearly 3,000 pages of testimony of which child health amendments formed only a small part. More individuals or organizations commented on the costs of the program than on any of the other three issues that would determine the shape of the future program. However, those testifying were confused as to who was to foot the bill, Title V or Title XIX. HEW had suggested $100 million extra for Title XIX earmarked for children and $15 million extra for Crippled Children under Title V. Some of the Title XIX money (or perhaps much of it) was supposed to go toward encouraging states to expand their programs to include any kind of services to children, not just the preventive ones (U. S. Congress, 1967b: 125-126). George Meany welcomed the President's proposals for "an increase of $100 million in federal financial participation for needy children," but added that the amounts authorized for child health were the "absolute minimum required" (U. S. Congress, 1967b: 584-585). The American Parents Committee (U. S. Congress, 1967b: 2006) and the American Academy of Orthopedic Surgeons (U. S. Congress, 1967b: 2351) supported the $10 million increase (presumably for crippled children), which would pay for additional case finding and increased medical costs. Other organizations were less certain that the amounts asked for would be adequate to carry out the additional case finding and payment for increasing medical costs. The American Cerebral Palsy Association (U. S. Congress, 1967b: 2237) said that $18 million extra was needed. The Founda-

tion for the Blind (U. S. Congress, 1967b: 2242) and the State of Illinois Commission on Children (U. S. Congress, 1967b: 2416) both
objected that CC is closed-ended funding and would limit the kinds
of services that could be provided. Title XIX funding is open-
ended. The strongest request for additional support for the CC program came from those who administered it, the Association of
State and Territorial Health Officers. Under a 1965 law the CC programs would have to pay "reasonable cost" for hospital services
and without the provision of additional federal funds, this "greatly
increased cost is working a tremendous hardship on these programs. . . . There is every possibility that they will result in a reduced amount of care given" (U. S. Congress, 1967b: 2263).

The concerns for the funding of this new program stemmed
from confusion over whether it was a Title V or Title XIX program,
or rather, whether it was a health or a welfare program. At the
federal level, Title XIX was administered by the Medical Services
Administration (MSA) of the Social and Rehabilitation Service
(SRS); Title V by the Children's Bureau, which at the time was part
of SRS but was soon to be dismantled and transferred to the newly
created Health Services and Mental Health Administration
(HSMHA). This separation was paralleled at the state level, where
the Title XIX programs were usually administered by welfare departments and Title V programs by health departments. The confusion was not clarified in commentary on the administrative
framework for the program. HEW Secretary John Gardner (U.S.
Congress, 1967b: 98) called for agreements between the Title XIX
and Crippled Children (Title V) agencies. Martha M. Eliot (U. S.
Congress, 1967b: 2267), former head of the Children's Bureau,
"heartily" approved of this relation. The American Nursing Association (U. S. Congress, 1967b: 2229) felt that the purpose of the
legislation was to broaden the base of the Children's Bureau Title
V programs, and ignored the role of the Title XIX agency.
Representative James A. Burke (U. S. Congress, 1967b: 1964) of
Massachusetts was the only one to comment on the ambiguity, saying: "it is a program that should be administered by the Department of Public Health. . . . It is not a welfare program. It is a health
program." The issue of whether health or welfare should implement a health program for welfare children was not resolved during
these or subsequent hearings; it has continued to plague all those
charged with implementing the program.

The issue of which children were to be served or which ones were eligible for the proposed program also received scant attention and produced conflicting points of view. Secretary Gardner (U. S. Congress, 1967b: 190), like the President, had suggested that 500,000 additional children would be screened furing the first year of operation, and within three to five years, the program would extend to five million children.[7] Whether these were children to be served under the CC or the Title XIX program was not clear. The American Parents Committee (U. S. Congress, 1967b: 2007) also picked up this 500,000 children figure and assumed the case finding for these low-income or medically indigent children would take place within the context of the CC program. Not only was there question of how many children would or could be served, but who would be eligible for the new program. There was pressure to expand state CC services to include children with vision or hearing problems and there was concern that specialized services not available through the private sector would no longer be available to middle-income families if the present program were carried out. Under the Title XIX program economic eigibility was the only criterion. The repercussions of this unresolved conflict would be felt down to the implementation of the programs within the state.

Except for the comment that vision and hearing screening should be included, no one testified at these or at later hearings on the scope or extent of screening or preventive care to be carried out in the proposed program. These details were to be prescribed by the Secretary.

Phase 2—Same Provision; New Bill

The three EPSDT amendments remained essentially unchanged when the Social Security amendments of 1967 were incorporated into H.R. 12080, which was reported out of the Ways and Means Committee in August 1967. The many major changes which affected the rest of the Social Security Act affected EPSDT only in-

[7]During 1968 before EPSDT, the CC program served 475,000 children while Medicaid served 5,574,000 children. The CC program had been serving over 400,000 children since 1964. No data are available on the children served by Medicaid during its first two years, 1966 and 1967 (HEW, 197la: Table 1; HEW, n.d.: Table 2).

directly.[8] One of the changes was to consolidate all the funding for Title V into one authorization of $250 million, of which half was to go for Maternal and Child Health and Crippled Children's Services combined. If the shares were divided equally, the CC program would receive an authorization of $62.5 million, a few million dollars less than had been proposed in H.R. 5710.[9]

The date on which screening was to become effective, July 1, 1967, was removed from the EPSDT amendment to Title V because the date was already past. July 1, 1969, remained as the effective date for the program in the Title XIX amendment. With the EPSDT amendment to Title V written into a new consolidated Title V, the two EPSDT amendments to Title XIX were called "conforming amendments.[10]

The question of administrative authority was immediately raised in the Ways and Means Committee's report which emphasized that the EPSDT provisions were to bring about more aggressive case-finding by the CC programs; however, the committee then obscured its intent: (U. S. Congress, 1967c: 127)

> Organized and intensified case-finding procedures will be carried out in well baby clinics, day care centers, nursery schools, Headstart centers in cooperation with the Office of Economic Opportunity, by periodic screening of children in schools, through follow-up visits by nurses to the homes of newborn infants, by checking birth certificates for the reporting of congenital malformation and by related activities. Title XIX (Medical Assistance) would

[8]One major issue debated throughout the 1967 Social Security Amendments was whether the eligibility levels for medically needy should be limited to 133 1/3 percent of the public assistance levels under the categorical programs. Both the states and the federal government were anxious to cut Medicaid costs by limiting the number of people who would be eligible for the medically needy category. Congress decided to apply this limitation only to the AFDC program. Consequently the number of children eligible for EPSDT through Title XIX was curtailed by this action.

[9]In fact, the MCH and CC shares, as they were allocated by the HEW Secretary, were not quite equal. The CC program received slightly more than the MCH program.

[10]SRS administrators later, when writing regulations for Title XIX, wondered whether the Title V amendment took precedence because the Title XIX amendments were "conforming." They were reassured by HEW General Counsel that juridically this had no meaning and they could proceed with regulations for Title XIX.

be modified to conform to this requirement under the formula grant program.

The legislative mandate was only for the CC and Title XIX programs, but the committee was suggesting that all other federal, state, and local programs be asked to cooperate as well, with neither the funding nor the administrative framework provided for them. Much of the screening work around the country was at the time being supported by the MCH program, but it was not mentioned in the commentary.

Although administration was to be in the hands of the CC program, case finding would also be carried out by the Title XIX program. A dual system of administration was being proposed, with the Title XIX agency expected to provide reimbursement to the Title V agency (U. S. Congress, 1967c: 195). CC's funding for this massive expanded program was limited to about $7.5 million more than its previous authorization, while there was no mention of the funding to be availble to Title XIX for the program. Thus the program was not likely to open the way for increased services by the MCH and CC programs (usually the health departments) in the states. The open-ended funding of Title XIX gave that program greater flexibility.

Finally, the committee did not mention the number of children to be helped by this expanded program nor the extent of services to be provided.

When H.R. 12080 passed the House in August and was sent to the Senate, the cost of EPSDT, the eligible population, the extent of care and how the program was to be administered, had not been clarified. The latter two questions were left for the Secretary of HEW to prescribe in regulations. Presumably, the Senate hearings would provide insight into the intent of the legislation, but this was not to be.

Phase 3—Senate Hearings and Passage

Hearings were held before the Senate Finance Committee during August and September 1967. The EPSDT provisions were unchanged from the hearings before the Ways and Means Committee on H.R. 5710, so most of those who testified did so on other controversial issues without reference to EPSDT. No special mention of EPSDT was made by either HEW Secretary Gardner or Under-Secretary Wilbur Cohen. Nor did senators raise questions. Among the hundreds of witnesses and communications that were incorporated into these hearings, only one witness, Dr. Donald C. Smith of the American Academy of Pediatrics, stressed the need for preventive health measures in childhood and asked that the high quality of CC programs be maintained. He therefore recommended an amendment that would *require* cooperation between state agencies administering Crippled Children's Programs and those administering Title XIX programs (U. S. Congress, 1967d: I, 201). No such requirement was added. Congress retained the more ambiguous wording of the amendment that state Title XIX agencies provide for "entering into agreements" with Title V and other agencies.

H.R. 12080 was a complex bill with titles relating to Public Assistance, Medicare, Medicaid, and Child Welfare. The Child Health Act of 1967 was only eight and a half of the 112 pages, and EPSDT took up only the three paragraphs described earlier. Provisions on AFDC stimulated the most comment. Early periodic screening and treatment, if not ignored, at least was not uppermost in people's minds. In retrospect, this lack of concern seems odd because so much time and energy during these hearings were devoted to restricting the costs of Medicaid. This new program would greatly increase Medicaid costs. Perhaps those who proposed the program were aware of its high potential cost and also of the jurisdictional dispute it would engender and therefore deliberately underplayed financing and administration.

The three amendments which became known as EPSDT passed the Senate unchanged from the House version. After a Senate-House conference, they then passed the two houses as part of the Social Security Amendments of 1967 or PL 90-248, and were signed into law by President Johnson on January 2, 1968.

The United States had just enacted its first policy mandating preventive health services for needy children, a kind of health insurance for the poor. All states with Title XIX programs[11] would have to provide such services for all eligible children. In addition, the Crippled Children's Program would also have to carry out early periodic screening for those who were eligible under its plans. Yet, despite the broad mandate, during its eight-month legislative his-

---

[11] By 1970, this would include all states but Alaska and Arizona.

tory, EPSDT's details were scarcely touched on. The scope of screening and the eligible population were hardly mentioned. Estimates of cost were applied separately for the CC and Title XIX programs with no public discussion on how these costs would be worked out. Nor was it discussed whether health or welfare agencies were to be responsible for this health-welfare program. Thus, the Secretary's office was faced with a formidable task in understanding legislative intent when it came to writing regulations.

Development of Regulations and Guidelines[12]

Although the EPSDT provisions had become law in January 1968 with the stipulation that they be implemented by July 1, 1969, final regulations and guidelines did not appear for four and a half years. Proposed regulations were issued in December 1970; after lengthy discussions final regulations appeared in November 1971 and final guidelines in June 1972. Meanwhile, the final implementation date for all age groups had been deferred until July 1, 1973. This four-and-a-half-year period was filled with discussions within HEW as to what direction rule making should take. Many people were involved—administrators and planners for the Title V and Title XIX programs in Washington, senators, representatives, Congress as a whole, the state Title XIX and Title V agencies, which were for the most part welfare and health departments, the HEW regional offices, the National Welfae Right Organization (NWRO), the Medical Assistance Advisory Council (MAAC), and professional groups such as the American Optometric Association. The law was interpreted and reinterpreted; the scope of services under EPSDT was broadened, narrowed, and then broadened again. Opposing forces used HEW as a battleground for issues which had not been resolved during the program's legislative history. The administrative framework, costs, eligibility, and scope of the program all had to be clarified before regulations and guidelines could be published and the program implemented.

[12]I am grateful to the many officials of the Social and Rehabilitation Service and the Maternal and Child Health Services who generously gave of their time to provide much of the information upon which the following pages are based. Their generosity should not be confused with responsibility for the way their information has been used.

Regulations and Guidelines—Administering Agency

Congress had given EPSDT both to Title XIX and to the CC program of Title V, without clarifying which agency was to administer the progrm. The CC program which was administered by the Maternal and Child Health Services (MCHS) was not asked by HEW Secretary Wilbur Cohen to develop regulations, even though the legislation called for them. This charge was giveninstead to Medical Services Administration (MSA) in the summer of 1968.[13] Even though MSA wondered at first what the implication was of the dual administration in the legislation, it worked out a draft whereby the state agencies would make firm agreements with one another, and this approach was coordinated with Dr. Arthur Lesser, the director of MCH Services. MSA proceeded to draft regulations and assume its role as the administrator for the EPSDT program, while using MCHS as consultants.

After proposed regulations for the EPSDT program were published in December 1970, states began to question how this cooperation would work.[14] The Medicaid program was to provide for (U. S. Federal Register, 1970b: 18879):

> . . . identification of those eligible individuals who are in need of medical or remedial care and services furnished through Title V grantees, and for assuring that such individuals are informed of such services and are referred to Title V grantees for proper care and services, as appropriate.

In most states, Title V agencies were in health departments while Title XIX agencies were in welfare departments. The greatest con-

---

[13]Writing regulations was a new procedure for MSA. Prior to 1968, Title XIX programs had provided all guiding material to the states through its *Handbook of Medical Assistance—Supplement D.* Since these guidelines gave no way for the public or interested parties to be heard, and since several different agencies had been placed together during the 1968 reorganization of HEW, their policies were standardized and regulations had to be written. H.R. 12080 required that regulations be written for use of skilled nursing homes as well as for EPSDT, and both these regulations were several years aborning.

[14]Proposed regulations for cooperation between Title V and Title XIX agencies had been published earlier that year but had elicited little comment from the states, possibly because the states did not know what the scope of the program would be (U. S. Federal Register, 1970a: 8664).

cern was duplication of effort between the two agencies, but one state official pointed out that this relation would result in more competition and misunderstanding between the programs than already existed. Neither Congress nor HEW had taken into account that these two agencies might not work well together on the state level. The MCHS pressed for greater details on the relationship in the guidelines, while state and regional officials asked why other agencies, such as Visiting Nurses Associations and home health agencies, had not been mentioned.

The question of reimbursement provided the major conflict and source of confusion for the Title XIX and Title V agencies. Early in 1970, MSA had received the legal opinion that the regulations called for total reimbursement for all Title V services and the Title XIX agency would have no control over the numbers of children screened, or the amount of reimbursement except as these items might be covered in the written agreements, nor could reimbursement be limited to children referred by the Title XIX agency. But the confusion persisted, perhaps because the state Title XIX agencies were not happy that they would be paying for Title V services which hitherto had been free to recipients. The following year MSA had to issue another clarification, slightly weakened by this time, that Title XIX payment could include both diagnostic and treatment services "as appropriate." It noted that responsibilities for payment were program decisions rather than those of legal prerogative. MSA was trying to force the states to work out their own relationships, but the state Title V and Title XIX agencies kept appealing to their respective HEW agencies for support. The next year another memorandum reiterating the previous position was sent out. The reimbursement issue was particularly difficult because in many states the Title V programs provided the major public screening services through child health conferences, and the major public diagnostic and treatment services through the Crippled Children's program. However, their funding had not increased and consequently they had trouble maintaining their programs.

Between 1968 and 1972, MSA gradually clarified its role as the sole administrator of the EPSDT program, while MCHS took a more and more consultative role.[15] MSA's involvement in its new

[15]Regulations for the Title V EPSDT amendment were finally issued in 1974 (U.S. Federal Register, 1974).

role of providing for health services was so strong that by 1973 it was letting contracts for EPSDT program evaluations and for the development of screening standards. These contracts, which were part of MSA's surveillance and evaluation responsibility, did not differ much from contracts which were let by MCHS for evaluation of its programs. Meanwhile, the MCHS were not entirely pleased to see MSA moving into the field of health services. This tension at the federal level was reflected within the state agencies, either because of the existence of an MSA and an MCHS encouraged their state counterparts to square off against one another, or because the two federal agencies could not control them. One MSA administrator wondered at the time whether MSA had a policy of encouraging interagency relations, because the guidelines did not reflect this. The issue always came to a head over whether Title XIX would reimburse Title V for its services. States were hard hit by inflation and were looking for ways to avoid spending money. When these issues had to be settled, Title V agencies (usually the health department) and Title XIX agencies (usually the welfare department) would buck the issue up to the federal level. The administrative issue had been resolved in one sense, but as soon as the states began implementing the program, all the tension between a health agency and a welfare agency which was running a health program erupted, and this ambiguity continued to plague all those charged with implementation.

Regulations and Guidelines—Costs and Funding

The administrative decision which made EPSDT a Title XIX program resolved the issue of who was to pay for it. Title XIX reimburses from 50 to 83 percent of states' costs. Theoretically no limits existed for the development of the EPSDT program, but experience with Title XIX had shown that generally states like California and New York took advantage of the program, while smaller, poorer states did not.[16] As Stevens and Stevens noted (1970: 365-378), when states did spend a great deal of money, as New York and California did in the early years of Medicaid, then Congress got upset because costs were too high.

---

[16]In 1969, these two states alone accounted for 45 percent of Medicaid expenditures (HEW, 1972b: Table 7).

During the first two years of regulation drafting, cost estimates were not made because, according to MSA and state officials, available data were so poor. However, by August 1970 someone had come up with a first-year cost of $45 million. This large sum must have alarmed HEW, for by December of that year it had advised the Senate Finance Committee that it had delayed issuance of regulations for EPSDT because of the "great cost" it would entail for both the federal and state governments. HEW then asked Congress for legislation to phase in the program slowly (U. S. Congress, 1970: 169), but Congress refused. Meanwhile, Senator Abraham Ribicoff and the Medical Assistance Advisory Council (MAAC) continued to press for regulations.

When proposed regulations were published in December 1970, the states responded vehemently and very rapidly on the question of cost. Eighteen out of the 22 states responding said the program would place a financial burden on the state beyond its capacity. In case HEW should miss the point, one southern state had its entire congressional delegation send letters of alarm. Part of the reason states could not estimate costs was that the federal guidelines were still not available.[17]

During the spring of 1971, the Nixon administration had committed itself to a reduction of federal Medicaid costs for fiscal 1972,[18] and by May HEW, following suit, decided it would allow states to implement the program in phases starting first with children under six in order to soften the financial impact on the states. The softened financial impact on the federal government was implicit. Costs continued to concern HEW; one official estimated EPSDT would cost $400 million by 1973 and this would create a sizable drain on the Treasury. HEW decided to narrow the scope of services and also to concentrate on slowly phasing in children by age groups. In September, HEW decided that the program would cost only $25 million the first year. When this sum was approved by the Office of Management and Budget in the fall of 1971, the final regulations could be published.

[17]One small midwestern state which had looked more carefully at costs than others estimated they would have 15 to 20 children eligible for kidney dialysis at $30,000 each.

[18]The administration was at the time proposing the ill-fated Family Health Insurance Plan (FHIP), and EPSDT was held up while HEW studied how they fit together. Officials in the secretary's office even considered getting legislation to eliminate EPSDT altogether.

The states through their concern for their own costs had managed to stave off for nearly three years the implementation of a law passed by Congress.[19] The power of the states in this case illustrated the limitations of federal aid programs. Since the incentive was not great enough, and since financial needs were sufficiently pressing, the states did what they could to hinder implementation. HEW was caught between the congressional groups which had favored EPSDT and the state welfare agencies who were its clients. HEW deferred making a choice by offering the states a few years' respite by phasing in the program slowly. This respite was only temporary, and eventually the states would have to come to terms with the financial burden of EPSDT, unless they could convince Congress to repeal it completely.

Regulations and Guidelines—Eligibility

The eligibility issue was also resolved when EPSDT became solely a Title XIX program. Under Title XIX any child who was eligible under the state plan was eligible for EPSDT. However, state plans varied considerably. By 1971, 48 states had Medicaid programs under which all children receiving AFDC welfare payments were eligible. In addition, 25 states offered Medicaid services to any low-income child who fell within the income guidelines (HEW, 1971c: 2-3). Arizona and Alaska had no Medicaid services. However, states varied considerably in their eligibility requirements. For example, in 1968 while New York was providing medical payments for 206 children per 1,000 inhabitants, South Carolina was providing for only two per 1,000 (HEW, n.d.: Table A). In all it was estimated that approximately 10 million children would have been eligible for EPSDT, or 12 percent of the United States child population of 80 million.

During the development of regulations and guidelines restrictions on eligibility arose from the need to cut back costs and one way to do this was to cut down on the eligible population and to allow states to serve first children under six years and not serve older children until 1973. This phasing-in approach met at first with some skepticism from the HEW general counsel, but it was finally ac-

[19]Two states, Virginia and Mississippi, were exceptions and had supported the program and were implementing the program before February 1972.

cepted. The eligibility restriction was supposed to be temporary but states were in fact slow to phase in the over-six population.

Regulations and Guidelines—Scope of Services

From the earliest drafts of the regulations, MSA understood that the amount, duration, and scope of services was to be comprehensive and this thinking was reflected in the proposed regulations published in 1970 (U. S. Federal Register, 1970b: 18879; emphasis added).

> Effective January 1, 1971 (or earlier at the option of the State), that early and periodic screening and diagnosis to ascertain physical and mental defects, and treatment of conditions discovered *regardless of the limits otherwise imposed under the State plan* on the type and amount of such care and services. . . . will be available to all eligible individuals under 21 years of age.

In the 48 states with Medicaid programs at the time, state plans were by no means comprehensive. All states included the five basic services: inpatient care, outpatient care, laboratory and X-ray services, skilled-nursing home services for those over 21, and physician services, but here the similarity ended. One state, Minnesota, provided the full range of services available; others like Kansas, Nebraska, North Dakota, and New York provided all but one or two services; still others like Mississippi and Missouri offered only three additional services. Eighteen states did not provide dental services and 18 did not provide eyeglasses; eight states did not provide prescribed drugs (HEW, 1971d). In fact, in five states the content of Medicaid programs was determined by state statutes, and since screening for eye defects or provision of eyeglasses, as well as other services, were not included, the above regulation would require a change in law. Thus to be comprehensive any federal regulation would have to go outside the bounds of state plans.

The states objected vigorously to providing unlimited amounts of services for unlimited periods regardless of the limits of the state plan. They said the regulations were contrary to the intent of Title XIX and federal-state grant programs because they took away from the state control over the scope of their programs. Some state officials also said that the state simply did not have the medical manpower to carry out such a comprehensive plan, implying that government should not try to provide services to low-income people until resources are available. Another state official suggested more directly that periodic screening was an outmoded concept largely abandoned by public health and the medical profession.

Strong support for the regulations came from the director of the National Legal Program on Health Problems of the Poor, who also lobbied effectively with other groups, particularly welfare rights groups, to support the EPSDT program. He asked that the regulations specify the types of care included, such as eyeglasses and hearing aids, and dental fillings.

During the long period between the proposed and final regulations, state and federal concern for EPSDT costs was rising. The result was that MSA regretfully curtailed the scope of services required of the states under EPSDT. The final regulations asked the states to provide EPSDT "within the limits of the state plan on the amount, duration and scope of care and services" (U. S. Federal Register, 1971: 21410). This constituted a major blow to the comprehensiveness of the treatment segments of the EPSDT services. As mentioned before, states were uneven in their provisions for treatment. The welfare rights lobby had had some effect, however, for the regulations included three treatment services which had to be included by states regardless of the limits of state plans:

> . . . eyeglasses, hearing aids, and other kinds of treatment for visual and hearing defects, and at least such dental care as is necessary for relief of pain and infection and for restoration of teeth and maintenance of dental health. . . .

These three treatment services, plus early and periodic screening, thus became the EPSDT program as it emerged from the federal regulations.

In writing guidelines, MSA tried to help states develop as comprehensive a program as possible. The MCHS which over the years had developed a body of information on quality health services for children provided valuable consultation. Other groups like the American Optometric Association, speaking in the interests of its own profession, asked specifically that visual screening and restorative services be included. The final guidelines reflected these interests, and detailed the case-finding procedures, screening tests to be performed, and diagnosis, treatment, and therapeutic services to be made available to eligible children (HEW, 1972a).

All these services, however, had to be carried out within the limits of the state plan.

To those who had viewed EPSDT as a major innovative comprehensive health program for needy children, the regulations were a disappointment. Treatment was not comprehensive. To those with a "toe-in-the-door" philosophy of federal policy making, it was an encouraging first step for the care of children. Certainly more poor children would get more types of care under this program than they had before. In one state, where the scope of the program had the potential of being comprehensive, an official commented wryly that the same services were not available to middle-income children.

Conclusion

The advent of EPSDT legislation provided the United States with the first major federally sponsored program for comprehensive health services for 12 percent of America's children. It could have been a prototype for health insurance for all children, but congressional intent for the program was so ambiguous that considerable energy had to be exerted to resolve the questions it posed. During the development of regulations and guidelines interest groups used what leverage they could to accomplish their ends. These conflicting interests used HEW as a battleground and compounded the task of program implementation. Some individuals and groups, such as community organizations, the MAAC, and the National Legal Program on Health Problems gave fairly steady, general support to the program, but factions tended to cluster around particular issues: administration, costs, and scope of services.

MSA emerged as the administrator of the EPSDT programs and found itself providing for health services for children, something that had been the province of MCH services. The factions within HEW managed to adjust to these new roles, but implementation of the program would create new tensions between health and welfare agencies at the state level. Ambiguity in legislative intent gave no one federal or state agency full responsibility for carrying out the program. Thus, the administering agencies were unable to build a bureaucratic constituency behind the program. Responsibility was divided between health and welfare agencies with most going to the latter. On the federal level, MSA showed yet greater commitment than MCHS. In the states, neither health nor welfare agencies could become committed and build up the solidarity needed to carry out the program.

Costs were another issue which brought several factions into conflict over a program variously described as costing anywhere from $15 to $400 million. President Nixon had pledged not only to reform the welfare system, but also to cut costs, yet he had inherited one of the most far-reaching health programs the nation had ever undertaken. Congress, although also committed to lowering welfare costs, and particularly Title XIX costs, managed to live with its ambivalence toward the EPSDT program and mandated its implementation while attempting to cut back on other programs. The states were the hardest hit by the program's staggering potential (though never defined) costs. During the development of regulations and guidelines they tried to discourage HEW from asking them to carry out the program, and when they had to implement, they moved very slowly. States were angered by the heavy costs and lack of lead time they had been given. One state official suggested that states should have been given the same amount of time for implementation as HEW had had to write regulations.

While most of those who grouped around the issue of costs wanted to cut back or eliminate the program, those concerned with the eligible population and scope of services strongly favored the program's development. County and national welfare rights organizations, with the support of MCH services, had shown their strength by the well-thought-out and comprehensive array of tests and screening mechanisms that became available to low-income children (at least those eligible for Title XIX under state plans). However, the states and federal government in their concern for costs succeeded in cutting back the scope of services available under the program.

The absence of discussion surrounding EPSDT's intent is not unique in the history of federal health policy. Title V when presented to Congress in 1935, received scant notice because attention was drawn to the major provisions of the Social Security Act. EPSDT's predecessor and umbrella program, Medicaid, slipped into the 1965 Social Security Amendments to fill the gaps left by Medicare. When it was passed, it was called the "sleeper" of the Amendments because no one had foreseen that the costs of this program would rise from \$2 billion to nearly \$9 billion in a few years and that by 1971 it would be serving nearly 20 million people.

The experience of Title V, Medicaid and EPSDT exemplify the toe-in-the-door procedures of federal policy making. Congress seems to assume that once a worthy policy is passed, its implications can be worked out later, and the program expanded when necessary or desirable. This had not always been the case. Title V was never expanded. Its funds were increased over time, but the program never became a national program for child health services. Since the sixties other programs such as Head Start and Neighborhood Health Centers and, of course, EPSDT have been added to supplement Title V rather than integrated. Medicaid was viewed as a stop-gap measure for those not eligible for Medicare. It did expand, but its unexpected high costs did little to endear to the American public the principle of publicly financed medical care. To compound the problem of poorly thought-out policy, EPSDT was added to Medicaid before its implications were studied.

What can one learn about ambiguous toe-in-the-door policy making from the experience of EPSDT and its four-and-a-half-year delay in implementation? First, that Congress and the executive agencies are unable or unwilling to come up with reliable cost estimates for health and welfare programs. One wonders whether accurate cost estimates were actually unavailable to Congress or whether no one in Congress or HEW was willing to face the costs the program would entail. At any time Congress or HEW could have gone back to the 1966 Program Analysis and discovered that the cost of screening five million children was \$150 million. It may be true that no politician can sell an expensive health program to his constituents, but unrealistic costing leads to a public that may become increasingly disenchanted with federal health programs which cannot live up to the expectation placed on them by Congressional and Executive rhetoric.

Second, ambiguity in administrative assignment lessens bureaucratic solidarity and thereby a program's chances for success. Had Congress given responsibility for EPSDT to one single agency, it would have been easier to build bureaucratic solidarity behind the program to smooth its implementation. The division of responsibility between health and welfare split the program between agencies with differing philosophies and goals.

Third, establishing federal child health policies through the mechanism of federal-state grant-in-aid programs increases the ambiguity of the final policy. Medicaid and EPSDT are officially state programs. And the states can put up formidable barriers to their implementation. They can protest vigorously to HEW as they did when the proposed EPSDT regulations were issued. In addition, they can refuse to implement the program at all; they can limit eligibility; or they can limit the scope of the state plan. Since states in fact have used all of these ways to limit the economic impact of the Medicaid and EPSDT programs, it is not an encouraging precedent. Even the threat of lawsuits and federal penalty have failed to move some states.

Finally, the role of health and welfare interest groups in urging HEW to carry out EPSDT should be noted. The welfare rights groups lobbied to get regulations to emerge from HEW. The continued role of these groups in bringing lawsuits against states for failure to implement EPSDT indicates that such groups may be taking the leadership which states have been unwilling to exercise in implementing federal policy.

Congressional intent in EPSDT legislation, as in much legislation which is born in compromise, had resulted in ambiguity. If Congress was ambiguous in its intent for EPSDT in 1967-68, it continued to be so. While trying to cut welfare and Medicaid costs on the one hand, in 1972 it reaffirmed its intent to maintain the EPSDT program by adopting a penalty for states which failed to carry out the program. This ambiguity encouraged many groups to work for the program's early demise. Compromises made during the development of regulations and guidelines placated, at least temporarily, the states, interest groups, and administering agencies, and thereby assured the program of a continued, albeit tenuous and unsatisfactory existence.

Anne-Marie Foltz, M.P.H.
Yale University
School of Medicine
Department of Epidemiology and Public Health
60 College Street
New Haven, Connecticut 06510

Valuable suggestions and criticisms of an earlier draft of this paper were provided by James W. Bjorkman, Jean Hoodwin, Lucille Reifman, George A. Silver, Rosemary Stevens, and Robert Stevens. Research was made possible through Department of Health, Education and Welfare Grant #5-RO1-HS-00900.

References

Cooper, Barbara S., and Mary F. McGee
  1971   ''Medical care outlays for three age groups.'' Social Security Bulletin
          (May).

Georgetown Law Journal
  1971   ''Comments: child health care: unresolved dilemma of Section 1905
          (a)(4)(B) of the 1967 Social Security Amendments.'' Volume 59, No. 4
          (March): 965-990.

HEW
  1957   Maternal and Child Health Services in 1955. Children's Bureau
          Statistical Series, Number 38.

  1966   Maternal and Child Health Care: Program Analysis (October).

  1967   Section by Section Analysis and Explanation of Provisions of H.R.
          5710. U. S. Government Printing Office.

  1970   Characteristics of State Medical Assistance Programs under Title XIX
          of the Social Security Act. Public Assistance Series No. 49.

  1971a   Children Who Received Physicians Services Under the Crippled
          Children's Program. MCHS Statistical Series, No. 3.

  1971b   Maternal and Child Health Services of State and Local Health Depart-
          ments, FY 1970.

  1971c   Medicaid Children; Who are They? Social and Rehabilitation Service.
          MSA-804-71.

  1971d   Medical Services State by State. Social and Rehabilitation Service
          (March): MSA-801-71.

  1972a   Medicaid: Early and Periodic Screening Diagnosis and Treatment for
          Individuals under 21. Social and Rehabilitation Service, MSA-PRG
          (June 28).

  1972b   Numbers of Recipients and Amounts of Payment Under Medicaid.
          National Center for Social Statistics, Report B-4 (CY69).

  1972c   Numbers of Recipients and Amounts of Payments Under Medicaid,
          1970. National Center for Social Statistics, Report B-4 (CY70).

  1974   ''Field Staff Information and Instruction Series, FY 74-75, Summary
          of Status of Implementation of EPSDT for Quarter Ending December
          31, 1973.'' Social and Rehabilitation Service.

  n.d.   Numbers of Recipients and Amounts of Payments Under Medicaid,
          1968. National Center for Social Statistics, Report B-4 (CY68).

Ingraham, Elizabeth A.
  1926   ''Connecticut's need for child hygiene work.'' Connecticut Health
          Bulletin, Volume 40, No. 5 (May): 115-118.

Minnesota Systems Research, Inc.
1972   ''The provision of health care to children: current programs and proposed legislation.'' Project Report Series 2-3(7) (March 15).

Schlesinger, Edward R.
1967   ''The Sheppard-Towner era: a prototype case study in federal-state relationships.'' American Journal of Public Health 57, 6: 1034-1040.

Sinai, Nathan, and Odin W. Anderson
1948   EMIC: A Study of Administrative Experience. Ann Arbor: University
of Michigan.

Stevens, Rosemary, and Robert Stevens
1970   ''Medicaid: anatomy of a dilemma.'' Law and Contemporary
Problems: Health Care, Part I (Spring): 348-425

Tolchin, Martin
1973   ''Tri-state area is found lagging on U.S. health aid for children.'' New
York Times (December 9): 77.

U. S. Congress
1967a   Congressional Record (February 8): 2883.

1967b   Presidential Proposals for Revision in the Social Security System.
Hearings before the Committee on Ways and Means on H.R. 5710.
Washington, D.C.: U. S. Government Printing Office.

1967c   Social Security Amendments of 1967: Report of the Committee on
Ways and Means on H.R. 12080. Washington, D.C.: U. S. Government Printing Office.

1967d   Social Security Amendments of 1967: Hearings before the Committee
on Finance, United States Senate, on H.R. 12080. Washington, D.C.:
U. S. Government Printing Office.

1970   Social Security Amendments of 1970: Report of the Committee on
Finance U. S. Senate To Accompany H.R. 17550. Washington, D.C.:
U.S. Government Printing Office.

U.S. Department of Commerce
1940   Census

1956   Statistical Abstract of the United States

1970   Census

U.S. Department of Labor
1941   Services for Crippled Children Under the Social Security Act: Development of Program, 1936-39. Bureau Publication Number 258.

U.S. Federal Register
1970a   (June 4): 8664.

1970b   (December 11): 18878-9.

1971   (November 9): 21409-10.

1974   (July 22): 26692-26696.

III Local and Regional Governance

Representing Consumer Interests: Imbalanced Markets, Health Planning, and the HSAs

THEODORE R. MARMOR and
JAMES A. MORONE

Center for Health Studies,
Yale University;
Center for Health Administration Studies,
University of Chicago

THE PASSAGE OF THE NATIONAL HEALTH PLANNING and Resources Development Act of 1974, PL93-641, set in motion the establishment of 205 health systems agencies (HSAs) across the country. The aims of the legislation were ambitious—to produce planning "with teeth," to cut the costs of medical care, to rationalize access, and to do so with more attention to consumer interests than was the case under earlier health planning. Many commentators expected these efforts to produce little change. Yet in some state and local areas the tasks of health planning have been taken up with fervor. Our interest is the connection between consumer representation and these health planning institutions. Our focus is on the conceptual, legal, and administrative questions raised by efforts to create HSA boards dominated by actors "broadly representative" of the constituents of each local HSA. Our aim is to untangle some of the theoretical and political difficulties that have bedeviled PL93-641's efforts to improve consumer representation.

We first set a broad theoretical background, and show why concentrated interests (such as medical-care providers) dominate the politics of most industries. Representing consumers is cast as an important attempt to break this recurring pattern in decision-making about public choices.

In the core of the paper we analyze the concept of representation

Milbank Memorial Fund Quarterly/*Health and Society*, Vol. 58, No. 1, 1980
© 1980 Milbank Memorial Fund and Massachusetts Institute of Technology
0160/1997/80/5801/0125-41 $01.00/0

and such associated notions as accountability and participation. Understanding these concepts is important in explaining why the law's clumsy efforts at representing consumers have fostered legal challenges and will almost certainly continue to fail. We describe a number of these failures and prescribe in brief outline a remedy that seems conceptually more defensible and legally more practical.

It would be naive, nonetheless, to expect the Health Planning Act to achieve a major reorientation in American medicine, even if consumer representation were successfully instituted. We suggest reasons why this should be so, emphasizing the wildly inflated expectations characterizing PL93-641 and its rhetorical promises about planning's high technology and regulatory "teeth."

Our effort throughout is to describe, illuminate, and appraise one widely discussed policy strategy for controlling contemporary medical care: local planning agencies dominated by consumer representatives. While we discuss consumer representation, its potential and limits, current pitfalls and proposed adjustments, we are keenly aware that the health planning law is in flux, that we are appraising, so to speak, a moving target. But, if our analysis is correct, the movements toward controlling medicine through planning and consumer control are crippled by flaws in both the statute and the regulations. Explaining why that is so constitutes this paper's aim.

Representation and Imbalanced Political Markets

The puzzles of representation are exacerbated in circumstances that stimulate representation without explicitly structuring it—when there are no elections, no clearly defined channels of influence, or only murky conceptions of constituency. The politics of regulatory agencies or regional authorities provide examples. Though representatives of groups commonly press their interests within such contexts, there are no systematic canvasses of the relevant interests, such as geographically based elections provide. It is unclear who legitimately merits representation, how representation should be organized, or how it ought to operate.

Interest-group theorists address the problems of representation in precisely such political settings. In their view, interests that are harmed coalesce into groups and seek redress through the political system. Despite the absence of electoral mechanisms of representation, their conception of representation is systematic; every interest that is strongly felt can be represented by a group. At their most sanguine, group theorists suggest that "all legitimate groups can make themselves heard at some crucial stage in the decision-making process" (Dahl, 1964:137). Politics itself is characterized by legions of groups, bargaining on every level of government about policies that affect them. Government is viewed as the bargaining broker, policy choices as the consequences of mutual adjustments among the bargaining groups (Bentley, 1967; Truman, 1951; Dahl, 1961; and Greenstone, 1975:256).

The group model is now partially in eclipse among academic political scientists (McFarland, 1979; Salisbury, 1978). One criticism is significant here: groups that organize themselves for political action form a highly biased sample of affected interests. This argument recalls Schattschneider's (1960:34) classic epigram: "The flaw in the pluralist heaven is that the heavenly chorus sings with a strong upper-class accent. Probably about 90 percent of the people cannot get into the pressure system." Furthermore, that bias is predictable and recurs on almost every level of the political process. We refer to it as a tendency toward imbalanced political markets.

Political markets are imbalanced in part because organizing for political action is difficult and costly. Even if considerable benefits are at stake, potential beneficiaries may choose not to pursue them. If collective goods are involved (that is, if they are shared among members of a group, regardless of the costs any one member paid to attain them, like clean air or a tariff), potential beneficiaries often let other members of the collectivity pay the costs, and simply enjoy the benefits—the classic "free-rider" problem.

Free riders aside, the probability of political action can be expected to vary with the incentives. If either the benefits or the costs of political action are concentrated, political action is more likely. A tax or a tariff on tea, for example, clearly and significantly affects the tea industry. To tea consumers, the tax is of marginal importance, a few dollars a year perhaps. Clearly those in the industry, with their livelihood at issue, are more likely to organize for political action. And even such concentrated interests are not likely to act if the expected benefits do not significantly outweigh the costs. As Wilson (1973:318) has phrased it, "The clearer the material incentives of the organization's member, the more prompt, focused and vigorous the action." (See also Marmor and Wittman, 1976.) From de Toqueville to David Truman, observers of American politics have argued that threats to occupational status are the most common stimulants to political action. If the group model overstated the facility and extent of group organization, some of its proponents isolated the most significant element: narrow, concentrated, producer interests are more likely to pay the costs of political action than broad, diffuse, consumer interests.

Not only do concentrated interests have a larger incentive to engage in political action, but they also act with two significant advantages. First, they typically have ongoing organizations, with staff and other resources already in place. This dramatically lowers the marginal cost of political action. Second, most economic organizations have an expertise that rivals that of other political interests, even government agencies and regulators. Their superior grasp (and sometimes even monopoly) of relevant information easily translates into political influence. The more technical an area, the more powerful the advantage, but it is almost always present to some extent.

In sum, two phenomena work to imbalance political markets: unequal interests and disproportionate resources. The two are interrelated: groups with more at stake will invest more to secure an outcome. However, the distinction warrants emphasis for it has important policy implications. Attempts to stimulate countervailing powers, by making resources available to subordinate groups, are doomed to fail if they do not account for differing incentives to employ them. For example, even a resource such as equal access to policy makers—now the object of considerable political effort—is meaningless if the incentives to utilize it over time are grossly unequal. The reverse case—equal interests, unequal resources—is too obvious to require comment. But that clarity should not obscure the fact that imbalanced markets pose an even greater dilemma than the obvious inequality of group resources.

Naturally, diffuse interests are not always somnolent. There are purposive as well as material incentives to political action. A revolt against a sales tax might necessitate cuts in programs that benefit specific groups—scattered taxpayers defeating concentrated beneficiaries; tea drinkers may be swept into political action (even to the point of dumping the tea into Boston harbor). Both are examples of diffuse interests uniting for political action. Such coalitions tend to be loosely organized and are characterized by a grass-roots style of politics. Since sustained, long-term political action requires careful organization, they tend to be temporary. With the end of a legislative deliberation, the group disbands or sets out in search of new issues. Concentrated interests, however, carry on, motivated by the same incentives that first prompted political action.

The conception of imbalanced political markets is relevant to any level of government, but it is particularly appropriate in considering administrative agencies and bureaus. The problem is less nettlesome for legislatures. On a practical level, lobbying legislators appears only marginally effective; analysts have generally found that politicians are more likely to follow their own opinions or the apparent desires of their constituency (Schattschneider, 1935; Bauer et al., 1963; Marmor, 1973; Eulau and Prewitt, 1973). More important, there is at least a formal representation of every citizen. Of course, this does not minimize the complexities of electoral representation. But elective systems do afford a systematic canvass of community sentiment, however vague a guide it may be to concrete policy.

The advantages of organized groups—whatever their extent in legislative politics—increase after a policy's inception. Such groups can be expected to pursue the policy through its implementation and administration. Administrative politics are far less visible; they are not bounded by clear, discrete decisions, and are cluttered with technical details rather than with the symbols that are more likely to arouse diffuse constituencies. The policy focus of program administration is dispersed—temporally, conceptually, even geographically. Only concentrated groups are likely to sustain the attention necessary to participate.

Furthermore, when a bureau deals with a group or an industry over time, symbiotic relationships tend to form. A considerable literature documents the range of these clientele relationships and offers the following account of their life cycle: The industry groups typically have information vital to governing; their cooperation is often necessary to program success; and, as a bureau loses public visibility, the groups with concentrated stakes form a major part of its environment, applying pressure, representing their interests, interacting regularly with the agency (Bernstein, 1955; Noll, 1971).

In extreme cases, groups with intense, concentrated stakes can use a friendly agency to recoup legislative defeats. Important decisions are made in agencies and bureaus that define, qualify, even subvert original legislative intent. Administrative processes may even grow biased to the point that other affected parties are shut out from deliberations that concern them. For example, Congress included a consumer-participation provision in the Hill-Burton Act, but the implementing agency never wrote regulations for it. When consumers overcame the imbalance of interests and sued for participation, they were denied standing. Since the regulations had never been written, consumer representatives had no entry into the policy-making process (Rosenblatt, 1978).

As governmental administration becomes more important, the imperative of balancing political markets becomes more pronounced. The difficulties of doing so are intensified by the disaggregated character of the American political process. In contrast to the British case (McConnell, 1966; Lowi, 1969), congressional oversight of the regulatory and administrative agencies has in the past been uneven and often quite loose. This pattern illustrates imbalanced political markets and its extreme manifestation, agency "capture." The notoriously weak and undisciplined political parties in America contribute to this centrifugal tendency of authority within national government (Burnham, 1978).

The issue we address is how to balance political markets in administrative politics. How do we represent broad, diffuse interests, when all the incentives point to domination by a minority of intensely interested producers? The following discussion analyzes the details of the effort to achieve this balance in local health planning according to the strictures of the 1974 law and subsequent regulation: agencies governed by representative boards ostensibly dominated by consumers. We suggest how clearly understanding and properly institutionalizing the concept of representation can help formulate measures to overcome the tendencies toward imbalance that would normally subvert such efforts.

Consumer Representation and HSAs

The Health Planning Act addressed the issue of interest imbalance by mandating consumer majorities on HSA governing boards: between 51 and 60 percent of each board must be composed of "consumers of health care. . . broadly representative of the social, economic, linguistic, and racial populations" and of "the geographic areas" of the health service area.[1] The rest of the governing board is to be composed of health care providers. There was no means specified for conforming to this mandate in either the law or the regulations.

Administrators quickly discovered that achieving meaningful consumer representation requires considerably more than simply calling for it. Within two years of the law's enactment, a spate of lawsuits had been filed as various groups contended that they were not being represented; the law's ambiguity lent some plausibility to the claim of almost every group. Equally problematic was the question of who should count as representative of whom. And there were reports of public meetings attended only by providers, of consumers shut out of all meaningful deliberations, and of representatives overwhelmed by technical details (Clark, 1977). Such difficulties in the efforts to represent consumers were a major factor in the unexpected delays in certification ("full designation") of most agencies; confusion about or

[1] PL93-641 §1512(b)(3)(C)(i).

repudiation of consumer dominance has actually led to decertification in several instances. Not all the agencies have experienced such troubles, but where HSA success has been achieved, it occurs despite the federal law and its regulations.

Establishing representation requires making fundamental choices. Decisions must be made about the selection of representatives, what those representatives should be like, and the expectations that govern their behavior. Furthermore, the governmental structures within which representatives operate must be considered. Do they encourage or impede effective representation? Is the tendency toward political imbalance redressed? Finally, there is the issue of who is to be represented, a question particularly significant when geographic representation is supplemented or abandoned.

The character and success of consumer representation is contingent on how these questions get answered. Indeed, many of the difficulties that plague the Health Planning Act follow from a failure even to consider most of them.

Conceptual Puzzles and Consumer Representation

Three factors, central to consumer involvement in PL93-641, have been conceptually muddled, both in the law itself and in the analysis and litigation surrounding it. They are accountability, participation, and representation.

Accountability. Put simply, accountability means "answering to" or, more precisely, "having to answer to." One must answer to agents who control the scarce resources one desires. In the classic electoral example, officials are accountable to voters because they control the scarce resources officials desire. Public officials are accountable to legislatures, which control funds; to pressure groups, who can extend or withdraw support; or even to medical providers, who can choose whether to cooperate with an official's program.

The crucial element in each case is that accountability stems from some resource valued by the accountable actor. Accountability is thus not merely an ideal—such as honesty—that public actors "ought" to strive toward. Rather, the resources one cares about hang in the balance, controllable by the relevant constituency.

We call the means by which actors are held to account "mechanisms of accountability." These mechanisms can vary enormously in character and in the extent of control they impose on an actor. For example, voters can occasionally exert control with a "yes" or "no" decision, whereas work supervisors can regularly monitor a subordinate's work, enforcing compliance with specific demands.

There is often, to be sure, a give-and-take process in which actors try to maximize their freedom of action within the constraints of the formal mechanisms and thus minimize accountability. And those indifferent to the scarce resources in question (e.g., an official who has no desire to be reelected) are not, strictly speaking, accountable. But this illustrates the crucial point: in speaking of accountability one must be able to point to specific scarce resources, particular mechanisms that hold representatives to account.

Many of the HSA requirements that are touted as increasing accountability to the public are, in fact, irrelevant to it: a public record of board proceedings;[2] open meetings, with the notice of meetings published in two newspapers and an address given where a proposed agenda may be obtained;[3] an opportunity to comment, either in writing or in a public meeting, about designation,[4] or health system plans (HSPs)[5] or annual implementation plans (AIPs).[6]

These requirements might be said to facilitate public accounting, not accountability. Public participation and information can inform the exercise of accountability but, without formal mechanisms that force boards to answer to consumers, there is not what we call direct public accountability.

Well-defined mechanisms of accountability are central to the idea of

[2] 41 Federal Register 12812 (March 26, 1976) §122.114.
[3] 41 Federal Register 12812 (March 26, 1976), §§122.104(b)(1)(viii) and 122.109(e)(3).
[4] 41 Federal Register 12812 (March 26, 1976), §§ 122.104(a)(8) and 122.104(b)(7).
[5] 41 Federal Register 12812 (March 26, 1976), §122.107(c)(2).
[6] 41 Federal Register 12812 (March 26, 1976), §122.107(c)(3).

holding leaders to account. Propositions that substitute such notions as "winning over" or "working with" the community for an identifiable mechanism are much weaker, conflating the common-language usage of accounting for action with accountability to a constituency, a distinction pointed out by our colleague, Douglas Yates.

Suggesting that health systems agencies would be ineffective without public support is an equally weak conception of accountability to consumers. Every agency of every government expresses these expectations and fears. What is unique about representative government is that the citizenry—not the government agencies—is given the final say. And that say is not expressed by "inhospitality" or "lack of trust" or "written protests" but by an authoritative decision. What we term mechanisms of accountability are the institutionalization of that authoritative decision.

Accountability can be to more than one constituency. As health planning is now structured, the Department of Health, Education, and Welfare (HEW), state governments, local governments, consumers, providers, and numerous other groups can all attempt to hold an HSA accountable. These competing agents introduce significant tensions. One especially difficult problem is the conflict between accountability to local and to national government. There are indications that precisely this conflict is asserting itself as HEW, for example, drafts guidelines, and local communities protest that they do not apply in their specific situations. (Rudolf Klein [1979] has elaborated this argument in the British context, with elegant insight on the question of consumer participation.)

The emphasis on community control rests on Jeffersonian traditions, and has been seized upon by opponents of big government and centralized bureaucracies. Local communities, according to this view, understand their own needs best and ought, therefore, to be responsible for the policies by which they are governed.

The opposing position draws from sources as disparate as Marx and Weber, Madison and Hamilton. National needs require national solutions. What is good for individual communities (e.g., the best hospitals) may not sum to what is best for the entire nation (lower medical costs). This conception typically expresses egalitarian values—only a national policy can redistribute costs and benefits among states and regions.

Accountability in the Health Planning Act is only partially delineated, and is therefore geographically ambiguous. Since local communities establish their agency's modus operandi, the potential for local accountability is present. However, insofar as the law takes up the issue explicitly, it presses accountability to HEW.

HEW is responsible for reviewing the plans, the structure, and the operation of every designated agency at least once every twelve months (sec. 201515 [c] [1]). Presumably, renewal of designation (an important resource that HSA boards desire) is at stake. This is accountability in every important sense. But it can be traced to the public only through the long theoretical strand leading through the presidency. From this perspective, HSA boards are no more accountable to the public than is any other executive agency—certainly a far cry from the rhetoric that accompanied the enactment of PL63-641. As the law now stands, accountability to the public (either directly or through states and localities) is not prohibited or rendered impossible. But neither is accountability to the public instituted or even significantly facilitated.

Participation. In classical political thought, self-government meant direct participation by the citizenry in public decisions. In this context, Plato envisioned a republic small enough for an orator to address; Aristotle, one in which each citizen could know every other. Rousseau argued that democracy ended when participation did. For obvious reasons, such formulations are generally considered anachronisms in modern industrial societies. Representation has replaced direct participation as the institutionalization of the idea that "every man has the right to have a say in what happens to him" (Pitkin, 1967:3). From a theoretical perspective, it is surprising that a law as concerned with consumer representation as PL93-641 articulates so few guidelines regarding representation, and so many regarding direct public participation.

The earlier discussion of imbalanced political markets suggests why direct participation provisions tend to favor providers over consumers. First, their interest in health planning is far more concentrated and obvious. Planning decisions can directly affect their livelihood. Hospital administrators, officials of state medical associations, and other employed medical-care personnel are far more likely to pay the costs of participating in open HSA meetings. The general public—"the consumers"—are not likely to do so. After all, their stake in the proceedings is much smaller; planning does not usually affect their livelihood in as obvious a way.

Furthermore, the difficulties of fostering direct consumer participation are aggravated by the nature of health issues. Health concerns, though important, are intermittent for most people. They are not as clearly or regularly salient as the condition of housing or children's schools—situations that citizens confront daily. Consequently, it is far more difficult to establish public participation in HSAs than in renter's associations or school districts (Marmor, 1977).

We are not suggesting that provisions for participation are objectionable or should be stricken from PL93-641. Rather, without being carefully tied to some mechanism of accountability or broader view of representation, the provisions are, at best, marginally useful to consumers. They are most likely to be utilized by aroused provider institutions.

Representation.   Representation is necessitated by the impossibility of direct, participatory democracy in modern society. The entire population cannot be present to make decisions. Hence, institutions must be designed to "represent"—literally, "to make present again" or to "make present in some sense something which is nevertheless not present literally or in fact" (Pitkin, 1967:8).

Three aspects of representation are usually considered in the appraisal of representative institutions: formal, descriptive, and substantive features, a formulation originated by Griffiths (1960), and refined and popularized by Pitkin (1967).

By *formal representation* we mean the institutionalization of representation—the specific mechanisms by which representatives are selected and controlled. The mechanisms need have nothing to do with what representatives should be like (descriptive), or the way in which they should act (substantive). Yet they are crucial in defining the process of representation. They are the structure through which representation is established and carried on; they define constituencies and link representatives to them. Institutionalizing accountability rests in large measure on formal requirements.

One commonsense definition of representation is purely formal. Birch (1971:20), for example, suggests that "the essential character of political representatives is the manner of their selection, not their behavior or characteristics or symbolic value." To him, elections equal representation. Few theorists would agree to so starkly formal a view. More commonly, elections must not merely be held but must offer significant "choice"—they must be "free" (Swabey, 1969; Friedrich, 1950:266 ff.). Although empirical referants are often noted (elections in the UK, not in the USSR), theorists have had difficulty in specifying precisely what constitutes "free" elections.

The most important issue of formal representation relevant to PL93-641 is whether representatives should be selected in general elections, by organized groups, by officials, or by self-selection. Though in many cases accountability to the community is increased by general elections, we do not believe that is the case for HSAs.

The Health Planning Act leaves most formal representational questions to be answered on the local level. This is not necessarily unfortunate, as long as the applications for designation are carefully reviewed regarding the issues of formal representation. These issues can be stated in broad terms by asking what constituency a representative is tied to, and by what institutional arrangements.

Descriptive representation refers to the characteristics of representatives. Early formulations of representation held that, since constituencies could not be present themselves to make public choices, they should be "represented" by a "body which [is] an exact portrait, in miniature, of the people at large." The reasoning is straightforward. Since not all the people can be present to make decisions, representative bodies ought to be miniature versions or microcosms of the public, mirroring the populations they represent. The similarity of composition is expected to result in similarity of outcomes; the assembly will "think, feel, reason (and, therefore) act" as the public would have (John Quincy Adams, cited in Pitkin, 1967:60).

A number of difficulties confront this formulation. First, "the public" is a broad entity. What aspect of it ought to be reflected in an assembly? The map metaphor is telling in this regard: Do we want the kind of map that shows rainfall, or altitudes? Topography? Trade regions? Dialects?

John Stuart Mill argued that opinions should be represented; Bentham and James Mill emphasized subjective interests; Sterne, more ambiguously, "opinions, aspirations and wishes"; Burke, broad fixed interests. Swabey suggested that citizens were equivalent units, that if all had roughly equal political opportunities, representatives would be a proper random selection and, consequently, would be descriptively representative. Whichever the case, a failure to specify precisely what characteristics are mirrored reduces microcosm or mirror theories to incoherence.

Even when the relevant criterion for selecting representatives is properly specified, mirroring an entire nation is chimerical. Mill's "every shade of opinion," for example, cannot possibly be reconstructed in the assembly hall on one issue, much less on all. One cannot mirror a million consumers, no matter which sixteen or eighteen consumers are representing them on the HSA governing board. Competing opinions or interests can of course be represented. But the chief aim of microcosmic representation is mirroring the full spectrum of constituencies. Pitkin notes that the language in which these theories is presented indicates the difficulty of actually implementing them. The theorists constantly resort to metaphor—the assembly as map, mirror, portrait. They are all unrealistic in more practical terms.

Mirroring the populace may be as undesirable as it is infeasible. Many opinions are idiotic. The merriment that followed Senator Hruska's proposal that the mediocre deserved representation on the U.S. Supreme Court suggests a common understanding of the foolishness of baldly descriptive views.[7]

Furthermore, if representatives are asked merely to reflect the populace, they have no standards regarding their behavior as repre-

---

[7] For notable formulations of this common idea, see Edmund Burke, "The English Constitutional System," in Pitkin (1969); or James Madison, "The Problem of Faction in a Republic," in *The Federalist,* Modern Library edition, 1937.

sentatives. Descriptive representation tells us only what representatives are, not what they do. Opinion polls would be more appropriate mechanisms for identifying public views.

Though microcosm theories are neither realistic nor achievable, descriptive (if not precisely mirror) views are relevant to the operation of modern legislatures. Legislators are commonly criticized for not mirroring their constituents' views or interests. In fact, Adams's formulation might be recast as one guideline to selecting representatives—members of the public vote, essentially, for candidates who appear to "think, feel, reason, and act" as they do. Thus, descriptive qualities inform the operation of formal mechanisms. But surely such very generally conceived descriptive representing is entirely different from the utopian endeavor of forming a microcosm of the populace in the assembly hall.

One contemporary manifestation of microcosm views is what Greenstone and Peterson (1973) refer to as "socially descriptive representation." Rather than mirroring opinions or interests, this conception proposes mirroring the social and demographic characteristics of a community's population. A precarious link is added to Adams's already rickety syllogism: If people a) share demographic characteristics, b) they will "think, feel, and reason" like one another and, consequently, c) act like one another. This is both bad logic and pernicious to the substantive representation of consumer interests.

The problems with mirror views, enumerated above, are all relevant to this version. Demographically mirroring a populace in an assembly is even more unlikely than mirroring their opinions. Obviously, not all social characteristics can (or ought to) be represented; the problem of discriminating among them is particularly vexing. Common sense rebels at representing left-handers or redheads. What of Lithuanians? Italians? Jews? The uneducated? Mirror views provide no guidelines for drawing such distinctions. Their central conception—the microcosm—is flawed, impossible. It is necessary to look beyond the logic of descriptive representation to choose the social groups that ought to be represented.

Even when the categories to be mirrored are specified, problems remain. Not all individual members of a social group will, in fact, "think, feel, and reason" alike; and they will not act with equal efficacy. Yet, in itself, mirror representation does not distinguish among members of a population group—one low-income representative, for example, is interchangeable with any other. As long as the requisite number of a population group is seated, the society is represented—mirrored—in the appropriate aspect. Such actors are not truly representatives but are mere instances of population groups.

Socially descriptive representation is pernicious because it removes the necessity of recourse to the constituency. The need for formal selection mechanisms and accountability is obviated. Skin color or income, for example, marks a representative as acceptable or not acceptable, regardless of what the constituency thinks. The result is that any member of the group is as qualified a representative as any other. This is a situation that almost begs for "tokenism." If the only requirement is that a fixed percentage of the board must be drawn from a certain group, there is nothing to recommend blacks, elected by fellow blacks or selected by NAACP, or women, elected by women or selected by NOW, over blacks and women "drafted" onto a board because they will "not rock the boat." Precisely this logic operated in New York litigation (*Aladmuy* v. *Pirro,* discussed below), where the judge found that, as long as the "quota" of minorities and poor was filled, there was nothing for him to do. He would not distinguish among them.

It has been suggested that socially descriptive representation might be effective if the representatives were tied to the groups they represented by some kind of pressure, some sort of oversight. Such representation then moves beyond mere socially descriptive representation. The selected agent is then a representative, not merely as an instance of a group's features, but because he or she is acceptable to that group. Thus, we return to a formal conception of representation—the constituency selecting a representative who "thinks, feels, reasons, and acts" as it does.

PL93-641, as it currently stands and has been interpreted in the New York and Texas district-court cases, does not provide for this. It requires only that the composition of the board be a statistical microcosm of the constituency's racial, sexual, and income distribution. The Health Planning Act does attempt to expand the health role of often overlooked groups. But, to be successful, it must mandate more than proportional representation on the HSA board; it must require that groups select and monitor their representatives.

Still, for all its difficulties, there is a kernel of truth (as Birch points out) within the theory of socially descriptive representation. Often social categories are related to interests; and, as we will argue in the following section, interests are what ought to be represented. Thus, religious affiliation bespeaks definite interests in Northern Ireland, race affects interests in America, poverty defines specific interests everywhere. And although the actual representation of interests may be subtle and complicated to evaluate, the social categories that are attached to them are almost correspondingly easy.

The choices regarding formal and descriptive representation must be made with the objective of furthering genuinely representative behavior, or *substantive representation*. This is an analytic category by which representatives can be guided and evaluated.

The central question about representative behavior is whether it is in the interest of the constituency. This raises the hoary problem of defining "interest" (Barry, 1965; Balbus, 1972; Flatham, 1966). Is it to be understood as objective fact or subjective choice? The answer determines whether representatives should be considered "messengers," simply conveying constituent desires and acting on constituent requests, or "guardians," doing what the representatives consider to be in the constituents' interest, without consulting them. Substantive representation fits neither of these extremes. Though certain choices are surely in a constituency's objective interest, regardless of their opinions, liberal institutions are ultimately structured on consent. Representatives may pursue their own understanding of constituent interest, but at some point the constituency must make a judgment. The directness of the judgment depends on the formal representation mechanisms, but that there is judgment is crucial.

There is always a danger of drift from substantive representation to simply a guardian or messenger role. In PL93-641, the former can occur, for example, when an organized group selects a representative and exerts too much control over his or her behavior. But drifting toward the guardian role is the greatest danger for consumer representatives.

Health issues are often viewed as technically complex; PL93-641 encourages that view in its emphasis on expert scientific planning. If consumer representatives are to be successful, they will need to develop expertise regarding health and planning issues, either through interaction with the HSA staff or by other means. However, as consumer representatives become sophisticated, their tendency may be to drift toward a guardian role, defending a consumer interest that is thought to be incomprehensible to the consumer constituency. This development may be aggravated when the perception of crisis gives representatives more latitude, at the expense of representational ideals such as accountability.

A related issue is the identity of the constituency. Should governing board representatives be working for the good of the community as a whole? Of the consumers as taxpayers? Of all black (female, poor) consumers? Some answers may be implicit in the formal mechanisms. The general model underlying HSA boards implicitly follows the liberal ideal of getting all the narrow, self-interested parties together and making them thrash out policy choices among themselves. Each representative works for his narrow interest group; yet, through the compromise and bargaining necessary to get his group anything, answers acceptable to all will emerge. If this is the model, then it is important that all groups be in on the bargaining process.

When, for example, lawyers for one HSA emphasize the importance of getting a board that is not segmented, they are incorrect. Ironically, the model calls for a highly segmented, even contentious, board, for a board on which every health interest is vigorously represented will be more contentious than one that is captured or dominated by a single interest.

It is also important that representatives affect policy outcomes. All representatives have some symbolic function; but insofar as they have no other, they are not substantively representative, for they give the public they represent no say over policy (Edelman, 1967; Pitkin, 1969: n.10, chapter 10).

By this logic it is clear how some representatives can represent their constituency better than others: they not only perceive what is good for—in the interest of—their constituency, but also have the ability to act successfully on that perception. An eloquent speaker, a successful operator, a person who is not easily duped, an individual with important contacts or serving on important committees, therefore provides more substantive representation than one with the same opinions but without the same capacities. There are many relevant examples from the community action programs (CAPs) of precisely this phenomenon—boards that were relatively more successful because of the political skills, experience, and intelligence of some of their members (Greenstone and Peterson, 1973).

A representative's effectiveness, then, generally flows from a mixture of position and ability. An able person may affect policy, even from a relatively weak position. An incompetent one may fail to do so, even in a position of authority. The point is that substantive representation necessitates both knowing and successfully pursuing the constituents' interests.

Conceptual Puzzles Reconsidered. Substantive representation is the effective pursuit of the interests of the constituency. Ultimately it is the goal of all democratic representation. However, the final judge of representation must be the represented; either directly or indirectly the represented must control some scarce resource their representative wants (e.g., votes). Only then can we properly speak of a governing board as accountable to its constituency.

The Health Planning Act gives these issues little consideration. There is no systematically mandated accountability and little evidence of it as a concern. A representative's orientation is considered only in terms of socially descriptive representation. This approach patronizes the relevant groups. It will ineffectively advance consumer representation unless it is linked to effective mechanisms of accountability by which the members of those groups can evaluate the substantive quality of the representation received.

Effective Consumer Representation

This section suggests ways in which adequate consumer representation can be facilitated and effective mechanisms of accountability created. The task, as pointed out earlier, is balancing the health-planning political market, rather than just getting consumers on boards.

The HSA staffs are one resource that could help consumers

achieve political parity. Staffs generally have considerable expertise in issues of medical care and health. Occupying full-time positions in health planning, they have a concentrated interest in the industry. Is there any reason to believe that they will typically support consumers when there are conflicts of interest?

The evidence thus far shows wide variation in staffs' views. In New England, some play an outspoken proconsumer role (Codman, 1977). In many other areas they have allied with providers, often seriously undermining consumer representatives who cannot match the combined expertise of providers and staff (Clark, 1977:55). Generally the support of the staff appears to be essential to an active consumer role on HSA boards. The problem is systematically harnessing the staffs' market-balancing potential to consumer interests.

The most direct approach is to restructure the health systems agencies so that part of the professional staff is placed under consumer control—to be selected by and accountable to them. The staff's tasks could be specified in any number of ways, but its critical function would be providing professional (i.e., expert, full-time) support to the consumer effort.

Another potential for balancing the health planning market lies in organizations that already exist within the consumer population. Political scientists generally agree that the "basic units . . . of polity or political process are groups formed around interests" (Schmitter, 1975). The very existence of these groups attests to a commitment to improve the life circumstances of some part of the population. Furthermore, they have already paid the costs of organizing. We can expect their attention to issues to be high and relatively sustained. They can often overcome lack of expertise by redeploying their staff (Berry, 1977; Nadel, 1971; McFarland, 1976).

Organizations can meet a problem with more resources and in a more sustained way than isolated individuals. It is telling that much of the litigation challenging HSA boards comes from organizations formed to further the rights or general circumstances of certain disadvantaged groups within the consumer population. Existing "reform" organizations have potential, then, for balancing the health-care political market; we believe that they can play an effective role in selecting and monitoring consumer representatives.

The experience of the community action program (CAP) provides some support for this claim. Selection by groups tended to produce the most independent and competent boards. Moreover, where more than one organization wanted to select representatives for the same population or interest, elections were held among the groups. Organizations representing the poor in parts of New York City, for example, competed fiercely to gain support of the community—a far cry from the apathy that greeted general elections, and the alienation and cynicism that accompanied selection of representatives by officials (Greenstone and Peterson, 1973).

We recommend, therefore, that those charged with selecting members of consumer boards select not the members themselves, but groups organized around health-care interests. If more than one group seeks to select a representative for the same interest, a special election would be called. It is crucial that the interests themselves (e.g., poverty, race) be specified by HEW. Competition among groups representing an interest is acceptable, even desirable; competition among interests to be represented is not. (The logic of choosing what interests merit representation on HSA boards will be discussed below.)

A potential gap always exists between an interest felt and a group's articulation of that interest; however, groups that have overcome the obstacles to organization are the most likely promoters of a particular interest. Representatives from these groups will have clearly defined constituencies, experience in organizational politics, and resources at their disposal. These attributes will help them both in identifying group interests and in pursuing them, regardless of their other characteristics. (Even minorities suing for represention in Texas were willing to accept whites to represent blacks, for example, if the NAACP selected them.)

The experience of the CAPs indicates that representatives selected in this way tend to be the most able, show a universalistic orientation, and are least likely to be co-opted.

A group can be expected to monitor its representatives more carefully than will the general public. Thus, as long as the representatives are chosen for a fixed term, accountability is increased. Representatives should be allowed to serve out their term (without recall) so as not to bind them too tightly to the selecting organization (Lipsky and

Lounds, 1976:107); they should be permitted reelection so that they are not bound too loosely.

Ideally, then, the imbalanced political market in health planning will be tempered by two mechanisms, one internal to the health systems agency (staff assigned to the consumer representatives), the other external (selection of representatives by groups). We expect the former to facilitate organization and expertise among the consumer representatives, the latter to improve representation and heighten their accountability.

Of course, in some locations and for some interests it will be impossible to find appropriate groups. In these cases, another, less desirable, mode of selection (or formal representation) will be necessary. We evaluate two others: general election, and selection by officials.

General Elections. Various reform groups have called for election of consumer representatives in a model roughly based on that for the selection of school boards. The surface plausibility of the proposal should not be permitted to obscure its difficulties. One problem with direct election of representatives to HSA boards stems from the failure of most Americans to consider themselves part of an ongoing health-care community. They typically seek care sporadically, and do not conceive of health care in terms of local systems. Both factors distinguish health planning from education or housing issues, where specific elections may be more effective.

Evidence from the CAP poverty programs supports the view that elections are problematic; fewer than 3 percent of the eligible population voted for local CAP boards in Philadelphia, fewer than 1 percent voted in Los Angeles. Those who did vote were moved to do so by personal, not policy, considerations. Overwhelmingly, they voted for their neighbors and, presumably, personal acquaintances. The consequent policy formulated by these representatives was, predictably, overwhelmingly particularistic. It helped their friends, not the community or the interests they ostensibly represented. Representatives generated little community interest or support. They tended to be ineffective advocates and operators.

Since the public chooses its health planning representatives directly, the representatives can theoretically be held accountable with relative ease. However, in practice, low incentives and marginal visibility will undermine elections.

It is important to note that "antiparticipation" city officials, who could not control the selection of CAP boards, preferred elections as the alternative. They apparently felt that this formal mechanism would not threaten their interests by generating energetic, aggressive representation of the interests of poor people—an outcome they feared from selection by groups.

Selection by Local Officials. This mechanism leaves accountability to the public very tenuous. The constituency is left with no direct control over its representatives, but must hold the selector of the representatives to account. In the worst cases, the selector is not directly accountable to the public either. Boards selected by local officials are accountable to, and presumably controlled by, local government; they will be as accountable as any other local agency. Yet they operate within a program that promises direct consumer participation. When a health planning issue becomes highly visible, we expect this mismatch of rhetoric and reality to cause public frustration and alienation.

Since officials can choose whichever member of a group they desire, many will choose ones that "make no trouble." Thus descriptive representation (what representatives "think, feel, and reason") will probably be low even when socially descriptive representation is high.

Substantive representation will generally be low. The HSA, over time, will become indistinguishable from other agencies in the local health-care bureaucracy.

Who Should Be Represented?

We now turn from the means of securing effective consumer representation to the issue of who should be represented. Which elements of the consumer population merit health representation?

The notion of dividing up the consumer population for the purpose of representation implies that there are subgroups of the consumer population with distinctive health care interests that ought to be represented.

Only one subcategory has been precisely delineated in PL93-641—those individuals who live in nonmetropolitan areas. Their representation on the board must reflect the proportion of nonmetropolitan residents in the health service area.[8] As for the rest, PL93-641 says only that consumers should be "broadly representative of the social, economic, linguistic, and racial population" of the area.[9]

Unscrambling the present confusion about representation requires an assessment of what consumer involvement is intended to accomplish. Presumably, the goal is to facilitate the articulation and satisfaction of the health care needs in American communities. If so, what is required is substantive representation, not hollow tokenism. Different health care interests in the area must be identified and selected for special attention through representation. The reason for including such groups as minorities, low-income persons, and women on the board should not be to mirror the community's population on the boards; that, we have argued, is foolish and impossible. Rather, certain groups—minorities, low-income people, and women—should be included insofar as they have different and important health interests that the political system ought to consider. The argument is most compelling when it refers to interests that are often overlooked in local political processes. Moving from mirror representation to the effort to improve representation of specified interests requires changing the language of the law requiring that consumer representatives be "broadly representative of the . . . populations" of the health service area, to language requiring them to be "representative of consumer health interests" of the health service area.

The obvious question, then, is what specific consumer health interests should be represented? The answer is not easy because interests vary by issue. Regarding questions of access to health care, the current debate has identified various groups with legitimate claims. For example, access problems are different for rural and for urban populations, or for the chronically as opposed to the intermittently ill. At the same time, there are groups that, while part of the population (and therefore potentially included on a board constituted on the microcosm principle), do not genuinely have health care interests peculiar to their own group. For example, it is not clear that those with little formal

---

[8] PL93-641, §1512(b)(3)(C)(iii)(II).
[9] PL93-641, §1512(b)(3)(C)(i).

education have specific health care needs or interests in the same way as the low-income or the aged populations.

As issues change, so do the interests that claim the right to a spokesman. The infirm could claim a representative for every type of disease, when the issue of new facilities arises; so could every ethnic group with specific genetic diseases that disproportionately or exclusively afflict them (blacks, Jews, Italians, for instance). The possible list is very long. However, to avoid an infinite round of litigation, HEW must make the difficult choices and specify the various consumer subgroups with recognizable health care interests that ought to be represented on the HSA boards. In this way, the present, almost infinitely broad, mandate would be replaced by one that is highly specific.

To illustrate, HEW could specify that groups reflecting the following interests be provided representation on the HSA board in approximate proportion to their number in the health service area: a) the poor; b) women; c) the aged; d) racial or linguistic groups comprising significant portions of the population; e) area of residence (the Codman Report [1977] breaks health service areas into hospital service areas—essentially, these are large catchment areas corresponding to the distribution of hospitals within a health service area. We suggest such a division of all health service areas, getting representatives from each subdivision in approximate proportion to its percentage of the total population of the health service area); f) groups that pay for medical care, such as insurance companies or unions; g) other identifiable groups that the secretary of HEW recognizes as having a health care interest and forming a significant segment of the population. Examples are migrant workers, black-lung victims, persons exposed to occupational hazards. These groups should be specified by the secretary either on the recommendation of the state or by appeal of that group.[10]

The specification of interest we propose will not only curtail the

---

[10] For a similar list, see Georgia Legal Services Program, "Proposed Amendments to PL93-641," Dec. 9, 1977, #3. To avoid litigation, regulations should make clear that this is a residual category to be filled at the discretion of the secretary, not a sweeping general provision mandating representation slots for all identifiable groups having significant health care interests.

stream of litigation that has sprung from the microcosm view, but will also help insure the representation of important interests. As the law stands, a great deal of discretion regarding who is represented is left to state and local political games. And while it is appropriate to maximize the competition among groups on the board regarding health care issues, it is important to minimize the competition over which interests get on the board in the first place to compete over these issues. The danger is that groups will try to take over the boards, shutting out other legitimate interests. The vagueness of the current law and regulations as to who is to be represented increases the possibility of conflict—and some of the litigation indicates that fear of further conflict is not groundless.

While the preceding discussion resolves a practical problem, it introduces a theoretical one: there is no systematic rationale by which HEW can make those "difficult choices" among affected interests. No matter which interests are selected, not all individuals are equally represented, or even equally enfranchised. How, under such conditions, can HSAs claim legitimacy as authoritative community decision-makers?

The answer is clear when there is a macrotheory of objective interests spanning the entire citizenry, such as class analyses include. However, liberal theory offers no comparable vision of fixed systematic interests. Pluralism brilliantly avoided the issue by assuming the link between subjective interest felt and group formed. Bentley is clear and adamant on this issue: "To state the raw materials of political life [—] the groups directly insisting on [a policy] . . . those directly opposing it, and those more directly concerned in it—is much more complete than any statement in terms of self-interest, theories or ideals" (Greenstone, 1975:244). Market conceptions provide little help. Although the populace is, theoretically, divisible into consumers and providers, regarding any functional area, those labels press a horde of often competing interests under a single label. As shown earlier, seating "consumer" representatives is a difficult mandate, regardless of the infelicitous mandate that boards be "broadly representative." Finally, the choices we have urged HEW to make are plausible, not Platonic ones.

This does not mean that we are without a rationale for selecting interests. Emerging groups can be legitimated or strengthened as political actors by this type of quasi-corporatist program. The most important of these may be advocacy groups speaking for broad consumer constituencies and organizations such as unions and industrial associations. They are organized and have a clear, relatively concentrated interest in the politics of medical care. Such groups are promising market balancers. Other interests (minority groups, poverty groups) can be included for similar reasons, or because it is reasonable, necessary, or prudent to include them, given the objectives of the program. Anderson's (1977) elaboration of this argument helps clarify the problem of the legitimacy of the HSA boards.

For various reasons, HSAs are structured to improve public accountability and representation. However, that structure is not relevant to the legitimacy of these agencies qua governmental units. HSAs must be viewed as a supplement to, rather than a substitute for, geographic representation. As administrative agencies, their legitimacy flows not from representational schemes, but from a legislative mandate—from Congress.

Litigation and Representation

PL93-641 was enacted in January 1975. By December 1977, it was the subject of eighteen lawsuits, five of which included the issue of consumer representation. These five cases are analyzed below in light of the preceding discussion of representation and accountability.

Aladmuy, et al. v Pirro, et al., C.A. No. 76-CV-204 (N.D., N.Y., April 7, 1977). The plaintiffs were dissatisfied with the minority representation on the Syracuse-Onandaga County (N.Y.) Planning Agency. The court ruled against plaintiffs because the representation of minorities was numerically adequate. With respect to the selection of certain minority members over others, the court stated that it would not find an abuse of discretion by the secretary of HEW except where the secretary's action was "so arbitrary as to be clearly wrong."

The case is an illustration of the application of the view of mirror representation. The court found no criterion in either the law or the regulations by which to judge representatives except for descriptive characteristics (in this case, "minority" status). Since both the representatives selected for the HSA board and their challengers satisfied that criterion, there was no way to choose between them. It was not possible to select one minority group member as any better, or more "representative," than any other. Since PL93-641 and its regulations say nothing about formal representation, challengers have no recourse and courts have no reason to insist on accountability if the criterion of socially descriptive representation is minimally satisfied.

Three companion cases can be considered together:

The Louisiana Association of Community Organizations for Reform Now (ACORN), et al. v New Orleans Area/Bayou Rivers Health Systems Agency, et al., C.A. No. 17-361 (E.D. La., filed March 15, 1977). ACORN is an association of low- to moderate-income citizens claiming that the New Orleans HSA is not "socially or economically" representative of the area. ACORN states that of thirty-nine consumer members of the board, only four have incomes under $10,000.

Rakestraw, et al. v Califano, et al., C.A. No. C77-635A (N.D. Ga., Atlanta Div., filed April 22, 1977). Plaintiffs assert that there is inadequate representation of low-income individuals and families as well as of the handicapped and women.

Califano is cited, not only for conditionally designating a board with inadequate representation of the above-mentioned groups, but for failing to "propose and promulgate regulations dealing with the composition . . . and selection process" of HSA boards. The court is asked to require Califano to devise a method of selecting consumer representatives that renders them accountable to the public.

Texas ACORN, et al. v Texas Area V Health Systems Agency, et. al., C.A. No. S-76-102-CA (E.D. Texas, Sherman Div., March 1, 1977). The plaintiffs argued that only three of the forty-one consumer representatives have incomes below the median for the area ($10,000). They argued that if people with income above the median are to represent lower-income consumers ("under specific circumstances"), then the burden of proof is on the defendant HSA to indicate how some or all of the board members with over $10,000 incomes would represent the poor.

They contend that representatives of the "public at large" do not count as representatives of the poor; this is a consequence of the model underlying their notion of HSAs, one of pluralistic bargaining among interests.

The federal defendants replied that it is not necessary to be poor to represent the poor; but they conceded that the federal regulations were inadequate, with regard both to the selection of the consumer representatives and to the representation of consumers on the board. (Note that these are precisely the charges in *Rakestraw*.)

The district court a) enjoined the defendant HSA from acting as an HSA or expending HSA funds, and b) ruled that between sixteen and twenty-five of the forty-one representatives must have incomes below the mean. Thus a strictly mathematical delineation was made, with a little "give" in it to make it "broadly" rather than "precisely" representative.

Defendant HEW has asked for a stay in the case until regulations can be developed; it will then be determined whether the Texas HSA conforms to the regulations.

Once again we find HEW mired in attempts to enforce socially descriptive representation. In bringing suit, the ACORN organizations use the mirror conception of representation to their advantage. But they recognize that it alone will not suffice to produce adequate representation of consumer interests over the long run. This realization—although present in all three cases—is most explicit in *Rakestraw*. There, HEW is sued not only regarding the "composition" but also regarding the "selection" of boards. The suit asks HEW to consider what we describe as the formal aspect of representation. Furthermore, plaintiffs demand not mere specification of a formal mechanism, but a mechanism that guarantees accountability to the public. They are, to some extent, willing to waive socially descriptive requirements in favor of accountability engendered by the selection process. The trade-off is illustrated in the Texas ACORN brief, with the suggestion that a white selected by the NAACP would be acceptable from the perspective of black interests.

Texas ACORN et al. v Texas Area Health Service Area, et al., 559 F2nd 1019 (U.S. Court of Appeals, 5th Cir., Sept. 23, 1977). On appeal, a broader view of the case was taken. The district court's undifferentiated mirror view was rejected and a full evidentiary hearing, in which HEW demonstrated precisely how board members were representative of the low-income or demographic population, was mandated. The view that one must be a member of those groups was explicitly rejected.

This ruling shows a far greater sensitivity to the issues of representation. There is cognizance of questions regarding the representatives' relations to their constituencies and the necessity of various skills relevant to achieving substantive representation. In sum, there is awareness that a mindless adherence to the mirroring ideal can undermine the effective (or—in our terms—substantive) representation of a constituency's interests.

Amos, et al. v Central California Health Systems Agency, et al. C.A. No. 76-174 ci (E.D. Calif., filed Sept. 10, 1976). Plaintiffs charged that Whites were underrepresented on the board because Fresno and Kern counties were underrepresented. HEW has sent the defendant agency a letter, noting that its governing board is not composed in conformity with the requirements of PL93-641, so this case will probably not be settled in court. The race issue was not directly dealt with by HEW but subsumed under the criticism that the representation of metropolitan and nonmetropolitan areas was not fixed in exact proportion to the population. About race, HEW said only: "The ethnic representation on your board can be reasonably readjusted when you correct its composition in terms of nonmetropolitan/metropolitan distribution."

The *Amos* case illustrates two other difficulties. First, the charge that minorities "captured" this HSA board, as the plaintiffs claimed, points out the distinction between a) giving contending groups a place on the board to dispute policy questions, and b) letting groups contend for the places on—or control over—the board. The latter defeats the purpose of representative boards: to allow local consumer interests to thrash out local health issues with each other as well as with providers.

A second difficulty follows directly from the first. Precisely who is being represented is not made clear by a law and regulations that merely mandate broad representation of the "social, economic, linguistic, and racial populations" of the health service area. Who is to determine what is "broadly representative"? We have argued that the concept of "broadly representing" (i.e., mirroring) a community is a meaningless guide to consumer representation. Instead, the interests or groups that merit representation must be specified precisely. That specification must be made with a fuller understanding of representation than is at present evident in PL93-641.

Health Policy, Health Plans, and the HSAs

HSAs face insurmountable problems completely apart from that of representing consumers. The Health Planning Act has generated expectations for reshaping American medicine that no HSA can meet. The health systems agencies are simply not equipped to control inflation, solve problems of inadequate access, or rationalize the health services of a community. In discussing why, we shall point particularly to the factors that were expected to distinguish this planning effort from previous ones—"teeth" and sophisticated technology.

Authority and Health Planning

Serious planning involves choosing goals for the future and the ways of arriving at them. One must distinguish between this sense of planning—manipulating a system toward particular goals in a specified fashion—and the writing of (often unreadable) documents termed "plans." The former requires the capacity for authoritative decisions about the allocation of resources.

How nations in fact plan for health—that is, make allocative decisions regarding future goals—is not exhaustively illuminated (indeed, sometimes not seriously touched on) by studies of how official planning bodies operate. Put another way, we have two subjects: the process of operational health planning, and the process of health planning organizations (Marmor and Bridges, 1980). The key element is the connection between choosing goals and the capacity to pursue or "implement" them. When the connection is loose—when plans are isolated from the process of resource allocation and, more generally, from authority—planning can become a smokescreen, a symbol, or simply frustrated wheelspinning.

At the same time, de facto plans will be either the choices of those who in fact allocate resources (the connection between authoritative choices based on financing arrangements and system control holds true under most conditions—including laissez-faire), or a result of the incentives operating within ongoing arrangements. The latter may be termed "change without choice" (Marmor, 1976), but it ought not be confused with the "change without influence" that is implicit in homeostatic—antiplanning—market conceptions. Such arrangements tend to be characterized, not by the theory's self-regulating market, but by the domination of identifiable actors—hospitals, nursing homes, physicians—with an unrelentingly clear incentive: "more." Thus, the well-known incentives of an American hospital are more high technology, more modernization, a fuller range of services and, therefore, more prestige, more first-class physicians, and so on. The consequences of this system are impressive technologies, rising costs, and a frustrating lack of corresponding change in health status indicators (Sidel and Sidel, 1977; Marmor and Morone, 1979). An HSA that overcomes some of the problems described above and plans for "less," will need more than its "plan" to deflect that hospital from the incentives that ideology, financing, and provider expectations have generated.

The American suspicion of centralized authority is well documented (Hartz, 1955; Shonfield, 1965). Even the sweeping expansion of government legitimacy in the 1930s included only fleeting relaxation of this resistance. Intellectually, the hostility has been expressed in two major ways: in arguments that authoritative planning or control is tyrannous (Friedman, 1962; Hayek, 1944; von Mises, 1962), and that it is not realistic (Lindblom, 1959). The Health Planning Act and its HSAs fit obviously into this tradition. Their mission is overstated, their role ambiguous, their authority and political capacity highly circumscribed. They are certainly no match for the grandiosity of their plans. Most of what occurs in local health markets is beyond their jurisdiction: the terms of reimbursement, the closing of facilities, the positive choices of places to expand. The powers they are given are widely qualified: they review certificates of need, but can only make recommendations; they are supposed to conduct "appropriateness review," but the sanctions of inappropriateness are unclear (indeed, the regulations guiding this task remain unpublished).

In sum, HSAs do not have the authority—"teeth" is the current metaphor—necessary for the tasks, such as taming medical inflation, that have been assigned to them.

The difficulties of limited authority are compounded by the uncertain relation between HSAs and the rest of government. Indeed, the brief history of the law reads like a catalogue of contemporary confusions in American federalism: local governments are spurned for the—partially new, partially redundant—HSA structures; states and counties fight for influence within the framework of the law (Iglehart, 1973). Federal guidelines are promulgated with little clarity about how seriously they will (or indeed ought to) be taken in the communities. To the confusion of the now traditional "marble cake" metaphor (M. Grodzins, cited by Sundquist and Davis, 1969:7) we can add the impermeability of "picket-fence federalism" (Hudson, 1979). Unclearly stated regulations, interagency jealousies, lack of hierarchical support, and a growing, bureaucratic, self-generating political sector (Beer, 1978) lead to confusion, and ineffective governance and planning. Within the confusion, both governmental accountability and authority are dissipated.

We are not sanguine about the HSA successes that have been reported. Logic rebels at the peculiar idea that a planning agency without sufficient authority can scheme, scold, and cajole a dynamic system into compliance with plans that run contrary to all that system's incentives. On their own terms, HSAs will achieve varying levels of success. But they will not achieve the foolish expectations that have been thrust upon them. They simply do not have the authority or the resources.

The Technological Fix

The present health planning effort promised more "teeth" than its failed predecessor (comprehensive health planning), but added few. Another well-publicized innovation was scientific planning. The Health Planning Act was presented as the marriage of community participation and scientific planning. The success of the law was seen to hinge to a large extent on the latter.[11]

The reliance on the technology of planning is the most recent manifestation of a recurring alchemy in American politics: the effort to derive objective solutions from political choices. This impulse was very much a part of the Progressives' search for the "public interest"; relatedly, the "best way" was a kind of grail for scientific managers preoccupied with achieving measurable efficiency (McConnell, 1966; Taylor, 1971).

There are of course legitimate—perhaps pressing—data needs in health delivery. Indeed, data are notoriously poor, and tend to be monopolized by provider institutions, which are predictably reluctant to share them with regulators. And, clear data sometimes have clear policy implications. For example, one Philadelphia study showed that people admitted on Fridays have longer hospital stays than those admitted on Mondays and Tuesdays with the same ailment. Furthermore, a quarter of the hospital days in the same sample were taken up by patients suffering from alcoholic and nervous disorders, both more effectively (and economically) treated on an outpatient basis (*Business Week*, 1979).

The policy implications of such findings are relatively clear, but difficult to implement. Furthermore, there generally remains the policy leap between facts and political choices—where to build a hospital, how to allocate limited resources, or, more dramatically, "who shall live." Even problems that seem objectively solvable (where to close down hospital beds) are intensely political. Ignoring the realities of political interests and value choices without some fundamental—and unlikely, undesirable—system changes is a naiveté that will result in irrelevant plans and frustrated planners.

The difference between data analysis and political choices is reflected in the odd disjunction of commentary on health planning: from Washington and academia flows an apparently steady stream of

---

[11] See, for example, the report by the Committee on Interstate Commerce and Foreign Commerce on the National Health Policy, Planning and Resources Development Act of 1974. Report No. 93-1382, Washingtin, D.C.: Government Printing Office, Nov. 26, 1974.

methodologies, simulations, and data processing advice. At the same time, reports from the HSAs deal with the different world of power struggles, influence peddling, and political choices. The language of science seems strikingly distant from the realities of local health planners.

There are some fundamental political and philosophical conflicts that the language of technology obscures. Two such conflicts are apparent in the Health Planning Act.

Federalism. The conflict between national demands and local desires was referred to earlier. When a national program invites local participation, the community will generally want to make alterations. Local residents see a different set of needs, for their perspective is different, and community politics—to recall a classic variant—involves a different cast of political actors. The conflict is resolved neatly when de facto responsibility for each part of the program is fixed at one level of government, however much the symbols or rhetoric of the program may distract attention from the outcome.

The structure of the Health Planning Act exacerbates this tension rather than resolving it. The law stimulated wide-ranging community participation, local discretion in agency design, and goals and purposes so vague that they appeared to promise significant local autonomy. However, set expectations, fixed goals, and stringent guidelines followed. With it came a furor that reflected the conflict between local participation and national goals.

Scientific planning cannot relieve this tension. Selecting problems requires choosing between values, as does the series of increasingly narrow decisions that follow. And participants on various levels of government must hammer out agreement about what those choices are. The vision of objective solutions, replicable from place to place (in the manner of scientific experimentation) is, in this context, a vacuous one.

Efficiency. A second formidable conflict lies between representing community interests and program efficiency. The constant juxtaposition of representation and scientific planning reiterates the hope that representative boards can somehow be made efficient with an infusion of "science." In reality, the phrase is an oxymoron—the juxtaposition of opposites.

The point is illustrated nicely by the Common Cause official (cited by McFarland, 1978) who was told that his organization was not sufficiently democratic and participatory. He responded that if it were any more so its efficiency at achieving policy objectives would be hampered. He was correct for a number of reasons.

First, inducing wider representation introduces conflict. This may be desirable, indicating the articulation of various interests and perspectives, but it is not administratively efficient. And much of the conflict is irrelevant to the agency's tasks, often reflecting long-standing community animosities, personal agendas, and the like.

Second, the essence of administrative superiority is the skillful gathering, use, and even monopolization of information. The resulting expertise and technical skills are complicated—often undermined—by the introduction of nonprofessional participants, particularly when they are accountable to outside constituencies rather than to agency superiors. The logic of representation emphasizes a principle directly contrary to the logic of efficient organizational management on this point.

Third, administration will be more time-consuming. Representatives reexamine first questions and basic values; they may need to consult with constituencies, delaying the decision-making process. Such problems particularly complicate long-term planning where objectives must remain fixed over time. The starts and stops of a volunteer-governed agency can make the planning process considerably rougher than one run by professional staff.

The result is that representative institutions are inherently less efficient than bureaucratic ones, even when they are properly institutionalized. In the case of HSAs, the inefficiency is more apparent because amateurs are asked to plan and regulate a technical system that has been highly resistant to almost every sort of government intervention. The litany about marrying representation and science is useless in this regard. And it even undermines the HSA effort. For each argument against the efficiency of representation is a hurdle that must be overcome if representation is to survive. And insofar as the myth of science distracts from serious consideration of a proper volunteer role, it contributes to the antirepresentational impulse grounded in the exigencies of efficient administration and planning.

Though expanded interest-representation makes administration less efficient, it is worth pursuing. There are numerous reasons for this choice, though all finally point to the permeability of policy-making institutions by the public.

First, Weber's efficient bureaucracy may not be desirable for policy bodies. The reevaluation of fundamental values, the limitations on technical vocabularies, the brakes on routinization and standard operating procedures, all make such agencies more accessible to public groups.

Furthermore, when limits to bureaucratization are removed, imbalance is facilitated. Bureaucratic agencies tend to tug issues out of politics and resolve them administratively. The bargaining process remains, but entry qualifications grow so high that only concentrated interests are likely to meet them. Administrators, with their expertise and their specialized vocabulary, grow inscrutable to any but provider (expert) groups. Public accountability is difficult, legislative scrutiny unlikely.

Finally, an open process makes it less likely that groups will be completely shut out—like the consumers suing by participation in Hill-Burton. A market open to all health system actors is more difficult to manage because conflict is introduced; the planning process grows more complicated and time-consuming. However, in a time of dwindling resources, forging a consensus among all health system actors is important to planning success.

In an increasingly bureaucratic age, representation is a more fragile value than efficiency. If the Health Planning Act accomplishes nothing more than introducing and legitimating potential market balancers on an ongoing basis, it will have achieved considerable success.

Conclusion

The vision of representation in the National Health Planning and Resources Development Act is impossibly flawed, but not irretrievably so. We have suggested one plan for achieving reasonably effective consumer representation and balancing provider dominance. But representing consumers, overcoming imbalance, even discerning the public interest on HSAs will not alter the American health system in any profound fashion. The HSA mandate—limiting costs, expanding access, and improving the quality of health—reaches far beyond the agency's capabilities. Measured by these standards, the act's program is trivial, more symbols and rhetoric than significant improvement.

Rather, the law's significance lies in its stimulation of a broad range of consumer interests. Viewed as an effort to organize communities into caring for their own health systems, it is the largest program of its kind. And one that could influence health politics long after its particular institutional manifestations—HSA planning boards—have been forgotten.

References

Anderson, C. 1977. Political Design and the Representation of Interests. *Comparative Political Studies* 10 (April):127–152.

Balbus, I. 1972. The Concept of Interest in Pluralist and Marxian Analysis. In Katznelson, I., et al., eds., *The Politics and Society Reader.* New York: David McKay.

Barry, B. 1965. *Political Argument,* chapter 10. London: Routledge and Kegan Paul.

Baur, R.A., Pool, I., and Dexter, L.A. 1963. *American Business and Public Policy.* New York: Atherton Press.

Beer, S. 1978. Federalism, Nationalism and Democracy in America. *American Political Science Review* 72 (March):9–21.

Bentley, A. 1967. *The Process of Government.* Cambridge, Mass.: Harvard University Press.

Bernstein, M. 1955. *Regulating Business by Independent Commission.* Princeton, N.J.: Princeton University Press.

Berry, J.M. 1977. *Lobbying for the People.* Princeton, N.J.: Princeton University Press.

Birch, A. 1971. *Representation.* New York: Praeger.

Business Week. 1979. August 6:54.

Burnham, W.D. 1978. American Politics in the 1970s: Beyond Party? In Fishel, J., ed., *Parties and Elections in an Anti-Party Age.* Bloomington, Ind.: Indiana University Press.

Clark, W. 1977. Placebo or Cure? State and Local Health Planning

Agencies in the South. Southern Governmental Monitoring Project, Southern Regional Council, Atlanta.

Codman Research Group. 1977. The Impact of Health Planning and Regulation on the Patterns of Hospital Utilization in New England. Executive Summary, DHEW Contract 291-76-0003. Final Report, Year 1, September.

Dahl, R. 1961. *Who Governs?* New Haven: Yale University Press.

————. 1964. *A Preface to Democratic Theory.* Chicago: University of Chicago Press.

Edelman, M. 1967. *The Symbolic Use of Politics.* Urbana: University of Illinois Press.

Eulau, H., and Prewitt, K. 1973. *Labyrinths of Democracy.* Indianapolis: Bobbs-Merrill.

Flatham, R. 1966. *The Public Interest.* New York: Wiley.

Friedman, M. 1962. *Capitalism and Freedom.* Chicago: University of Chicago Press.

Friedrich, C.J. 1950. *Constitutional Government and Democracy,* 266 ff. New York: Blaisdell.

Greenstone, J.D. 1975. Group Theories. In Greenstein, F., and Polsby, N., eds., *The Handbook of Political Science,* vol. II. Reading, Mass.: Addison-Wesley.

————, and Peterson, P.E. 1973. *Race and Authority in Urban Politics: Consumer Participation and the War on Poverty,* chapter 6. Chicago: University of Chicago Press.

Griffiths, A.P. 1960. How Can One Person Represent Another? *Aristotelian Society,* supplementary vol. 34 (6):187–208.

Hartz, L. 1955. *The Liberal Tradition in America.* New York: Harcourt, Brace, and World.

Hayek, F. 1944. *The Road to Serfdom.* Chicago: University of Chicago Press.

Hudson, R. 1979. A Bloc Grant to the States for Long Term Care. Waltham, Mass.: University Health Policy Consortium, February 2.

Iglehart, J. 1973. Health Report: State, County Governments Win Key Roles in New Program. *National Journal,* November 8.

Klein, R. 1979. Control, Participation, and the British National Health Service. *Milbank Memorial Fund Quarterly/Health and Society* 57 (Winter):70–94.

Lindblom, C.E. 1959. The Science of Muddling Through. *Public Administration Review* 19 (Spring):79–88.

Lipsky, M., and Lounds, M. 1976. Citizen Participation and Health Care: Problems of Government Induced Participation. *Journal of Health Politics, Policy, and Law* 1 (Spring):106–109.

Lowi, T. 1969. *The End of Liberalism.* New York: Norton.

Marmor, T.R. 1973. *The Politics of Medicare.* Chicago: Aldine Press.

———. 1976. Welfare Medicine: How Success Can Be a Failure. *Yale Law Journal* 85 (July):1149–1159.

———. 1977. Consumer Representation: Beneath the Consensus, Many Difficulties. *Trustee* 30 (4):37–40.

———, and Bridges, A. 1980. Comparative Policy Analysis and Health Planning Processes Internationally. Prepared for the director of the Bureau of Health Planning and Resources Development, DHEW, May 1977. Revised for *Journal of Health Politics, Policy, and Law.* In press.

———, and Morone, J.A. 1979. Innovation and the Health Service Sector: Notes on the U.S. In Altenstetter, C., ed., *Innovation in Public Services.* Berlin: Internationales Institut für Management und Verwaltung.

———, and Wittman, D. 1976. Politics of Medical Inflation. *Journal of Health Politics, Policy, and Law* 1 (Spring):69–83.

McConnell, G. 1966. *Private Power and American Democracy.* New York: Knopf.

McFarland, A. 1976. *Public Interest Lobbies.* Washington, D.C.: American Enterprise Institute.

———. 1978. "Third Forces" in American Politics: The Case of Common Cause. In Fishel, J., ed., *Parties and Elections in an Anti-Party Age.* Bloomington, Ind.: University of Indiana Press.

———. 1979. Recent Social Movements and Theories of Power in America. Paper delivered at the American Political Science Convention, August. Washington, D.C.

Nadel, M.U. 1971. *The Politics of Consumer Protection.* Indianapolis: Bobbs-Merrill.

Noll, R. 1971. *Reforming Regulation.* Washington, D.C.: Brookings Institution.

Pitkin, H.F. 1967. *The Concept of Representation.* Berkeley: University of California Press.

———, ed. 1969. *Representation.* New York: Atherton Press.

Rosenblatt, R. 1978. Health Care Reform and Administrative Law: A Structural Approach. *Yale Law Journal* part 2:264–286.

Salisbury, R. 1978. On Centrifugal Tendencies in Interest Systems:

The Case of the U.S. Paper delivered at the International Sociological Association, Uppsala. August 17.

Schattschneider, E.E. 1935. *Politics, Pressures and Tariff.* Englewood Cliffs, N.J.: Prentice-Hall.

———. 1960. *The Semisovereign People,* 34. Hinsdale, Ill.: Dryden Press.

Schmitter, P.C. 1975. *An Inventory of Analytical Pluralist Propositions.* Unpublished monograph. University of Chicago.

Shonfield, A. 1965. *Modern Capitalism.* New York: Oxford University Press.

Sidel, V., and Sidel, R. 1977. *A Healthy State.* New York: Pantheon Press.

Sundquist, J., and Davis, D. 1969. *Making Federalism Work.* Washington, D.C.: Brookings Institution.

Swabey, M.C. 1969. The Representative Sample. In Pitkin, H.F., ed., *Representation.* New York: Atherton Press.

Taylor, F. 1971. Scientific Management. In Pugh, D.J., ed., *Organizational Theory.* New York: Penguin Books.

Truman, D. 1951. *The Governmental Process.* New York: Knopf.

Von Mises, L. 1962. *Liberalism and Socio-Economic Exposition.* Kansas City: Sheed, Andrews, and McMeel.

Wilson, J.Q. 1973. *Political Organizations.* New York: Basic Books.

Acknowledgments: We want to thank Brian Barry particularly for his careful reading and constructive criticisms. Various other colleagues at the Institution for Social and Policy Studies, Yale University, and the Center for Health Administration Studies, University of Chicago, have been challenging, and helpful. And our thinking was advanced, particularly at the outset, by the writings and comments of Rudolf Klein and Charles Anderson. Julie Greenberg deserves great credit for improving the successive drafts of this article.

Earlier versions of the paper were presented at seminars at Yale, Harvard, and the University of Chicago; the penultimate draft was read at the American Political Science Association's Convention, 1979. The topics here discussed are more fully dealt with in part of Morone's forthcoming dissertation on "Consumer Representation, Public Planning and Democratic Theory."

Address correspondence to: Theodore R. Marmor, Ph.D., Chairman, Center for Health Studies, and Professor of Public Health and Political Science, Yale University, 15A Yale Station, 77 Prospect Street, New Haven, Conn. 06520; or James A. Morone, Bustin Research Fellow, Center for Health Administration Studies, 5720 South Woodlawn Avenue, Chicago, Illinois 60637.

Milbank Memorial Fund Quarterly/*Health and Society, Vol. 57, No. 1, 1979*

Control, Participation, and the British National Health Service

RUDOLF KLEIN

School of Humanities and Social Sciences,
University of Bath

I N JULY, 1978, THE BRITISH NATIONAL HEALTH SERVICE (NHS) celebrated the 30th anniversary of its birth. But the debate about how to run the NHS organization—the issue of democratic control, in its widest sense—continues. This suggests that it is far easier to create the organizational framework for a national health care system than to solve the problem of making it socially accountable and responsive. This paper explores the history of the debate and the policy options currently being canvassed to delineate the dilemmas inherent in designing a national health service, whether in the United States or any other society that subscribes to the traditions of liberal Western democracy.

The British NHS is unique among Western health services in a number of respects. It is a *national* health service in the full sense, in that the Secretary of State for Social Services[1] is directly answerable to Parliament for its operations; the field authorities—regional and area health authorities—are his agents, responsible to him (Fig. 1). The NHS is financed by central government mainly out of general taxation; direct payments by users of the service are individually

---

[1]The Secretary of State for Social Services is the Cabinet Minister overseeing the Department of Health and Social Security (DHSS), which is responsible for the administration of the National Health Service in England.

0026-3745-79-5701-0070-25/$01.00/0 ©1979 Milbank Memorial Fund

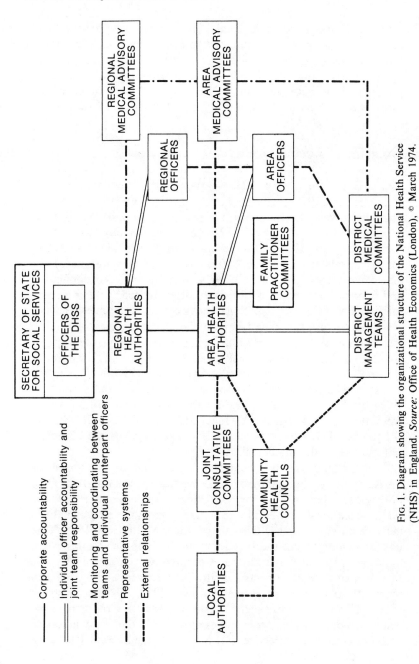

FIG. 1. Diagram showing the organizational structure of the National Health Service (NHS) in England. *Source:* Office of Health Economics (London), © March 1974.

small and unimportant in total. In contrast to Sweden, local authorities play no role; in contrast to France and Germany, there are no *caisses* or *kassen* to collect contributions or represent the consumer. Lastly, the British NHS is a near-monopoly health care provider; the private sector is small (Klein, 1979) and the great majority of the population look to the NHS for provision of health care.

Doctrine of Accountability

The architecture of the NHS—although modified by the reorganization of 1974—reflects, in its basic design, the egalitarian aspirations of its designer, Aneurin Bevan. The aim of the NHS, as he explained to Parliament in 1946 (*Hansard,* 1946a) was to "universalise the best, that we shall promise every citizen in this country the same standard of service." Hence the need, Bevan argued, for a *national* service—given the diversity, in terms of both population and financial resources, of local authorities. Indeed, it was precisely this decision to create a national service that represented Bevan's main innovation, diverging from the plans for a much more federal, local authority-based service that he had inherited from the wartime coalition government (Willcocks, 1967). Implicit in this approach was the assumption that distributional equity could only be achieved by means of central direction and planning. Nor was this surprising, given the history of public health care provision in Britain, which from the days of Chadwick (Finer, 1952) and Sir John Simon, (Lambert, 1963) had largely been a struggle against the parochial self-interest of the municipalities.

In actuality, central control did not lead to the hoped-for measure of distributional equity. In particular, the distribution of hospital resources—by far the most expensive part of the NHS—continued stubbornly to reflect the inherited inequalities between different parts of the country (Buxton and Klein, 1975). One of the main objects of the 1974 reorganization of the administrative machinery, carried out by a Conservative Government, was therefore to strengthen central control of resources and introduce a more effective planning system (Brown, 1973: 70–83). Although widely criticized as managerial in inspiration, this reorganization could also be, and was, presented as an attempt to make democratic accountability more effective. For how could the Secretary of State be accountable to Parliament if he did not exercise effective control over the execution of policy in the NHS?

The emphasis on central control, whether in the original 1948 model or in the revised 1974 model, has had a further consequence. Persons appointed to serve on the health authorities—the Regional Hospital Boards and Hospital Management Committees before 1974 (or on the Regional Health Authorities and Area Health Authorities thereafter)—were the creatures of the Minister of Health (or, as he later became, the Secretary of State for Social Services). It was constantly stressed that they were not to be regarded or to think of themselves as representatives of special interests, whether occupational or geographic. Just as the Secretary of State was accountable to Parliament for the expenditure of public funds, so they were accountable to him and to no one else. Accountability, in the NHS and in the British tradition of public administration, is a one-way street and does not permit dual loyalties.

The doctrine is clear; the practice turned out to be somewhat less so. At least one occupational interest was strongly represented in the service created by Bevan, even though there were no "representatives" in the most limited sense of that ambiguous word—men and women answerable to their constituency (Pitkin, 1967). The medical profession was strongly in evidence everywhere, excessively so in the view of the Guillebaud Committee, which reported in 1956 on the operations of the NHS (Ministry of Health, 1956). The Committee pointed out that in 1954–1955 almost one-third of all Regional Hospital Board members were doctors, and that the proportion exceeded two-fifths in one case. Similarly, the medical membership of the Hospital Management Committees was about one-quarter physicians, although it too reached two-fifths in some instances. Further, in the case of the Hospital Management Committees, the lay members were chosen precisely because they were active members of their local communities—often as elected councillors—although they were not, in any formal sense, chosen to represent those communities.

The element of syndicalism was more evident still in the case of the Executive Councils, which are the local bodies responsible for running the general practitioner, dental, pharmaceutical, and ophthalmic services. On these, under the terms of the legislation, doctors, dentists, chemists, and ophthalmologists had half the membership, thus perpetuating the strong position of the medical profession in the administration of general practice, first conceded in 1911 when health insurance was introduced (Klein, 1973). No doubt this form of organization largely reflected political expediency—the need to conciliate family practitioners, the most militant section of the medical profession. But Bevan's defense, or rationalization, is worth recalling (*Hansard*, 1946b):

> I have never believed that the demands of a democracy are necessarily satisfied merely by the opportunity of putting a cross against someone's name every four or five years. I believe that democracy exists in the active participation in administration and policy. Therefore, I believe it is a wise thing to give the doctors full participation in the administration of their own profession. . . . [W]e do not want the opposite danger of syndicalism. Therefore, the communal interests must always be safeguarded in this administration.

So although the theory of syndicalism was thus explicitly repudiated, the reality of professional representation was, in effect, conceded in this area of the NHS.

The 1974 Reorganization: Representation and Interests

The 1974 reorganization did not affect the composition of the Executive Councils, which changed only in name to become "Family Practitioner Committees" (see Fig. 1). Otherwise, however, the membership of the various authorities continues to reflect the hierarchic nature of the system of accountability. In the case of the 14 Regional Authorities, the members are appointed by the Secretary of State. To quote the 1972 White Paper that introduced the legislation (DHSS, 1972: 24):

> Their authority will derive from the selection and appointment of their chairmen and members by the Secretary of State, who will be required before making this choice to consult with the appropriate interested organizations including the Universities, the main local authorities and the main health professions.

In turn, the members of the 90 Area Health Authorities—the next administrative tier below the regions—are appointed by the regions, although the chairmen are directly nominated by the Secretary of State.

The 1974 reorganization had a number of other significant

features as well. In each Area, four members were to be nominated by the matching local authorities; one of the main aims of the reorganization was to align the administrative boundaries of the health authorities with those of the local authorities in order to promote the coordination of services. In addition, the membership was to include at least one doctor and one nurse, but it was stressed that they were not to have a representative role. They were to see themselves as being exclusively responsible for the management of services, not as being accountable to any interest groups. To the extent that there was to be any representative role for professional interests, this was to be performed by the various advisory committees with which the new health authorities were liberally festooned.

The representation of public interests was, in the 1974 reorganization model, to be the role of a new institution, the Community Health Council. There were to be 206 of these, one for each district of the NHS, i.e., they were the basic administrative unit below the area level. Half of their members were to be nominated by local authorities, one-third by voluntary organizations, and the rest by the regional authorities. The logic for choosing this composition was not entirely clear, and seems to have reflected a mixture of motives rather than explicit principles (Klein and Lewis, 1976: 19–20). In the outcome, however, it meant representation both for geographical communities (represented by the local authority nominees) and special health service client groups like the mentally ill, the elderly, and the handicapped (represented by the voluntary organization nominees). There was some ambiguity as to whether Community Health Councils should represent "the views of the consumer" or "the interests of the public in each health district" (ibid., 17). Both phrases were used by government spokesmen, as though the interests of the actual consumers of health care were identical with those of the community at large. But it was quite clear that the Community Health Councils should have an explicit, and indeed exclusive, representative role as spokesmen for the public—however defined. They were to have no managerial function whatsoever. Their powers were limited to the right to information, to access to health service facilities, and to kick up hell if their views were ignored.

The rationale for adopting this system of introducing community interests into the NHS was set out in the 1972 White Paper. This pointed out that:

The expression of local public opinion can be catered for in one of two ways. It can be done by including in the membership of the health authorities local people serving in a representative capacity. Or it can be done more directly, through bodies specially set up for this purpose.

The Government preferred the second option (DHSS, 1972: 27) because "it avoids a confusion between the direction of services and representation of those receiving them." This conclusion reflected two considerations. First, there was the doctrinal emphasis on the need for a clear hierarchy of accountability. Second, there was pragmatic evidence of the actual workings of the NHS, which suggested that lay members of the Hospital Management Committees tended to identify themselves with the interests of the service providers rather than those of the service consumers. This evidence had been elicited in the course of a number of inquiries into scandals in the neglected long-stay sector of the NHS (Klein, 1971).

Persistent Policy Aims of the NHS

There have been minor changes in the organization of the NHS since 1974, with the arrival of a Labour Government in office, but, in all its essentials, the administrative structure remains as described. It reflects an attempt to accommodate a number of policy aims that are worth reiterating before turning to the analysis of the on-going debate about community and worker representation and the issues raised by this.

First, there is the view that an *egalitarian* NHS requires effective central control over the disposition and use of centrally financed resources.

Second, there is the view that a *democratic* NHS requires both accountability to Parliament and responsiveness to local needs.

Third, there is the view that an *effective* NHS requires coordination with other social services operated by local authorities.

Fourth, there is the view that there ought to be a voice—of one kind or another—for those working in the NHS.

Lastly, to take up a theme that has so far not surfaced from the discussion but which will emerge strongly in the subsequent analysis, there is the view that an *efficient* NHS requires the basic units of administration to be large enough to provide reasonably comprehensive health care for most of its population for most of the time. Thus, the population of the majority of districts falls in the range of 150,000 to 350,000 (although the minimum is 86,000 and the maximum is 530,000).

It is precisely because these various policy aims do not necessarily point in the same direction—and may, indeed, conflict—that the debate about the future "ideal" structure of the NHS is still unresolved. Furthermore, it is precisely because the considerations involved raise general issues of principle, common to all attempts to devise a national health care system, that the experience of the British NHS is relevant to other countries as well.

Attempts to Square the Circle

In the discussions that have taken place both before and since reorganization about what is wrong with the NHS, one of the main preoccupations has been how to make it more "democratic." But, of course, democracy tends to be used as an emotive term of rhetoric (Klein, 1976). The definition of "democracy" depends on the values and preconceptions—seldom articulated explicitly—of those using the word. In analyzing the policy options that have been put forward or adopted in Britain, it may therefore be helpful to set them into the framework of theoretical assumptions that are implicit in the arguments of their advocates.

A Clash of Values: Centralism vs Localism

A helpful starting point is the distinction drawn by Robert Nisbet (1970: 70) between two streams of thought in European radicalism. On the one hand, there is the tradition stemming from Marx: "centralized, nationalist socialism." On the other hand, there is the tradition stemming from Proudhon: "decentralist, pluralist anarchism." The former "was as hostile to localism, community, and co-operation as was the line of utilitarian liberalism that reached from James Mill to Herbert Spencer." The latter rested "upon localism, with the small community—rural and industrial—the essential element." Leaving aside the much debated question as to whether the Marxian tradition represents a correct reading of Marx's views, we find that Nisbet's distinction remains a useful analytical tool for examining the different approaches to the issues of accountability, representation, and participation in a monopoly social service like the NHS.

The 1948 NHS was, as we have seen, a triumph of centralized socialism. So, too, was the 1974 reorganization—although perhaps it is possible to detect the influence of utilitarian liberalism, as well. The reorganization, in essence, was an attempt to make the NHS more effective in achieving the aims of the original model; centralization was emphasized because a more egalitarian and efficient use of resources was thought to be desirable. And, indeed, since 1974 a Labour Government has used the planning system to try to move toward developing "norms" for the distribution of resources (DHSS, 1976b), an approach that is also characteristic of the highly centralized Eastern European health services (Zhuk, 1976).

The critique of the NHS has, increasingly, come from those whose views stem (usually unconsciously) from the opposite tradition of localism and participative self-government. It can be seen as part of a wider reaction—drawing on support from both the Left and Right—against "big" government, against bureaucracy, and against professionalism. The critique is by no means limited to the NHS. Just as the 1948 NHS reflected a general move toward the centralization of power—as exemplified by the various nationalized industries like coal, electricity, and gas—so the current critique of the health service reflects a more general disillusionment with what is perceived to be a "technocratic solution" to social and political problems.

So, in effect, there is a clash of values. What is being stressed, on the one side, are the values of egalitarianism (fair rations for all, decided nationally) and efficiency, and, on the other side, the values of self-determination and democracy-as-participation. And, as the ongoing debate about the organization of the NHS shows, the problem of designing a national health service derives from the fact that different values imply different organizational solutions.

The present NHS represents a monument to the liberal definition of democracy as accountability. Without necessarily accepting the criticisms of Pateman (1970) and others of this definition, it must be conceded that the practice of accountability has, in fact, lagged behind the theory. The capacity of Parliament to call the Secretary of State to account for all that happens in the NHS is circumscribed. MPs can, and do, ask questions about specific cases or issues. But their ability to influence policy is limited. Parliamentary committees—in contrast to Congressional committees—have virtually no staff (Klein, 1977b) and are therefore in no position to carry out a systematic surveillance of policy-making and policy execution. This is not to argue that Parliamentary influence is non-existent, or that accountability is a fiction. It is to argue, however, that accountability is bound to be erratic and spasmodic, given the sheer size and heterogeneity of the NHS. Moreover, the system of centralized accountability tends to have pathological side-effects. The fact that the Secretary of State is in theory answerable for everything that happens in the NHS means that the center has to exercise detailed control over the periphery, with a consequent growth in bureaucracy (DHSS, 1976c).

Constraints on Local Democracy

One much-canvassed option for dealing with the problem of over-centralization is to transfer control over health services to the local authorities. These, in Britain, already administer most of the social services: education, housing, and social care. And, indeed, this transfer was the policy advocated by the Labour Party in the debates preceding the 1974 reorganization (*Hansard,* 1973). However, no Labour Government has adopted this solution in office. And the reason for this is not simply tactical; the fact is that the medical profession—and some of the trade unions representing health service workers (Confederation of Health Service Employees, 1977)—is opposed to such a transfer.

The main objection was spelled out by Richard Crossman (*Hansard,* 1970) when, as Labour's Secretary of State for Social Services, he explained why he did not include a transfer of responsibility in his own reorganization proposals. If the local authorities were given the power to run health services, he told Parliament, "No responsible Government could permit them to run those services with the degree of independence which they take for granted in running their other services." A health service, he stressed, must be planned nationally. In short, the values of egalitarianism—with all they imply for the distribution of resources and the equalization of access throughout the country—constrain the scope for local democracy in the shape of control by local authorities. In practice, central government can and does impose sharp limits on the freedom of local authorities, even in the case of the other services—like education—for which local authorities are responsible. So a strong measure of central control over locally administered services is possible. There are norms for the number of school teachers, just as there are norms for consultant posts in the hospital service. But, as a recent committee of inquiry has recognized (Department of the Environment, 1976), such central control blurs local accountability. Why should citizens bother to turn out to vote in local elections if all the important decisions are taken centrally? In fact, unsurprisingly, turnout in British local elections is very low. Widespread apathy seems to be the price paid for the emphasis on egalitarian values and the suspicion of diversity (Klein, 1977c). Moreover, in contrast to the other social services, the NHS is exclusively financed from national taxation—thus compounding the arguments against a transfer of control to authorities who would be making no financial contribution. Lastly, local authority boundaries were not determined with the needs of the health service primarily in mind; many of them can therefore not even begin to deliver a comprehensive range of health care.

Given these arguments against the decentralization of control in the NHS, it is not surprising that the main emphasis has been on ways of trying to square the circle. How best can the NHS be made responsive to the views, demands, and needs of the public? How can a national service include an element of local accountability? Different answers have been given to these questions, at different times and by different governments. But none of them has, as yet, come up with a wholly satisfactory solution.

Strategies for Modifying the NHS Structure

Community Health Councils: Advocacy, Adversary, and Authority. The 1974 reorganization introduced, as already mentioned, Community Health Councils. These translated the concept of consumer representation to mean consumer advocacy: they are, in effect, public bodies with the legitimacy to voice and promote the views of local interest groups—whether these interests are defined geographically or in terms of specific clients. But the experience so far suggests this approach raises a number of difficulties.

The first difficulty stems from the general lack of clarity about the concept of community. To quote the 1968 edition of the *International Encyclopaedia of the Social Sciences* (Sills, 1968: 157):

> Little attention has been devoted in contemporary community power research to the problem of defining a community ... For the most part, a conventional perspective has been adopted and a 'community' has been defined as a population living within legally established city limits.

Indeed, often the term "community" appears to be used as though it were synonymous with "popular control," with no precise definition at all. In the case of the Community Health Councils, the community has been defined as "the population living within the legislatively established NHS districts." These, as already mentioned, range in size from 86,000 to 530,000. Yet, as shown by earlier research in Britain (Royal Commission on Local Government Control in England, 1969), community, as defined by the inhabitants' self-identification with a particular district, tends to be strongest in areas with a population of less than 30,000. It is therefore not surprising that many Councils have found it difficult to establish a constituency and to maintain contact with the public they are supposed to represent (Klein and Lewis, 1976: 116–119).

The second difficulty stems from the problem of not knowing whether a community should simply be seen as an aggregation of individuals who happen to live in a particular area or as an aggregation of interest groups. The membership of Community Health Councils embodies both concepts. It represents an attempt to bias the membership to ensure representation for disadvantaged groups whose interests might otherwise be swamped by a majoritarian view. In other words, the composition of the membership is a deliberately paternalistic attempt to load the democratic dice. As such, it is an interesting experiment in rigging the system so as to ensure a voice for weak minorities. But it is out of line with conventional one-man, one-vote democratic theory.

Lastly, and perhaps most important, there is the question of power. The Labour Government, which took office in 1974, gave the Community Health Councils some additional weapons, notably, the right to delay changes, such as the closure of hospitals, by health authorities. But, aside from the ability to obstruct and protest, the Councils have no formal decision-making powers, as already pointed out. This indeed is implicit in the advocate or adversary model. In practice, however, the Councils have sought to involve themselves in the decision-making process; they have actively sought the responsibilities, and inhibitions, of authority. In the outcome, therefore, their members often perceive their role in much the same way as the appointed lay members of the Area Health Authorities (Brown, Griffin, and Haywood, 1975: 100). The assumption that representation can be externalized from the running of the NHS—to avoid contamination and absorption by professional and technocratic values—has, in reality, turned out to be an over-simplified concept.

Area Health Authorities. Alternatively, then, is it possible to make the members of the Area Health Authorities themselves more representative? This, in fact, was the course adopted by the 1974 Labour Administration. As part of its proposals for "Democracy in the National Health Service" (DHSS, 1974), it increased the proportion of Area Health Authority members nominated by local authorities. Similarly, and introducing a new theme for the first time, it proposed that each Area Health Authority should include two members drawn from the NHS staff: a proposal which, at the time of this writing, has yet to be implemented because of a continuing argument as to how these two members should be chosen. This argument revolves around both the machinery of election and the question of eligibility to vote (DHSS, 1976a).

Such changes in the membership of the Area Authorities cannot solve the dilemma of central accountability. The collective responsibility of the Authorities for the management of the NHS means, by definition, that they cannot be representatives of, in the sense of being accountable to, local interests. Local councillors may, by virtue of their office, bring with them a wider knowledge of local problems and the experience born of contacts with their constituents. But, unless democracy is defined in terms of "communication," it is difficult to see how the presence of local councillors makes health authorities more "democratic." A similar consideration applies to Authority members nominated, in one way or another, from the NHS staff. If there are Authority members drawn from the ancillary and clerical workers in the NHS, they will—like the doctors and nurses who are already present—bring a different view to bear on decisions, simply by the fact of their own experience and background. But they will not represent their constituency, and thus will not be able to speak with the authority of the formal representatives of the trade unions acting through the normal channels of industrial negotiations.

Evaluation of Modification Strategies.   These attempts to modify the existing structure of the NHS thus suggest that there are severe constraints on any strategy designed to meet radical critiques within a framework that reflects the values of "centralized, nationalist socialism." The circle obstinately refuses to be squared. The next, and concluding, section therefore analyzes some of the options that become available—and their implications—if the assumptions about desirable values and policy aims are changed. In particular, it examines the problems that would arise for an institution like the British NHS—or indeed any national health service—in trying to translate the concepts of community control and workers' control into organizational practice.

Political Theories and Policy Options

The future design of the British NHS is currently being considered by a Royal Commission whose appointment reflected widespread dissatisfaction with the present administrative structure of the health service. A useful starting point for analyzing the options currently being discussed is therefore the evidence that has been submitted to the Commission: particularly the evidence coming from those organizations with a special interest in increasing involvement by the community (taking this word in its widest sense) and by the workers.

Labour Party Proposal: National Priorities and Local Execution

The evidence of the Labour Party (1977)—drafted by a working group under the chairmanship of Mrs. Barbara Castle, Secretary of State for Social Services from 1974 to 1976, and one of Bevan's disciples—states that one of the aims of any further reorganization should be to secure:

> [A] new surge of popular identification with the health service by making it accountable to the public which use it and the staff who work in it.

But, having made this pronouncement of principle, the Labour Party's document then candidly discusses the difficulties involved in trying to translate it into practice. These will be familiar from the earlier discussion. Taking the view that "central government must retain ultimate control over national priorities," the Labour Party recognizes the problems involved in handing over responsibility to local authorities. For example, it argues (Labour Party, 1977: 52–59):

> The fair distribution of manpower—particularly highly skilled and talented professionals—would be much harder to achieve without imposing central government controls. The present mechanisms need to be not just maintained but considerably strengthened.

So, recognizing the dilemma while yet striving to move toward control by elected representatives at the local level, the Labour Party document concludes by tentatively suggesting a new solution. This is that, while central government would continue to direct service strategy and to decide on priorities, the execution of policy would be left to local health authorities "with one third of the members being elected by all the staff in the NHS, one third directly elected by the local electorate and one third nominated by the Secretary of State in recognition of the fact that the service was wholly financed by central government."

Unfortunately, the document does not explain how financial accountability to central government would be reconciled with electoral accountability to workers and community. Nor does it address itself to the crucial question of why there should be local interest in participating in elections if there is not also freedom for local health authorities to differentiate themselves in terms of the policies they pursue (Monsen and Downs, 1971). If their main responsibility is to execute *national* priorities, then, by definition, there is going to be only limited scope for discretion by elected members, and little incentive to invest time and interest in participation.

National Union of Public Employees Proposal: Limited Devolution

The same difficulty is raised by the proposal submitted by the National Union of Public Employees (NUPE) (1977: 15–20), whose membership includes many of the less-skilled ancillary workers in the NHS. Again, the proposed solution is to maintain a national service with administration devolved to locally elected district committees. Only, NUPE proposes that half the membership should be elected "from and by all grades of NHS staff," while the other half should be elected by the voters.

Confederation of Health Service Employees Proposal: Consensus Management

Taking a somewhat different line, the Confederation of Health Service Employees (COHSE) (1977: 38–40), whose membership includes the less highly qualified nurses and some of the semi-skilled workers in the NHS, argues for the formal representation of trade unionists on Community Health Councils. This, COHSE argues, would "enhance the experience and working ability" of these Councils, who could then "act as a valuable bridge for staff to become aware of public feeling about the service."

More interesting, still, is COHSE's position concerning another problem inherent in worker representation. Its document (ibid.) states: "We take the view that staff who become members of an employing authority will not be (and should not be) accountable to the staff for their actions." Consequently, COHSE stresses, "[T]here is room for worker-participation in the sense that there must be full involvement of staff *before* decisions are taken which are likely to affect them." This is, in effect, a different theory of participation, namely, participation through direct involvement in the decision-making process, as an implicit right, rather than through more representative managerial bodies.

The theory is not developed explicitly in the COHSE statement, but, clearly, it is suggested as an alternative perspective on the problem of community and worker control in the NHS, and requires further analysis. The first difficulty inherent in this approach is that of knowing under what circumstances involvement can be equated with control. That, crucially, depends on the form of involvement. Like participation, involvement is a hold-all concept; it can, at one extreme, mean simply the right to be consulted, and, at the other end of the spectrum, veto power over all decisions (Klein, 1975). Thus, a strongly developed form of this theory might imply that all groups with a recognized interest in the operations of the NHS—whether as members of the public or as members of the staff—should have the right to veto any decision. This is the principle of consensus management in its most complete version. In turn, it raises some questions.

Costs of Consensus Management. The first set of questions is about the costs of introducing a fully developed form of consensus management that includes all the groups with a claim to involvement. Multiplying veto power also multiplies, by definition, the power to stop things from being done. It consequently strengthens the ability of the various groups to maintain the status quo when change threatens their interests. Thus, veto power may have a tendency to freeze the existing distributions of resources and make it more difficult to secure a more equitable distribution.

The point can be illustrated by the recent history of the NHS. As already noted, it has been Government policy to try to alter the inherited historical imbalances between different parts of the country by applying a formula designed to match funds to needs, as defined by a set of objective criteria (DHSS, 1976d). At the same time, Government has attempted to switch resources from specialties judged to have an excess of resources—notably, maternity, where the declining birth rate has produced a crop of empty beds—to those that have been relatively neglected, like geriatrics and mental handicap (DHSS, 1976b). Both operations imply—particularly under the current conditions of resource constraints in Britain—closing wards and hospitals in order to free resources for reallocation. But this has met opposition both from Community Health Councils, concerned with maintaining local facilities (Community Health Council, 1976: 26–30), and from workers, concerned with maintaining local jobs (National Association of Local Government Officers, 1977). In other words, creating more scope for involvement may also mean creating more opportunities for resisting change. These opportunities are precisely the kind that, in the first three decades of the NHS, have been exploited by the one group that has often had effective veto power over proposed changes—the medical profession (Klein, 1977a).

In opposition to this interpretation, it is argued that involvement creates a sense of responsibility; when people are engaged in the decision-making process, they become educated to take a less parochial, self-centered view of their own interests. This appears to be the belief of those who argue for a system of direct organizational democracy, as against the liberal democratic form of representative institutions. Thus, Pateman (1975: 22–23) argues that "parochialism and selfishness may be less likely" because participatory citizenship "would make explicit what liberal democratic formal separation of roles obscures—that individuals do belong to more than one stakeholder or interest group." Possibly this may be so, but the status of such an assertion is that of a declaration of belief or article of faith. What evidence there is points in the opposite direction, on British experience, although it can always be maintained that this is only because the participation is partial and inadequate.

The Scale for Consensus Management. The second set of questions is about the conditions necessary for introducing anything like a fully-fledged system of direct participation by workers or community, as distinct from strengthening representative institutions. For the theory of democracy as involvement depends crucially on the element of direct, personal participation. In doing so, its advocates—who come from a long line of political theorists running through Aristotle and Rousseau—stress the importance of small size. Direct involvement, they argue, is only possible in small units. Hence, of course, the interest in workshop democracy as the arena for precisely this kind of direct involvement on a scale that makes it feasible (Pateman, 1970: 67–103). As Weber pointed out (1947: 338), it would be possible to escape from the domination of bureaucracy "only by reversion in every field—political, religious, economic, etc.—to small-scale organizations."

Does, then, a national health service offer the necessary conditions for such a reversion to small-scale organizations? And what would be the implications of so doing? On the face of it, a health service would seem to provide precisely the right kind of laboratory conditions for democracy through direct participation. The delivery of health care is the responsibility of a multiplicity of individual hospitals and group practices of family doctors, although over the decades there has been a tendency to concentrate these resources in ever-larger units—whether larger hospitals or health centers. But this process of concentration already indicates one of the clashes of values (large size equals more equipment and more expertise) and participatory values (small size equals more democracy). For example, one of the achievements of the British NHS—as seen by those who took part in its creation (Godber, 1975: 17)—was precisely the physical concentration of specialist staff and resources into larger hospitals. This involved the elimination of small cottage hospitals where part-time surgeons had frequently put their patients at risk because of their lack of experience.

Professional Autonomy and Public Accountability

But, size apart, there are further problems about envisaging a health service as a series of self-governing republics as an alternative to the present highly centralized, inevitably bureaucratic, NHS. They stem from the fact that health services involve professionals who, like the doctors, insist on their own autonomy (Freidson, 1971) and organizational units that cannot be autonomous. In other words, the difficulty is how to reconcile the insistence of the medical and other professions that they must be free from any interference in the exercise of their craft and the organizational reality of health services, involving the coordination of a large variety of skills and institutions, the rationing of scarce resources, and the management of relations with other, complementary, social services.

Autonomy is indeed compatible with self-government. More than that, it may be argued to be the necessary condition for it (Dahl and Tufte, 1973: 21), for how is it possible to have self-government without the right to make one's own decisions? But whether such autonomy, for professionals and others, is compatible with the organizational aims of a health service is another matter. In the case of a factory, for example, the workers deliver a well-defined product, and, assuming its price and design appeal to customers, it does not matter how they organize their work schedule or whether they work an 8- or 24-hour day. Similarly, if they get their investment priorities wrong, it is their jobs that will be in peril.

In the case of a health service, however, it is precisely the way in which the organization is run that determines the quality of the service provided. And if the investment decisions are wrong, it is the patient who suffers. There is no market mechanism to mediate between workers and community, to translate signals about preferences and make the producers listen. Indeed, one of the characteristics of health service organizations—in contrast to most factories—is that many of the decisions are already taken by small autonomous groups: whether by the surgeon and his team or a small group of nurses running a ward for the mentally handicapped. And it is precisely the introverted, introspective nature of these teams—whose values may not necessarily be those of the community at large—which has caused criticism of excessive professional autonomy.

Imbalance in Worker and Community Interests

The theorists of democracy through direct worker participation have, admittedly, sought to introduce an element of community participation into their organizational schemes. More than 50 years ago, Cole (1920: 101–110) argued that all public services, whether health or education, should be based on self-government by the "smallest natural units of control." The service would thus be run by a series of "Health Guilds." But Cole recognized that "education and health are matters in which every citizen is intimately concerned, and upon which he must be assured of the fullest opportunity of bringing his opinion and influence to bear." So he proposed elected "Health Councils" to represent the community interest. The relationship between the Councils representing the producers and the consumers would, he believed, "be essentially not an antagonistic but a co-operative and complementary" one. And much the same optimistic assumption about a basic harmony of interests is made by recent advocates of organizational democracy.

But this approach fails to take account of the basic imbalance in worker and community interests, whether represented in elected bodies or in direct participation. The producer, by the very fact of working in the service, has total involvement in what is happening. Members of the community do not. The balance of incentives to invest in participation is therefore very different. By definition, those members of the community with the greatest incentive or capacity to invest effort in participation or representation will be atypical of the population at large (Klein and Lewis, 1976: 27–59). Additionally, and particularly relevant to the health service, any theory of participation that fails to recognize differences in knowledge is bound to be inadequate. To transfer theories of worker control from the factory setting to the health care setting, without taking into account the problem of the imbalance in incentives and information in the political market, is therefore to ignore the real issues involved.

So the paradoxical conclusion would seem to be that a system of worker control would only be compatible with community control in a health service based on a free market economy. If, in fact, members of the community were to buy their health care from whichever producer-cooperative provided the services best tailored to their requirements, then, of course, they would be able to signal their preferences. They could exercise control by virtue of their ability to take their patronage elsewhere. In fact, ironically enough, it would seem necessary to recreate something suspiciously like the present health care system in the United States. But, in practice, the logic of this argument is flawed. It assumes a symmetry of knowledge and bargaining power among producers and consumers, and the equal distribution of both among the latter. It is thus likely to be rejected on exactly the same grounds that the present U.S. system is so widely criticized.

Community Control or Consumer Control

In making this last point, community control has been discussed as though it can be identified with consumer control. In fact, the two concepts are distinct, if related. One of the problems about much of the discussion of community control is that it tends to conflate concepts of the public-as-citizens and of the public-as-consumers. In the former role, the public are presumed to be other-regarding, paying attention to what might be called "the general interest" insofar as this term has any meaning. In the latter role, the public are presumed to be self-regarding, paying attention only to their own self-interests.

The distinction is of more than theoretical importance. It has direct implications for any national health service, in particular, for the question of whether the aim of policy should be to create a national monopoly, thus narrowing or even eliminating the scope of the private sector (always assuming that the latter course of action is politically feasible or desirable). If the object is to encourage the public-as-citizens, then it can be argued that a state monopoly should be created. Only so will the public be forced to take an interest in the health service. If there is no opportunity to exit, then the incentives to exercise political voice are all the greater (Hirschman, 1970). If, on the other hand, the object is to encourage the public-as-consumers, then competition between the national health service and a private sector ought to be encouraged. For then the public will vote with their feet, and the private sector will act as an indicator of dissatisfaction.

In practice, the antithesis may be too neat. It may well be that the opportunity to exit into the private sector is a necessary condition for encouraging the use of voice in the public sector. Particularly in the case of Britain, where the opportunities to shop around among different doctors are limited by the increasing concentration of resources, as has already been noted, the use of voice may be constrained by the inability to exit (Birch, 1975). If the patient offends his doctor, or other health service personnel, in asserting his rights as a citizen to criticize or demand change, he may imperil his interests as a consumer. He may prefer to keep quiet for fear of retaliation. Hence, it would seem that a democratic health service—meaning an organization that is both sensitive and responsive to public demands—requires both the safety valve of a private sector and the existence of institutions like Community Health Councils, which can act as proxy for citizens, thus lowering the cost of political activity and protecting individuals.

The Dilemmas of Democracy

The aim of the analysis in the previous sections has been twofold. First, it has been to delineate the particular practical problems encountered in the British NHS in trying to achieve a satisfactory balance between centralized control and some elements of community and worker involvement. Second, it has been to demonstrate, using a more theoretical perspective, that these problems do not just reflect the special local situation of the NHS but also point out some more general dilemmas.

These dilemmas, to sum up, spring from the fact that a national health service embodies a variety of values, and fills a variety of functions, some of which may be incompatible with the values and organizational imperatives inherent in a move toward more community or worker control. If a national health service is seen as a device for rationing scarce national resources in an equitable and egalitarian manner, then immediately the scope for decentralization of power is inescapably limited. If a national health service is seen as a way of introducing national priorities, which may run counter to those embodied in the power structure of the professions and occupations within the system, then participation may be the enemy of the required changes. If a national health service is seen as part of a complex system of interrelated social services, then this may dictate that the size of any administrative unit should be determined by the needs of administrative coordination rather than by considerations of participatory autonomy.

So the ongoing debate about the structure and organization of Britain's National Health Service represents a necessary dialectic, and one which is likely to continue without any final resolution. Different aims of policy—embodying different values, all desirable in their own right but not necessarily compatible with each other—pull in different directions. In this situation, there may well be a constant reassessment of the weighting to be given to individual values, and their relationship with each other, but it is unlikely that everything will be sacrificed to the achievement of one particular objective to the exclusion of all others.

References

Birch, A. H. 1975. Economic Models in Political Science: The Case of 'Exit, Voice, and Loyalty.' *British Journal of Political Science* 5 (1): 69–82.

Brown, R.G.S. 1973. *The Changing National Health Service.* London: Routledge and Kegan Paul.

————, Griffin, S., and Haywood, S.C. 1975. *New Bottles: Old Wine?* Hull: University of Hull, Institute for Health Studies.

Buxton, M.J., and Klein, R. 1975. Distribution of Hospital Provision: Policy Themes and Resource Variations. *British Medical Journal* 1 (5943) (8 February): 345–349.

Cole, G.D.H. 1920. *Guild Socialism Re-stated.* London: Leonard Parsons.

Community Health Council. 1976. *Annual Report 1975–76.* London: St. Thomas's Health District.

Confederation of Health Service Employees. 1977. *Memorandum of Evidence to the Royal Commission on the National Health Service.* London: COHSE.

Dahl, R. A., and Tufte, E. R. 1973. *Size and Democracy.* Stanford, Calif.: Stanford University Press.

Department of the Environment. 1976. *Local Government Finance: Report of the Committee of Enquiry,* Cmnd. 6453. London: Her Majesty's Stationery Office (HMSO).

Department of Health and Social Security (DHSS). 1972. *National Health Service Reorganization: England,* Cmnd. 5055. London: Her Majesty's Stationery Office (HMSO).

_____. 1974. *Democracy in the National Health Service*. London: HMSO.

_____. 1976a. *Election of Staff Members: Consultative Document*. London: HMSO.

_____. 1976b. *Priorities for Health and Personal Social Services in England*. London: HMSO.

_____. 1976c. *Regional Chairmen's Enquiry into the Working of the DHSS in Relation to Regional Health Authorities*. London: HMSO.

_____. 1976d. *Sharing Resources for Health in England: Report of the Resource Allocation Working Party*. London: HMSO.

Finer, S. E. 1952. *The Life and Times of Sir Edwin Chadwick*. London: Methuen.

Freidson, E. 1971. *Profession of Medicine*. New York: Dodd, Mead and Company.

Godber, Sir G. 1975. *The Health Service: Past, Present and Future*. London: The Athlone Press.

Hansard (House of Commons). 1946a. 30 April, col. 45.

_____. 1946b. 30 April, col. 52.

_____. 1970. 23 March, col. 1001.

_____. 1973. *Standing Committee G: National Health Service Reorganisation Bill*. First Sitting, 5 April, cols. 6–12.

Hirschman, A. O. 1970. *Exit, Voice, and Loyalty*. Cambridge, Mass.: Harvard University Press.

Klein, R. 1971. Accountability in the National Health Service. *Political Quarterly* 42 (5): 363–375.

_____. 1973. *Complaints Against Doctors*. pp. 75–103. London: Charles Knight.

_____. 1975. *Notes Towards a Theory of Patient Involvement*. London: Centre for Studies in Social Policy.

_____. 1976. Political Models and the National Health Service. In Acheson, R. M., and Aird, L., eds., *Seminars in Community Medicine*. Vol. I, pp. 93–101. London: Oxford University Press.

_____. 1977a. The Corporate State, the Health Service and the Professions. *New Universities Quarterly* 31 (2): 161–180.

_____. 1977b. The Cumbersome Closed Shop Facing MPs Who Keep an Eye on Public Spending. *The Times*, 25 August 1977.

_____. 1977c. Democracy, the Welfare State and Social Policy. *Political Quarterly* 48 (4): 448–458.

_____. 1979. Ideology, Class, and the National Health Service. *Journal of Health Politics, Policy and Law* 4 (Forthcoming).

_____, and Lewis, J. 1976. *The Politics of Consumer Representation.* London: Centre for Studies in Social Policy.

Labour Party. 1977. *The Right to Health: The Labour Party's Evidence to the Royal Commission on the National Health Service.* July. London: The Labour Party.

Lambert, R. 1963. *Sir John Simon.* London: Macgibbon and Kee.

Ministry of Health. 1956. *Report of the Committee of Enquiry into the Cost of the National Health Service,* Cmnd. 9663. London: HMSO.

Monsen, R. J., and Downs, A. 1971. Public Goods and Private Status. *The Public Interest* 23 (Spring): 64–76.

National Association of Local Government Officers. 1977. Work-in to Stop Hospital Closing. *Public Service* 51 (10) (September).

National Union of Public Employees. 1977. *Memorandum of Evidence Submitted to the Royal Commission on the National Health Service.* February. London: NUPE.

Nisbet, R. A. 1970. *The Sociological Tradition.* London: Heinemann.

Pateman, C. 1970. *Participation and Democratic Theory.* Cambridge: Cambridge University Press.

_____. 1975. A Contribution to the Political Theory of Organizational Democracy. *Administration & Society* 7 (1) (May): 22–23.

Pitkin, H. 1967. *The Concept of Representation.* Berkeley and Los Angeles, Calif.: University of California Press.

Royal Commission on Local Government in England. 1969. *Research Studies No. 9, Community Attitudes Survey: England.* London: HMSO.

Sills, D. L., ed. 1968. *International Encyclopaedia of the Social Sciences.* Vol. 3. New York: The Macmillan Company and The Free Press.

Weber, M. 1947. *The Theory of Social and Economic Organization* (trans. Henderson, A. M., and Parsons, T.). Glencoe, Ill.: The Free Press.

Willcocks, A. J. 1967. *The Creation of the National Health Service.* London: Routledge and Kegan Paul.

Zhuk, A. P. 1976. *Public Health Planning in the USSR.* Washington, D.C.: U.S. Department of Health, Education, and Welfare.

Acknowledgment: In writing this paper I have drawn on many ideas which evolved in discussions with my former colleague, Dr. Janet Lewis. I gratefully acknowledge her help.
Address correspondence to: Professor Rudolf Klein, School of Humanities and Social Sciences, University of Bath, Claverton Down, Bath, BA2 7AY, England.

Inflation and
the Federal Role in Health
LOUISE B. RUSSELL

Cooper, B.S., and P.A. Piro
   1974   "Age differences in medical care spending, fiscal year 1973."
           Social Security Bulletin 37 (May): 3–14.
Cooper, B.S., N.L. Worthington, and M.F. McGee
   1973   Compendium of National Health Expenditures Data. U.S.
           Department of Health, Education, and Welfare, Social Security
           Administration.
Cooper, B.S., N.L. Worthington, and P.A. Piro
   1974   "National health expenditures, 1929–1973." Social Security
           Bulletin 37 (February): 2–19.
Davis, K.
   1973   "Rising hospital costs: Possible causes and cures." Washington,
           D.C.: The Brookings Institution, Reprint 262.
Feldstein, M.
   1971a   "Hospital cost inflation: A study of nonprofit price dynamics."
           American Economic Review 61 (December): 853–872.
   1971b   "A new approach to national health insurance." Public Interest
           23 (Spring): 93–105.
National Center for Health Statistics
   1973   Health Manpower and Health Facilities, 1972–73. U.S.
           Department of Health, Education, and Welfare, Public Health
           Service, June. Washington, D.C.: Government Printing Office.
National Institutes of Health
   1973   "Basic data relating to the National Institutes of Health, 1973."
           (February): 4–7.
Noll, R.G.
   1974   "The consequences of public utility regulation of hospitals."
           Paper presented at the Conference on Regulation in the Health
           Industry, National Academy of Sciences, Institute of Medicine,
           Washington, D.C., January 7–9.
Office of Management and Budget
   1973   Budget of the United States Government, Fiscal Year 1974:
           Special Analyses, p. 144. Washington, D.C.: Government
           Printing Office.
   1974   Budget of the United States Government, Fiscal Year 1975,
           p. 136. Washington, D.C.: Government Printing Office.
Russell, L.B.
   1975   "The effects of inflation on federal health spending." Medical
           Care (in press).

Russell, L.B., B.B. Bourque, D.P. Bourque, and C.S. Burke
 1974   Federal Health Spending, 1969–74. Washington, D.C.: National
         Planning Association.
Salkever, D.S.
 1972   "A microeconomic study of hospital cost inflation." Journal of
         Political Economy 80, No. 6 (November-December): 1144–1166.
Strickland, S.P.
 1972   Politics, Science, and Dread Disease, p. 249. Cambridge, Mass.:
         Harvard University Press.
U.S. Congress
 1974   "Health care, final phase IV regulations." Weekly Compilation of
         Presidential Documents, Federal Register 39, No. 16 (January
         23): 2697, Part II: Cost of Living Council.
U.S. Department of Health, Education, and Welfare
 1974   Monthly Statistical Report: Summary of Selected Price, Cost,
         and Utilization Data for the Health Care Market in the United
         States. Washington, D.C.: Office of Research and Statistics,
         Social Security Administration, October.
Waldman, S.
 1972   "The effect of changing technology on hospital costs."
         Department of Health, Education, and Welfare, Social Security
         Administration, Research and Statistics Note No. 4-1972.

Politics, Public Policy, and Medical Inflation
THEODORE R. MARMOR,
DONALD A. WITTMAN,
AND THOMAS C. HEAGY

This essay was written with the assistance of two institutions to whom we are greatly indebted: The Robert Wood Johnson Foundation provided financial support to Dr. Marmor and the Center for Health Administration Studies provided a helpful setting in which all of us could work. An early version was presented at a Center workshop and benefited particularly from the comments of Ronald Andersen, Odin Anderson, Rich Foster, and Joel May. Harrison Wagner and Rick Carlson gave us the benefit of their extended written comments for which we are very grateful. The staff of the Center for Health Administration Studies patiently and efficiently aided in the production of this paper, particularly Lynn Carter, Evelyn Friedman, Elaine Scheye, and Linda Randall. We want to warmly thank all of these colleagues while absolving them of responsibility for what we did with their assistance.

Alford, R.R.
  1974   Health Care Politics: Ideological and Interest Group Barriers to Reform. Chicago: University of Chicago Press.
Allison, G.T.
  1971   The Essence of Decision. Boston: Little, Brown & Co.
  1973   "Massachusetts medical school case." Public Policy Program, Harvard University.
Andersen, R., et al.
  1973   Health Service Use: National Trends and Variations— 1953-1970. Washington, D.C.: National Center for Health Services Research and Development. DHEW Publication No. (HRA) 74-3105.
Anderson, O.
  1972   Health Care: Can there be Equity? The United States, Sweden, and England. New York: John Wiley & Sons.
Andreopoulos, S., ed.
  1975   National Health Insurance: What Can We Learn from Canada? New York: John Wiley & Sons.
Bureau of Labor Statistics. Monthly Labor Review (various issues).

Chambers, J.
1975   A Diagrammatic Exposition of the Logic of Collective Action. Institute of Public Policy Studies, Discussion Paper No. 66.

Davis, K.
1976   "The impact of inflation and unemployment on health care of low-income people." This volume.

Davis, K., and R. Foster
1973   Community Hospitals: Inflation in the Pre-Medicare Period. Social Security Administration, Research Report No. 41. Washington, D.C.: Government Printing Office.

Feldstein, M.
1971   "A new approach to national health insurance." The Public Interest 23 (Spring): 93–105.

Fraser, R.D.
1974   "Overview: Canadian national health insurance." Paper presented at Conference of Canadian Health Economists, Queens University, Ontario, September.

Friedman, M.
1975   "Leonard Woodstock's free lunch." Newsweek 84 (April 21).

Ginsburg, P.B.
1976   "Inflation and the economic stabilization program." This volume.

Lave, L.
1976   "The effect of inflation on providers." This volume.

Lewin, L., and Associates
1974   Nationwide Survey of Health Regulation. NTIS Accession No. 236660-AS, September.

Lewin, Somers, and Somers
1975   "Issues in the structure and administration of state health cost regulation." Toledo Law Review Symposium, June.

Marmor, T.
1973   Politics of Medicare. Chicago: Aldine Publishing Co.

Marmor, T., T. Heagy, and W. Hoffman
1975   "Canadian national health insurance: Policy implications for the United States." Policy Sciences, special issue on cross-national policy studies, December, forthcoming. Also, in different form, in Spyros Andreopoulos, ed., National Health Insurance: What Can We Learn from Canada? New York: John Wiley & Sons.

Meyer, M.
1975   Catastrophic Illness and Catastrophic Health Insurance. Public Policy Studies No. 6. Washington, D.C.: Heritage Foundation.

Newhouse, J.P.
1976   "Inflation and health insurance." This volume.

Piven, F.F., and R.A. Cloward
1971   Regulating the Poor: The Functions of Public Welfare. New York: Random House.

Posner, R.
1974   "Theories of economic regulation." The Bell Journal of Economics and Management Science 5 (Autumn): 335-358.

Russell, L.B.
1976   "Inflation and the federal role in health." This volume.

Sattler, F.L.
1975   "Hospital prospective rate setting, issues and options." Working paper, SSA InterStudy Hospital Prospective Payment Workshop. Minneapolis: InterStudy.

Social Security Administration
1974   Background Information on Medical Expenditures, Prices, and Costs. Office of Research and Statistics, September.

Stevens, R., and R. Stevens
1974   Welfare Medicine in America: A Case of Medicaid. New York: The Free Press.

Stigler, G.
1971   "The theory of economic regulation." The Bell Journal of Economics and Management Science 2 (Spring): 3-21.

U.S. Department of Health, Education, and Welfare
1974   Report of the Conference on Inflation: Health, Education, Income Security and Social Services, September 19, 1974. Washington, D.C.: U.S. Department of Health, Education, and Welfare.

Wittman, D.
1975   "Political Decision-Making." In Morris Silver, ed., Economics of Public Choice. (In press.)

Index

355

for preventive health care, 85–86
in provider supply, 73–74
public finance assumptions for, 60–61
public utility model of, 75–78
Gramm, Congr. W. Philip, 210
Gramm Amendment, 210

Harm, subjective determination of, 7–8
Harm-to-others doctrine, 39–40
Health
  as absolute good, 9, 11
  as goal of government life-style reform, 4
  as instrumental value, 59
  social component in, 58
Health advocates, 79
Health behavior reform. *See* Life-style reform
Health care, 59–60
  personal health maintenance in, 60
  and socioeconomic status, 60
  technological factors in, 60
Health care expenditures. *See also* Costs
  in Canada, 151, 153
  in France, 151
  in Germany, 151
  in Great Britain, 153
  in the Netherlands, 151
  in Sweden, 151, 153
  in the United Kingdom, 151
  in the United States, 151, 153
Health insurance. *See also* National health insurance
  as cause of health sector inflation, 133–134
  major risk type, 144–145
  restructuring, as inflation cure, 137–138
Health maintenance, neglect of, 59
Health Maintenance Organization Act (1973), 158, 187
  amendments to, 167
  assessment of, 194
  consumer protection provisions of, 188–190
  difficulties with, 159, 166–167
  enabling provisions of, 190
  funding provisions of, 191
  as impediment to HMOs, 214
  minimum benefit requirements in, 214
  regulatory aspects of, 190–193
Health maintenance organizations (HMOs). *See also* Office of Health Maintenance Organizations
  as business enterprises, 161

Congressional action on, 208–210
consumer participation in, 80
definition of, 169n
enrollment in, 163
federal grants to, 163
federally qualified, 161, 163
  and HMO Act, 214
increase in, 162–163
issues in, 167
as market mechanism, 78
origins of, 203
rationale for, 169–170
self-sufficiency in, 160
Health maintenance organizations, growth of
  barriers to, 174
  in California, 171n, 172
  government policy conditions determining, 170
  legal conditions determining, 170, 172–174, 174–176, 178–183 (*see also* Medicaid; Medicare)
  market conditions determining, 170, 174–176, 178
  from 1969 to 1974, 171–172
  policy conditions determining, 177–178
Health Planning Act (1974). *See also* Health systems agencies
  accountability under, 293
  efficiency vs. representation under, 317–319
  litigation under, 309–313 (*see also* Consumer representation litigation)
  national demands vs. local desires under, 317
  and participation in health systems agencies, 283, 293–294
  representation under, 295, 298–299, 300, 301
  role of scientific planning in, 315–316
  significance of, 320
  and suspicion of centralized authority, 314
Health policy. *See* Government; Government intervention
Health services. *See also* Deinstitutionalization; Early and Periodic Screening Diagnosis and Treatment Program; Government funding
  as consumption and investment, 66–67
  federal funding for, 127–131
  as merit good, 69
Health Services Administration (HSA), 127, 128, 129

359

360

distinguished from fair distribution of burdens, 21n
goals of, 3, 4
as government policy, 2–4
and harm-to-others doctrine, 39–40
through health education, 25–27
through incentives, 27–29
means to, 25–30
as paternalism, 5–15
through regulation, 29–30
Litigation. *See* Consumer representation litigation
Loan programs, federal, 164n

Major risk insurance, 144
Market system. *See also* Political markets; Venture capitalism
government health policy in, 55–56, 73, 76
government intervention in, 61
and health care inflation, 144
HMOs in, 200–202
and political process, 202
professional autonomy vs. public accountability in, 342–343
reconciliation of worker and community interests in, 343–344
standard benefits in, 211–212
"third best" in, 215–216
wide-open, 211–212
Maternal and Child Health Services (MCHS)
in administration of EPSDT, 267–268, 273–274
and development of EPSDT regulations, 266
percentage of U.S. children in, 253
Maternity and Infant Care Projects, 252
Maternity leave, 58
McGovern, Sen. George, 69
Meany, George, 259
La médecine libérale. *See also* French health care system
cliniques as protectors of, 102
conflict with state of, 100
definition of, 92
prospects for, 111, 113, 114
retreat from, 98
Medicaid
children in, 253
costs of, 274–275
deinstitutionalization under, 234
federal funding through, 127, 128, 129
and health care inflation, 150–151
HMO participation in, 183–184

provisions of, 253–254
"unbalanced" strategy of, 57–58
Medical care inflation. *See* Inflation, health care
Medical services. *See* Early and Periodic Screening Diagnosis and Treatment programs; Government funding; Health services
Medical Services Administration (MSA)
and EPSDT program, 266, 267–268, 273–274
Medicaid administered by, 254
Medicare
deinstitutionalization under, 234
as example of upgrading benefits, 213–214
federal funding through, 127, 128, 129
and health care inflation, 150–151
HMO participation in, 184–187
unbalanced strategy of, 57–58
Mental disability. *See also* Deinstitutionalization
and drugs, 224, 231–232
nature of, 221–222, 225, 242–245
Mental illness hospitalization, 227
Merit goods. *See also* Market system
as basis for government intervention, 67–72
and categorical assistance programs, 69
medical services as, 69
and national health insurance, 70–72
non-market rationale for, 67–72
paternalistic explanation, 68, 69
redistribution explanation for, 69
Mill, John Stuart, 41, 42, 43, 47
Minimum benefit requirements
as aid to HMOs, 211
and costs, 214
effects of, 211–212, 214
in HMO Act, 190–193, 214
rationale for, 201
and upgrading of benefits, 215
Monopoly
as basis for government intervention, 63–65
natural vs. unnatural, 63–64
Moralism, 14, 30–31

National Academy of Science (NAS), and HMOs, 179
National Cancer Act (1971), 123
National defense, as public good, 63
National health insurance (NHI)
for catastrophic disruptions, 84–85
and competition, 195

Regional authorities, 284–285
Regulation. *See also* Government intervention
and health care inflation, 135–137
and life-style reform, 29–30
Regulation, federal
of health behavior, 47, 48
of HMO participation in Medicare, 185–187
Regulation, state, of HMOs, 172–174, 175–176. 178, 180–183, 184
Regulatory agencies, 284–285
Representation. *See also* Consumer representation
and accountability, 294–295, 301
descriptive, 295, 297
formal, 294–295
under Health Planning Act, 298–299, 300, 301
and imblanaced political markets, 285–288
interest group model of, 285
problems with 295–298, 299, 300, 306–307
substantive, 299
and technological efficiency, 317–319
in unstructured situations, 284–285, 289–290
Research, medical
funding for, 122–123
and health sector inflation, 134–135
Responsibility, and government life-style reform, 18–19, 20, 31

Sanitary Condition of the Labouring Population of Great Britain, Report on, 42
Scientific planning, in Health Planning Act, 315–316
Sheppard-Towner Act (1921), 251
Social-costs argument
application to public health of, 43
and balancing of costs and benefits, 48
and blanket prohibitions, 48
and coercive measures, 37, 38, 39, 42
completeness of, 49
and difficulty of determining net social costs, 45, 49
in federal laws, 48
and minimization of coercion, 46–48, 49
origins of, 42–43
problems with, 44–48
relation to harm-to-others doctrine, 43
Social Security Act (1935). *See also* Title V
Early and Periodic Screening Diagnosis and Treatment programs of, 250
1967 amendments to, 257, 264 (*see also*

H. R. 5710)
1969 amendments to, 183
1972 amendments to, 182, 183, 185, 208
Subsidies. *See* Incentives
Suicide, 11, 13
Supplemental Security Income (SSI) program, 235

Taxation
and fair distribution of health burdens, 20–22
life-style reform through, 4–5, 29
"Technological fix"
and political choice, 316–317, 318–319
and representation, 317
in use of drugs for mental disability, 232
Therapeutic nihilism, 2
Title V, of Social Security Act, 251, 252, 253, 254
Crippled Children program of, 251
and EPSDT, 263, 266–267, 268
Maternal and Child Health (MCH) services in, 252
percentage of U.S. children under, 253
Title XIX, of Social Security Act, 253, 254. *See also* Medicaid
and EPSDT, 254, 256–258, 260–261, 266–267, 268, 270, 271
percentage of U.S. children under, 253

Underserving, HMO Act protection against, 189–190, 194

Value pluralism, and paternalism, 9, 10–11, 12
Veit, Howard R., 159
Venture capitalism
features of, 159–160
as foreign to Department of Health and Human Services, 159
and government as high risk-taker, 163
as role of Office of Health Maintenance Organizations, 158
Veterans Administration, 124, 128, 130, 131

Welfare. *See* Public Welfare
"Warehousing" of mentally ill, 223
White Paper on HMOs, DHEW's, 177
Working conditions, as source of illness, 3–4

363